No. 15 IN THE PHYSICIANS' AND STUDENTS' READY-REFERENCE SERIES.

SYPHILIS

IN THE MIDDLE AGES

AND

IN MODERN TIMES.

BY

DR. F. BURET,

PARIS, FRANCE.

TRANSLATED FROM THE FRENCH, WITH NOTES, BY

A. H OHMANN-DUMESNIL, M.D.,

OR OF DERMATOLOGY AND SYPHILOLOGY IN THE MARION-SIMS COLLEGE OF MEDI-
LTING DERMATOLOGIST TO THE ST. LOUIS CITY HOSPITAL, TO THE ST.
E HOSPITAL; PHYSICIAN FOR CUTANEOUS DISEASES TO THE
AN BROTHERS' HOSPITAL; DERMATOLOGIST TO PIUS HOS-
PITAL, TO THE REBEKAH HOSPITAL, TO THE ST. LOUIS
POLYCLINIC AND EMERGENCY HOSPITAL, ETC., ETC.

"Syphilis To-Day and Among the Ancients." *In Three Volumes.*

VOLUMES II AND III.

"*Nihil sub sole novum.*"—ECCLES., i, 10.

PHILADELPHIA:

THE F. A. DAVIS COMPANY, PUBLISHERS.

1895.

Library of Congress Cataloging in Publication Data

Buret, Frédéric.
"Syphilis to-day and among the ancients."

Reprint of the 1891-95 ed. published by F. A. Davis, Philadelphia, which was issued as no. 12 and 15 of the Physicians' and students' ready-reference series.

CONTENTS: v. 1. Syphilis in ancient and prehistoric times.—v. 2-3. Syphilis in the Middle Ages and in modern times.

1. Syphilis—History. I. Title. II. Series: Physicians' and students' ready reference series; no. 12, 15.

RC201.4.B8713 1975 616.9'513 72-9627
ISBN 0-404-57422-X

Reprinted from an original copy in the collection of the University of Chicago Library

From the edition of 1895, Philadelphia and London
First AMS edition published in 1975
Manufactured in the United States of America

International Standard Book Number:
Complete Set: 0-404-57422-X
Volumes II & III: 0-404-57424-6

AMS PRESS INC.
NEW YORK, N. Y. 10003

PREFACE.

THAT syphilis has existed from the remotest antiquity is an historical point which it is no longer possible to doubt, and which Dr. Buret has done much to establish. The numerous proofs which he accumulates to the support of this way of seeing—drawn from the annals and even the legends the most ancient—are, for the greater part, irrefutable. It is an acquired fact, to-day, that the appearance of syphilis is lost in the twilight of time, and that that disease has no age. It is found described, in fact, among the most ancient peoples,—even among the Assyrians and Babylonians,—under pretty similar forms, by priests and poets rather than by physicians; but it must be admitted that the physicians, in these remote times, did not seem to enjoy the confidence which is accorded to them to-day.

In addition, documents which can hardly be called into question bring into light the existence of syphilis among the most ancient people of America,—in such a way that this disease, which has no age, neither has a country; it is of the remotest antiquity, and belongs to humanity in general.

That, in ancient times, its frequency should have been greater in Asia and in Europe than in the West Indies is susceptible of the most simple explanation; that was dependent, without a doubt, upon the degree of civilization. The more the latter advanced, the more syphilis spread; it is the same with this disease as with tuberculosis: it follows the progress of civilization or, if it be preferred, it extends with large gatherings of people.

Even to-day it is evident that syphilis is less spread among savage peoples than among the most civilized nations.

After a large number of proofs favoring the antiquity of syphilis, Dr. Buret has made it a point to give the counter-proof by devoting himself to the refutation of the opinion, accredited since Astruc, of the American origin of syphilis. The demonstration is of the most clear sort, and no one can doubt, to-day, of the existence of syphilis among the people of Europe before the first voyage of Christopher Columbus for America. The coincidence of an epidemic of syphilis which raged in Italy some little time after the return of this great captain has been the principal argument called forth to the support of the claim of the American origin of syphilis; but this argument, which rests upon the dictum, *post hoc, ergo propter hoc*, is without scientific value.

The syphilitic epidemic of the end of the fifteenth century, which Dr. Buret reasonably compares with former and succeeding epidemics, rather similar in character, easily explains under what peculiar circumstances Italy found itself, then invaded by several armies among whom hygiene was unknown. The agglomeration of large masses of individuals,—that is to say, the crowding,—joined with bad hygiene, constitutes the predisposition to the development and existence of all the diseases, including syphilis.

The study which this author makes of the numerous opinions which were current concerning the nature of syphilis and its treatment is as interesting for the clinician as for the historian; it shows how difficult are scientific discoveries and how slow is the progress of medicine. Few men, as a matter of fact, know how to see scientific questions in a just light, and misfortune decrees that, as long as a science is misunderstood, every one considers himself competent to speak upon it.

This is what formerly occurred in the case of chemistry and physics. Since those sciences rest upon certain data, they are no longer assailed by superior intellects. Will the same thing occur in medicine? Everything leads to this way of seeing; but the large number of works published each day shows conclusively that, despite the remarkable work of Claude Bernard ("Introduction à l'étude de la médecine expérimentale"), the time has not yet come, which means that medical science has not yet emerged from its empiric stage. From this point of view, as well as from many others, the work published by Dr. Buret will certainly be well received by the medical public, for it is a work of erudition and is scientific.

E. LANCEREAUX.

AUTHOR'S LETTER TO TRANSLATOR.

VOLUME II.

Au Professeur Ohmann-Dumesnil:

MON CHER CONFRÈRE,—Vous me faites savoir que votre intention est de traduire le plus tôt possible le second volume de mon historique de la syphilis. Je suis hereux de vos bonnes dispositions et je profite de la circonstance pour vous prier d'être mon interprète auprès de vos concitoyens. Remerciez pour moi vos lecteurs du bon accueil qu'ils ont fait à "La syphilis chez lez anciens," et faites part à toute la Presse Américaine de mes sentiments de gratitude pour les comptes-rendus bienveillants dont mon modeste ouvrage a été l'objet sur votre Continent. Permettez moi aussi, mon cher collègue, de vous féliciter pour la façon dont vous avez traduit mon premier volume; un auteur est toujours heureux de voir interpréter aussi exactement sa pensée. Je joins ma faible voix au concert d'éloges dont vous a gratifié à juste titre toute la Presse Médicale des Etats Unis d'Amérique.

Pour cette étude concernant le Moyen âge, j'ai suivi le même plan que pour celle de l'Antiquité; je me suis attaché à faire ressortir l'existence évidente de la syphilis à toutes les époques en suivant pas à pas les évolutions de la science et en produisant les documents d'après leur ordre chronologique. Toutefois cet ex-

To Professor Ohmann-Dumesnil:

MY DEAR COLLEAGUE,—You have informed me of your intention of translating, at the earliest possible moment, the second volume of my history of syphilis. I am much pleased at your kindly disposition and I take advantage of the circumstance to ask you to be my interpreter to your countrymen. Return thanks, in my name, to your readers for the kindly reception they have given to "Syphilis in Ancient Times," and communicate to the entire American Press my grateful sentiments for the kind reviews which my modest work has elicited in your continent. Permit me also, my dear colleague, to compliment you upon the manner in which you have translated my first volume; an author is always pleased to see his thoughts interpreted in such an exact manner. I join my feeble voice to the chorus of praise with which the entire Medical Press of the United States of America has justly gratified you.

In this study regarding the Middle Ages, I have followed the same plan as for that of Antiquity; I have confined myself to the task of making the evident existence of syphilis at all times show itself by following step by step the evolution of science and by introducing documents in their chronological posé a fait l'objet de deux chapîtres consacrés, l'un à la médecine, l'autre aux documents littéraires. Nos confrères d'Europe sont, pour la plupart, ralliés dès maintenant à notre cause; beaucoup sont fort ébranlés—je le sais de bonne source—mais ne l'avouent pas officiellement. Le présent volume est destiné à frapper le dernier coup; et malgrè l'accueil plutôt froid—sinon hostile—qu'a reçu mon dernier ouvrage à l'Académie de Médecine ou le syphiligraphe le plus en vue est un des défenseurs de la légende américaine, j'y présenterai encore hardiment celuici. Il faut que la vérité triomphe envers et contre tout!

J'ai consacré un chapitre entier aux circonstances qui ont accompagné la déconverte du Nonveaumonde par Christophe Colomb. Je crois avoir démontré, preuves en main que ses voyages n'ont jamais influé en quoi que se soit sur la propagation de la syphilis en Europe, ou cette maladie existait déjà. J'ai fait mon possible pour laver l'Amérique de la calomnie absurde qui veut en faire le berceau de la vérole, et, si je n'ai pas réussi, j'ose espérer que vos compatriotes me sauront gré de l'intention.

DR. F. BURET.

PARIS, 1er Novembre, 1893.

order. At all events, this *exposé* has formed the end in view of two chapters devoted, one to medicine, the other to literary documents. Our European colleagues are, for the greater part, rallied, from this moment, to our cause; many are strongly shaken, —I know it from good authority, —but do not acknowledge it openly. The present volume is destined to strike the last blow, and despite the rather cold reception—if not hostile—which my last volume received at the Académie de Médecine (of Paris), where the syphilographer of most prominence is one of the defenders of the American legend, I will boldly present this one. Truth must triumph in the presence of and against everything!

I have devoted a whole chapter to the circumstances which attended the discovery of the New World by Christopher Columbus. I believe that I have demonstrated, proofs in hand, that his voyages never exerted any influence, however slight it might be, on the propagation of syphilis in Europe, in which that disease already existed. I have done my utmost to clear America of the absurd calumny which strives to make it the cradle of syphilis, and, if I have not succeeded in this, I dare hope that your countrymen will give me credit for the effort.

DR. F. BURET.

PARIS, November 1, 1893.

TRANSLATOR'S PREFACE.

VOLUME II.

THE present volume is the second one of the trilogy which embraces a critical history of syphilis from prehistoric times up to the present day. The author, Dr. Buret, has happily finished his colossal undertaking, whose magnitude can only be appreciated after a careful perusal of his work. He has ransacked literature in his search for documentary evidence and he has been rewarded by finding some of the most valuable information buried in manuscripts which only an enthusiastic and learned bibliophile would ever succeed in unearthing.

Those who have read the first volume—"Syphilis in Ancient and Prehistoric Times"—will have perceived the argument laid down by the author. He traces the disease not only to the most ancient historic epochs; but he goes farther and clearly demonstrates the evidences of syphilis in prehistoric remains. He has, moreover, shown that antiquity did not limit venereal disease to one country, or clime, or epoch, but it manifested itself everywhere at all times with more or less intensity. Syphilis never died out and it never sprang into being *de novo*. It simply excited more attention at some times than at others, either on account of the keener powers of observation of some individuals or on account of its greater prevalence or intensity.

This naturally leads us to the disease in the Middle Ages. It existed, in a moderate way, until the time of the Crusades. The Crusaders, left to their devices in an Oriental country, became thoroughly debauched, and on their return disseminated venereal diseases—or leprosy, as it was called—so thoroughly that it became absolutely necessary to segregate them as lepers,—a treatment which, it will be confessed, was both practical and effective. However, plagues would occasionally manifest themselves, and these scourges decimated the population of different countries in Europe, as cholera now does those of the Indian archipelago. No particular attention was paid to these visitations of Providence until the time of the celebrated siege of Naples by the French. By some fortuitous chance an epidemic preceded the expedition of the army of Charles VIII into Italy, and Providence was abandoned as an explanation and the French army adopted as the scape-goat.

But we will not continue this synopsis. The author proves his point so well, and his arguments are so well supported by documentary evidence of contemporaneous writers, that it is thoroughly convincing. He conclusively shows that syphilis is not of American origin. He does not deny its existence in America at the time of its discovery; in fact, he insists that it had a pre-Columbian birth; but he proves that it did not act as the source of European syphilis. For this we are truly grateful from an historical point of view, for history should be exact and truthful. As Americans, we may be pardoned a certain amount of satisfaction in being vindicated of the charge of having infected Europe with a disease which, at one time, inspired so much horror and is still looked upon by the public as disgraceful and disreputable.

We have endeavored to give an exact and faithful translation of the original, which the author kindly sent in proof-sheets. This may account for a certain unevenness in some parts, but elegance of diction had to be sacrificed to clearness of interpretation, in order that the reader might not be led astray into any inaccuracies of apprehension. The author may, at times, appear irreligious, but he has merely given a reflex of the times of which he speaks, and gives a vivid portrait of the general depravity which then prevailed.

In closing this introduction nothing more need be said, unless it be that the reader will not judge too harshly of the efforts submitted in this volume by

THE TRANSLATOR.

AUTHOR'S PREFACE.

VOLUME III.

WE should be failing in our duty did we not begin by thanking the learned public for the good reception accorded the first volume of our work,—"Syphilis in Ancient and Prehistoric Times." This result is a good omen for the present volume, which completes our history of syphilis. The Press equally deserves our gratitude for the good-will with which it has noticed our efforts. Upon this occasion the managers of lay journals will not have occasion to fear on account of the prudishness of their readers; the word "syphilis"—the bugbear of M. Prudhomme—has been changed to "gros mal" in the title of our work. This expression, borrowed from the Middle Ages, whilst sufficiently vague not to frighten any one, suits the subject perfectly, since it was currently employed, even in law, in the fourteenth and fifteenth centuries.

Our work is divided into two parts[1]: the first includes the history of the disease during the whole period of the Middle Ages up to the siege of Naples[2]; the second is devoted to modern times, from the expedition of Charles VIII up to our days.[3]

We accordingly first examined the documents emanating from authors who lived in the first fifteen

[1] This preface was written to include volumes ii and iii.—O-D.

[2] Volume ii of the present series.

[3] The present volume.

centuries of our era. As progress is made in these investigations the advances are noted as more and more marked in clinical observation and especially in that which concerns venereal pathology. There are even certain descriptions so clear that every one would agree in recognizing them as applicable to syphilis, were they given over the signature of a modern author.

We have next made a retrospective study upon all the great epidemics which have made their mark in history; and, whilst dealing with them in as succinct a manner as possible, we have endeavored to separate, amid this multitude of morbid symptoms described in the method peculiar to each nation and to each epoch, the portion which is referable to syphilis. To bring about a proper understanding of the fact that the latter played a preponderating part in the epidemics of the Middle Ages, we have been brought to sketch a picture of the manners of that period which was amazing in so many different respects.

Coming to the famous epidemic of Naples, we have made an effort to pierce through this pathological mystery. We have wished to make understood how syphilis, known up to that time under different names corresponding to its symptoms, could appear as a new morbid entity in the eyes of the physicians of those times who were more enlightened than their predecessors. Then, reviewing the principal authors who have written upon syphilis since the fifteenth century, we have reproduced certain curious passages, rendered so by their form or testifying to simple beliefs, and we have studied step by step the progress of venereal therapeutics so slowly accomplished. There is nothing more curious than these scientific researches, nothing more attractive than this study which permits us to follow, during the centuries, the struggle of intelligence against the genius of obscurantism. One is a spectator, so to speak, of the efforts of men of science endeavoring to raise the veil which hides the truth. Each advance is marked by the loss of some celebrated name, but medicine has advanced a step. Men die, but science remains; and a day comes when the veil is entirely torn.

A disease unrecognized for centuries suddenly appears still enveloped in darkness; it is the venereal disease. It is classified; and no one suspects that the symptoms which are observed are due to three viruses which are essentially distinct: syphilis, chancroid, and gonorrhœa. It requires three centuries for the light to show itself. At first it is timid hypotheses which are warmly opposed. Then a man is met gifted with a great practical sense: it is Ricord. With the scientific scent which is characteristic of him, he rapidly knows how to distinguish true theories from false ones. He takes up discoveries which have remained in an embryonic state, puts them in relief, adds thereto his personal comment,—makes them his, in a word,—and the truth bursts forth in all directions!

We have also devoted a chapter to the examination of the best hygienic measures to adopt, with the object of preventing the extension of venereal diseases. We have not hesitated to arraign the coercive measures at present obtaining, convinced, as we are, of their uselessness, of their immorality, and of their injustice. They are useless because they fail in their object and do not reach contagious women in so small a proportion as 1 per cent. They are immoral because this hunt is made, as a rule, by the disreputable, and most often has no real effect, except against the unfortunate women who are unable to buy their liberty at the very moment, and with coin. They are immoral, in addition, because honest mothers of families are but too frequently the victims of the taunts and brutalities of hirelings for the greater part ignorant.

Besides, these methods are unjust because they are only applied to, and will never be possibly applied to more than, a very limited number of prostitutes. For prostitution is like a spiral; we cannot say where it begins nor where it ends. The woman filled with genesic sensations is only an exception; the nymphomaniac comes within the category of pathological cases; whilst the majority of *professionals* look for nothing beyond means of existence at first, of luxury later on. Besides, among these latter this mode of life is most often only temporary; very few furnish a complete career.

Must we not, also, count among prostitutes those working-girls who finish their day's work with the sale of their bodies, and sow as much more contagion as they are ignorant upon this matter? In what class will you place those married women who cause themselves to be *helped* in their toilettes, with or without the complicity of the husband? They are to be found from the foot to the topmost round of the social ladder; from the wife of the clerk to countesses and marchionesses,—and the latter do not even have the excuse of having suffered from hunger! Whether the sale be made for five francs or for a bill of twenty thousand francs paid at the dress-maker's, the fact remains the same: there is no State license which can erase the word "*prostitution*" from the alcove where the delivery of the goods has taken place. The name of the seller of delights, were it emblazoned on a coat of arms, would none the less have been dragged in the mire!

In conclusion, it has appeared useful to us to give some advice in regard to individual hygiene; after having noticed the different methods proposed with the object of avoiding contagion, we have pointed out a simple and easy procedure. Experience having proven that it is good, we have made it our duty to divulge it.

Now, what will be the conclusions of our work? That syphilis has prevailed in an undisputed manner during that entire period of a thousand years known as the Middle Ages. If the least doubt whatever could be retained in regard to antiquity, the above is no longer possible from the time that the works of physicians who lived from the twelfth to the sixteenth century are read. *Syphilis is a contemporary of the first ages.* Such is the conviction which six years of constant labor has given us,—labor in which we have only been sustained by our desire of knowing and wish to bring to a successful issue this work of spreading it.

In truth, we cannot say that we have only met in our path roses and encouragement. We still see, for instance, the face of the first publisher to whom we brought "Syphilis in Ancient and Prehistoric Times."

"That," he told us with a disdainful air, "is scarcely good for anything better than to pull down a prize at the Académie. . . . There is at least one year's work in that?"

"No, three."

"It's a pity! it's a pity! . . ."

And he returned us our manuscript. Let us hasten to confess that it would be in poor taste to bear him a grudge. He was logical from the very moment in which he did not believe in successful sales, and he could only pity an author influenced by any other object. Others, who are not publishers and do not even suspect of what value a scientific work is, simply call one a "chump"; in the world of vermicelli, of boots at 12 francs 50, or of stuffed crocodiles, it is the only epithet which is applicable to monsieur for whom the five-franc piece is not the only and constant object. Let us smile pleasantly and let them talk.

DR. F. BURET.

PARIS, October, 1893.

AUTHOR'S LETTER TO TRANSLATOR.

VOLUME III.

Au Professeur Ohmann-Dumesnil:

MON CHER COLLÈGUE,—J'apprends avec plaisir que vous avez achevé la traduction du troisième volume de "La Syphilis à travers les âges"; et, comme pour les deux premiers, je suis convaincu que j'aurai encore à vous féliciter pour votre profonde connaissance de la langue Française.

Il existe donc maintenant, en Amérique comme en France, un historique complet de la maladie vénérienne, tel que je l'avait conçut en 1886. Mon but est atteint, car c'est un de ces ouvrages qu'on ne fait qu'une fois. Vous voyez jusqu'où m'a entraîné ce travail que je pensais terminer en deux ans! C'est que les recherches se multiplient tous les jours dès qu'on a commencé; une trouvaille en amène une autre—fort heureusement—et l'on est en quelque sorte forcé de pousser ses investigations, sinon au hazard, du moins partout où l'on pressent un fil conducteur. Bien des recherches ont été ainsi pratiquées en vain: mais aussi quelle joie lorsqu'on peut mettre la main sur un document ignoré de tous!

Pour le présent volume ma tâche a été bien simplifiée. N'ayant plus à démontrer l'antiquité

To Professor Ohmann-Dumesnil:

MY DEAR COLLEAGUE,—It is with pleasure that I learn that you have completed the translation of the third volume of "Syphilis through the Ages"; and, in the same manner as for the two first ones, I am convinced that I shall once more have to congratulate you upon your profound knowledge of the French language.

So there exists now, in America as well as in France, a complete history of venereal disease such as I had conceived it in 1886. My object is attained, for it is one of those works which one never does but once. You see the point to which this work has led me, which I imagined I could complete in two years! It is because researches multiply daily, as soon as they are begun; one find brings on another,—very fortunately,—and one is, in a sort of a way, forced to push his investigations, if not blindly, at least in every direction in which one feels a guiding thread. Many researches have been vainly made in this manner; but, then, what joy when one can place his hands on a document unknown to all!

de la syphilis Européenne, il m'a suffi de lire les ouvrages parus depuis quatre siècles sur la grande Maladie. J'ai pu suivre pas à pas, sans aucune fatigue, les progrès péniblement réalisés de la thérapeutique vénérienne. J'en ai donné un résumé aussi complet que possible pour permettre au lecteur de s'initier, sans perte de temps, à ces essais bien instructifs.

En vénéréologie, comme dans les autres branches de la pathologie interne, il faut bien reconnaitre que nous ne sommes pas sortis de la phase empirique. M. Lancereaux est un des rares, parmis nos Maîtres de Paris, qui aient le courage de proclamer tout haut ce que les autres avouent tout bas. Je ne parle pas des nullités prétentieuses, ces "*erreurs de concours*" que le favoritisme nous impose ; ceux-là se figurent avoir tout découvert : ils ne confesseront jamais leur impuissance. Et cependant, pour ne prendre que la methode hypodermique, dans le traitement de la syphilis, qu'est-ce autre chose que de l'empiricisme ? Néanmoins, qui oserait, à l'heure actuelle, la déclarer sans valeur et digne des charlatans ?

Empiriques, les alchimistes de l'époque féodale ! Empiriques, les "*graisseurs de vérole*" de la fin du XVe siècle ! Pourtant, lorsqu'une syphilis grave résiste à des monceaux de pilules de bichlorure ou de protiodure hydrargyrique, n'a-t-on pas recours aux frictions

For the present volume my task has been greatly simplified. Having no longer to demonstrate the antiquity of European syphilis, it was sufficient for me to read the works which have appeared for the past four centuries on the great Disease. I have been enabled to follow, step by step, without any fatigue, the progress of venereal therapeutics, realized with so much difficulty. I have given as complete a *résumé* as possible, so as to permit the reader to introduce himself, without loss of time, to these very instructive attempts.

In venereology, as in the other branches of internal pathology, it must be certainly acknowledged that we have not emerged from the empiric phase. M. Lancereaux is one of the rare ones, among the Masters of Paris, who has the courage of proclaiming, in a loud voice, that which the others acknowledge in whispers. I do not speak of the nonentities who are pretentious, those "*competitive mistakes*" which favoritism forces upon us ; these gentry imagine that they have discovered all : they will never confess their impotence. And yet, to take up only the hypodermatic method, in the treatment of syphilis, what else is it but impotence ? Nevertheless, who would dare, at the present day, to declare it as without value and worthy of quacks ?

Empirics, the alchemists of the feudal era ! Empirics, the

mercurielles, et cela pour le plus grand bien du malade? Et ces gommes gangréneuses qui se cicatrisent après une injection de quelques centigrammes de calomel, lorsqu'elles on bravé iodures et frictions! Qu'on nous montre les lois thérapeutiques régissant ces cas—moins rares qu'on ne le pense—de la pratique courante! Donc empirisme partout, et nous serons tous empiriques jusqu'au jour où nous aurons un appareil assez sensible pour enregistrer l'intensité du virus syphilitique, comme nous avons des balances pour peser l'onguent napolitain, le calomel, ou le sublimé corrosif.

DR. F. BURET.

PARIS, le 20 Mars, 1894.
10 Avenue de l'Opéra.

"*anointers of the pox*" of the end of the fifteenth century! Yet, when a grave syphilis resists heaps of pills of bichloride or of protiodide of mercury, is recourse not had to mercurial inunctions for the greater good of the patient? And those gangrenous gummata which cicatrize after an injection of a few centigrammes of calomel, when they have resisted the iodides and inunctions! Show us the therapeutic laws which govern these cases—not so rare as is supposed—in current medical practice! Hence empiricism everywhere, and we shall all remain empirics until that day when we shall have an apparatus sufficiently sensitive to record the intensity of the syphilitic virus just as we have scales to weigh blue ointment, calomel, or corrosive sublimate.

DR. F. BURET.

PARIS, March 20, 1894.

TRANSLATOR'S PREFACE.

VOLUME III.

THE present volume completes the monumental work of Dr. Buret on the history of syphilis. The compilation of the data necessary to achieve the task was an herculean labor requiring no less than six years' unremitting researches of books, manuscripts, and documents, some of them almost inaccessible except to the most persistent inquirer after truth. The value of these researches cannot be overestimated, in view of the flood of light which they have thrown upon a scientific doubt which has existed for centuries. The entire work will stand for many years as a monument to its writer's energy and intelligence, and be as an incentive to others in the pursuit of investigations surrounded by presumably insurmountable obstacles.

Whilst the first two volumes were devoted to the proofs of the existence of syphilis, as derived from various sources, in the present we find a classified morbid entity to deal with, there being not the least shadow of a doubt as to its existence. This necessarily places the author in a superior position in the treatment of his subject and brings us into much closer touch with it. The various theories regarding the etiology, pathology, and treatment of venereal disease are sketched with a master-hand and in a manner as thorough as it is scientific.

Little remains to be said beyond the fact that the English translation is placed before its readers in the hope that it will prove both interesting and profitable reading. If elegance of diction be found wanting in certain parts, it was for the reason that clearness of statement was looked upon as more desirable. Gallicisms have been unavoidable, and untranslatable words and phrases have been paraphrased in the best manner possible under the circumstances. The intrinsic value of the work is such that indulgence is asked of the reader for any shortcomings upon the part of

THE TRANSLATOR.

TABLE OF CONTENTS.

VOLUME II.

CHAPTER III.

CHAPTER IV.

CHAPTER V.

CHAPTER VI.

APPENDIX A.

APPENDIX B.

TABLE OF CONTENTS.

VOLUME III.

SYPHILIS

IN THE MIDDLE AGES.

CHAPTER I.

SCIENTIFIC DOCUMENTS.

Syphilis in Europe in the first fifteen centuries of our era.—Documents obtained from the works of the physicians of the Western Empire, of the masters of the Arabian school, and of the Arabists and their successors.—The *asafati* of the Arabians.—The leeches, or physicians, of the Middle Ages; manuscripts relating to sexual pathology.—The symptoms of syphilis described in scientific works since the tenth century.—What the authors of that epoch understood by the word *leprosy*.—The *thick* (crustaceous) *itch* and its treatment by mercury before the epidemic of Naples.—A discovery by Broca in an ancient cemetery of Paris.—M. Lancereaux at the Catacombs.

From a purely historical point of view, that period which extends from the fall of the Roman Empire up to the end of the fifteenth century is generally designated as the Middle Ages. But, for the study which we have set before us, it was difficult to confine ourselves exactly within the limits imposed by the dates which have marked the destiny of nations. It is for this reason that, in our first volume, in looking up works relating to syphilis, which emanated from the authors of antiquity, we did not exhaust the list of physicians of the school of Galen. The powerful Roman Empire expired A.D. 312, being replaced by what we have called the Western Empire, which disappeared, in its turn, in the middle of the fifteenth century.[1] The Greek school still lives, but it throws its last rays to leave permanently, five centuries later, its place to the Arabian school represented by Alexandria and Bagdad. We will, therefore, pass in review the principal masters who, inspired by the doctrines of Hippocrates and Galen, professed either in Greece or in Italy. Next we will study the Arabians and Arabists to arrive to the school of Salernum, which shone in full in the midst of the Middle Ages; and, finally, to the authors who were best known in the fourteenth and fifteenth centuries. These last, breaking with the traditions of antiquity, marked a new era in the healing art, which caused their epoch to be known as the *age of renovation.*

From the stand-point of our subject, the quotations furnished by the works of the successors of Galen do not differ much from each other. All, as Renouard remarks,[2] copied each other with an abandon which they did not always take pains to conceal. It would therefore be fastidious to reproduce to satiety, under divers labels, the parts of sentences which we have extracted from Galen, Dioscorides, Areteus, Oribasius, and others. Besides, being given the rich collection of proofs furnished by the Greek and Roman poets, we believe it almost useless, as we have already said, to continue to make efforts to demonstrate the antiquity of syphilis. The question is lost or it is won: if it is lost, the new documentary evidence which we can bring will not save it; if, on the other hand, it be won, the reader will be

[1] The last ruler of the empire (second Greek Empire) was Constantine Poleologos Dragoses, who bravely fell fighting in the streets of Constantinople on the day that the Sultan Mahomet II captured that city (1453). The Eastern Empire—which was then almost reduced to the city of Constantinople—fell under the dominion of the Turks from that time.

[2] Hist. de la médecine. Paris, 1846. History of Medicine.

grateful to receive interesting accounts unaccompanied by commentaries which have become stereotyped. So that, assuming the problem to be solved, let us complete our task by bringing up some few original points, but without entering into an argument which carries itself beyond the limits of our vision.

After Oribasius, the most remarkable Greek physicians were Aëtius, Alexander of Tralles, and Paulus Ægineta, who made the sixth century illustrious. But long before them, during the first three or four centuries of our era, other less-renowned physicians lived, whom we have not yet quoted, but whose works have equally reached us. They are more or less servile reproductions of the medical treatises of their predecessors, but occasionally there are to be found some passages which attest to a slight progress in clinical observation, and it may be seen that venereal diseases, in proportion as the centuries succeed each other, are the subject of descriptions becoming less and less vague. In these authors of secondary prominence there may be found, here and there, an instructive phrase which has not been formerly read. All describe fissures, rhagades, and condylomata of the anus; pimples of the vulva, and chancres of the yard, etc.

Scribonius Largus, a Roman physician of the first century, speaks of a *tumor*, of an *unhealthy ulcer* of the penis (*veretri tumorem sordidum*). Sextus Placitus Papyriensis (fourth century), besides the affections we have just mentioned, speaks of *figs* of the anus (*ficos qui in ano nascuntur*) and describes *chancres* and *corns* of the penis (*carbunculos, callos in veretro*). Without dilating any further, we beg to remark that these *corns* of the penis can scarcely be referred to anything but the induration which sometimes persists after the cure of the infecting chancre. Celius Aurelianus, the translator of Soranus (second century), Moschion (second century), Marcellus Empiricus (fourth century), and others give descriptions identically similar. This Marcellus the Empiric, a Roman citizen, practiced medicine at Bordeaux under the Emperor Gratian (about A.D. 380). He relates that Soranus had undertaken to cure, in Aquitania (Gascony) alone, two hundred persons affected with *mentagra* and *filthy scales* which repercussed themselves all over the body.[1]

Aëtius was celebrated toward the end of the fifth century; he studied at Alexandria and located in Constantinople. Like his predecessors, in his works he speaks of rhagades and condylomata of the anus, but he states that these condylomata may be soft and without irritation, at other times *hard*, *irritated*, and *painful.* There did not exist, at the anal orifices of his time, simple vegetations alone. Speaking of *thymi* (θύμοι), so called on account of the analogy which exists, from the stand-point of color, between certain small syphilides and the flower of thyme, he gives the following description:—

Excrescentiæ turgidæ, asperæ, subrubræ. Frequens est hic morbus circa sedem, pudenda et femora; invadit tamen quandoque et faciem.[2]	Turgid excrescences, rough, reddish. This disease is frequently found at the *margin of the anus*, on the *genital organs* and *thighs;* however, it sometimes also involves the *face.*

It is useless to attempt to demonstrate that this description alludes to papular syphilides, and in nowise to the ordinary cauliflowers. Besides, Celsus had already stated that the *condylomata of the anus* were ob-

[1] Dufour, Hist. de la prostitut. Paris, 1851. History of Prostitution.
[2] Tetrabibl.

served in sodomites. When they are larger, adds Aëtius, these growths assume the name of *sycoses* (σῦκα). Like all the others, he designates the word *acrochordon* as applied to a simple vegetation (*verruca*), and speaks of *formica* of the genital organs; of *unclean ulcers* of the vulva, of the prepuce, and of the glans; of *chancrous ulcers* (carbunculosa ulcera) of the vulva, etc. Farther on a chapter is devoted to fissures of the prepuce, of the anus, and of the genital organs of women (*ad præputii, ani, et muliebrium pudendorum rhagadas*); so it was not always the simple anal fissure. Finally, he notes the *eruptions* which suddenly appear in the sexual regions (*pudendorum spontanea exanthemata*). In the works of Alexander of Tralles, not a word is found referring to venereal diseases.

Paulus Ægìnita, who flourished at the end of the sixth century, has left important works in which a real progress in the medical sciences may be observed. Venereal diseases are treated of in a much more detailed manner than by his predecessors. He gives the description of *figs:* "ulcerating, roundish eruptions, slightly indurated, of a reddish color."

Ficus nominent eruptiones ulcerosas, rotundas, subduras, rubicundas . . .[1]

Farther on he recommends an inert powder for the syphilitic pustules of the head and chin.

Ad ficos in capite ac mento pustulas medicamentum siccum.

These are not the ordinary vegetations, for he devotes a paragraph to warts of the sexual parts (*verrucas in pudendas*). He evidently refers to the urethral chancre, so often unrecognized, in this phrase: "If it should happen that an *ulcer of the glans* is situated in the in-

[1] Paulus Æginita, De re méd., iii, p. 3.

terior of the meatus urinarius, and *should not have been observed,"* . . .

Si vero in cole intra pudendi foramen inconspicuum ulcus fiat . . .

In fine, to sum all in a word, it was he who gave to syphilis its true name, that of "*universal ulcer*,"—the only one which it should have retained. Under the name of *diopter* he describes an instrument which is nothing else than our actual *speculum.*

In a manuscript of the ninth century, which may be found in the "Bibliothèque Nationale," of Paris, a passage may be seen which testifies to a relation existing at that time between certain morbid growths of the anus and ulcers of the genital organs. The anonymous author claims to have observed, at the very orifice of the anus, fissures, holes, tumors, vegetations, etc., "and *pustules* of divers sorts, as large as beans, peas, or even filberts, and sometimes elevated to such a degree that they seemed to close that orifice." . . .

. . . et ibi pustias diversorum genera, in magnitudine granorum fabæ vel pisi, aliquando ut avellanæ fiunt, aliquando eminens ut ipso orificio clandere videatur. . . .

What Latin! But that is not the question; let us hear the end :—

. . . Non solus anus tumefit, sed et alia membra quæ prope sunt; et veretri immunda vulnera et sordida vel maligna inde fiunt, si medici propter turpitudinem vel fetorem ipsas immunditias non extergunt diligenter curando.[1]

. . . Not only is the anus tumefied, but also the adjoining organs; this state may even become the *starting-point of sores* which are foul, infected, or *malign of the penis*, if physicians, either on account of the *shameful* nature of the disease or of its fetidity, have not diligently hastened to clean out these impurities by well-directed treatment.

[1] Fol. 101, cap. 89.

Then comes the Arabian school, which completely eclipses that of Greece. This school is represented first by Rhazes, a Persian in origin, and who was celebrated in Bagdad toward the end of the ninth century; then Ali-Abbas, also of Persian origin, and who lived toward the end of the tenth century. Rhazes describes venereal papules, which he calls *bothor;* and he defines "bothor" as an itching followed by a rising (tumor) on the vulva or penis, as a result of coitus. Then come Mesue, Isaac, Avicenna (this last born A.D. 980), Avenzoar, Averroes, Albucasis (1100), of the tenth to the twelfth centuries, who all give about the same details on venereal diseases. These authors speak of bothor, apostems, of pustules of the penis and of the vulva, and republish what we are already acquainted with. However, Mesue tells us that the Persian fire (*ignis Persicus*) was of the nature of chancres (*carbunculorum*); that *formica* (μυρμήκιον of the Greeks) was an apostem of the skin capable of degenerating into a putrid ulcer (*ulcus putridum*). The *saphati* or *asafati*, of which Avicenna and his successors speak, was something analogous. Isaac, after the apostems of the penis, describes the *nodes* which arise at the anus as they do on the vulva (*nodi in ano ut in vulva nascuntur*). Avenzoar speaks of *red pustules* which originate at times upon the glans (*pustulæ rubræ in capite virgæ*), and which are called, in Arabic, *alohumbra.*

We come to the school of Salernum, which shone for nearly five hundred years; its most illustrious teacher was a monk of the name of Constantine the African (of Carthage), who lived about the year 1080. The physicians of this school, known under the name of Arabists, teach us, for the most part, nothing more than their predecessors, so far as the subject in hand is concerned. For this reason we will quote but a few.

We are come to the thirteenth century. In a chapter entitled *De cancris et fistulis et aliis pustulis in genitalibus consurgentibus* (Of chancres, fistulas, and other pustules which arise on the genital organs), Roland, an author of this epoch, advises an emollient treatment for excoriations of the frenum followed by œdema and induration: "But if it should come to pass that the string becomes *excoriated* and spoils, then *swells* and *becomes hard*, oil of violets is to be used." . . .

Si autem excoriari filumque corrumpi contingat, unde inflatur et tumet, atque durescit, oleum violarum. . . .

Is not this the œdema and induration which are pathognomonic of the infecting chancre, already noted by Celsus?

We find in Michael Scot,[1] who lived from 1214 to 1291, a phrase which is extremely interesting in connection with the heredity of venereal disease:—

Si mulier fluxum patiatur et vir eam cognoscat, facile sibi virga vitiatur. Sciendum est quod, si erat fluxus quando erat facta conceptio, creatura concipitur vitiata.

When a woman has a discharge, if a man have intercourse with her, he has many opportunities of contracting an affection of *bad nature* on his *penis*. In addition, it should be known that, if conception take place at that time, *the product will be tainted* with the disease.

This discharge from the woman could be menstrual,[2] gonorrhœal, leucorrhœal, but with syphilides or a chancre which were invisible (*inconspicuum ulcus*); or else

[1] De procreat. homin. Physionomia, cap. vi. On the Procreation of Man.

[2] This etiological factor was sufficient for the physicians of the Middle Ages to explain venereal diseases in men.

the discharge from vulvar mucous patches mixed with the uterine fluid, syphilis always bringing on a certain amount of metritis. What is undeniable is that a contagious and hereditary virus is clearly defined. You may say that it was leprosy. Yes, if by that name you understand the leprosy of the authors of the Middle Ages who so designated venereal diseases, and notably classic syphilis; no, if you allude to true leprosy.

August 13, 1889, Dr. Zambaco,[1] a physician of Constantinople, declared to the Paris Académie de Médecine that for nine years he studied leprosy in the East; the conclusions of the learned Pasha are that if leprosy is hereditary, on the other hand, it is *in no way contagious.* But our college friend, Professor Leloir (of Lille), in his remarkable work, declares himself a partisan of the contagiousness of leprosy,[2] agreeing on that point with Vidal, Besnier, and Hillairet. On the other hand, our colleague, Springer, says, in his interesting paper on "The Lepers in Norway,"[3] that "contagion, after having been proclaimed by all, is to-day questioned by a great number of physicians, and even denied by a few of those upon whom the care of lepers devolves."

The discovery of the bacillus of leprosy, studied since then by Hansen, has restored the doctrine of contagion to favor. Nevertheless, Professor Cornil, al-

[1] The nationality of Dr. Zambaco often gives rise to errors, in both newspapers and medical journals, which it would be well to correct once and for all. Some say that he is a Turk, others a Greek; more rarely he is believed to be an Italian. The truth is that he practices medicine in Turkey with a reputation that is as well known as it is extensive, that he is of Greek origin, and his name is Genoese; but, what very few are acquainted with, is the fact that Dr. Zambaco-Pasha, officer of the Legion of Honor and national corresponding member of the Paris Académie de Médecine, is a French citizen.

[2] H. Leloir, Traité théorique et pratique de la lèpre. Paris, 1886. Practical and Theoretical Treatise on Leprosy.

[3] "Les lépreux en Norwége," Bulletin Méd., November, 1888.

though having reported cases favorable to this last opinion, remains in an hesitating attitude. "Contagiousness," says he, "is very difficult to establish, for direct and irrefutable proofs are wanting." M. Leroy de Méricourt is also of the opinion that the proofs are insufficient. It is the opinion which predominates in Norway; and, in Christiania, it has for its principal upholders Danielsen, Kaurin, and Bidenkap. On the other hand, success should have attended the inoculation of a criminal condemned to death.[1] Was heredity at fault? asks Springer, from whom we have borrowed the major part of our facts. It is presumable; for Neisser, Damsh, and Hansen, who have made numerous experiments on animals and on *the human being* with bacilli and morbid products, have *never* succeeded in producing leprous infection.

Springer, who does not clearly commit himself,—and we can understand his reserve,—seems inclined to contagiousness, for he confesses himself much shaken by the fact that isolation caused a fall in the number of Norwegian lepers from three thousand to twelve hundred in thirty years. Such a reduction would seem to be very slow for a disease clearly contagious; and we feel inclined to ask our colleague if he does not think that this phenomenon is rather due to the impossibility of reproduction for individuals who are confined? It must not be forgotten that leprosy is considered hereditary by the majority of specialists. Finally, the physician-in-chief of the hospital of Bergen, where leprosy is treated,

[1] The author evidently refers to the case of the Sandwich Islander, Keânu, who was reported to have been successfully inoculated with leprosy. A critical study of his case revealed the fact that he not only was descended from a markedly leprous family, several of whom are to-day suffering from the disease, but it is doubtful if he were not already suffering from the trouble at the time he was inoculated.—O-D.

has not personally observed, for *thirty years past*, a single case in which contagion was established. It is Springer, again, who acquaints us with this fact. The observations of the Norwegian dermatologist confirm those of Zambaco in the East.[1]

It will be seen from this short *résumé* that the problem is far from being solved. For us, in whom it would come with bad grace to decide a question upon which the most authoritative masters are disagreed, we desire to humbly propose to verify an hypothesis which is, perhaps, not far removed from the truth.

Let us reason a little. Here we see Norwegian physicians, who have been treating lepers for many years, clearly stating that leprosy is not contagious. A physician of our army and Dr. Zambaco, who have studied leprosy in the Orient, say the same thing. Dr. Ramboldi, who was physician-in-chief of the hospital of San Remo for twenty years, where lepers coming from the Piedmont are treated, states that leprosy is not contagious, and that it is only transmitted hereditarily. On the other hand, our most eminent dermatologists uphold the possibility of contagion. To tell the truth, the distinguished practitioners of the Hôpital St. Louis see but a very limited number of lepers. But Professor Leloir went to study the disease where it occurs; that is to say, in the north of Italy and in the leper-hospitals of Bergen. His observations, embracing a large number of patients, have necessarily more weight. Besides, the discovery of the bacillus of leprosy is a theoretical support for the possibility of inoculation followed by success. For this

[1] We may add that a number of superintendents of leper-asylums in the Windward Islands, Brazil, etc., who daily see cases, operate on them, and make post-mortem examinations, have been doing so for years, and, so far, we have failed to hear of any case of contagion occurring in any of them.—O-D.

reason, whilst not positively denying the contagiousness of leprosy in a radical manner, why could it not be regarded as a constitutional parasitic disease, analogous to tuberculosis, whose direct transmissibility would only take place under exceptional circumstances and in an already well-prepared soil?[1] Let us admit the idea for a moment that a learned bacteriologist should some day demonstrate to us the bacillus of cancer, which Virchow claims to have outlined dimly, and succeed in implanting it on a healthy individual. Everything is possible, especially in bacteriology. Well, would an attempt be made from that to assert that the *ficus* of the Romans was nothing but a common epithelioma? We hope not. In the same manner a well-demonstrated case of transmission of leprosy—independent of all hereditary principle—would not prove that the disease, as we know it to-day, flourished alone, under that name, in the Middle Ages. It would be childish to find, in an inoculation followed by success, the explanation of that terrible contagion which all authors of the time have noted; the description given in all works is that of venereal affections, to which leprosy, before the siege of Naples, served in reality as a convenient label.[2]

It was thus that we wrote in September, 1889, but,

[1] The same idea has been advanced, in analogous terms, by a few authors since 1889, the time at which these lines were penned. The chapter containing them should have formed a part of our first volume; but a question as to the size of the book forced us to reserve it for the second volume. [In regard to the soil, which the author mentions above, there is no doubt that certain races are refractory to leprosy, whereas others appear to be exceedingly susceptible. Thus, we know that the Sandwich Islanders acquired leprosy very easily, and it spread with astonishing rapidity. Zambaco-Pasha states that, in Turkey, those of Hebrew descent are more easily infected than the others.—O-D.]

[2] Many writers on skin diseases even to this day designate psoriasis by the old name, *lepra*, or *lepra alphos*, reserving these terms, of course, for the list of synonyms. Still, it indicates that leprosy was a term not entirely confined to one disease.—O-D.

since the intervening four years, very interesting new publications have appeared on this subject. Well, despite the real talent shown by the authors in combating or defending the contagiousness of leprosy, and the tone of conviction which pervades their works, we have resolved to retain the foregoing paragraph; for we do not feel ourselves as yet disposed to modify—we will not say our way of seeing the matter, but at least our first impression in regard to the manner in which this horrible disease is transmitted.

For example, we have read, with the greatest interest, the remarkable memoir[1] of Dr. Le Grand, a surgeon of the first class of the French navy. Our distinguished *confrère* reports numerous cases, which have been thoroughly studied, in which leprosy seems to have been transmitted by contagion. It seems to us that the author, carried away by his belief, has left in the shadow the question of predisposition, which is one that certainly ought not to be neglected.

No more than in 1889 will we seek to deny the direct transmissibility of leprosy; but, in the cases reported by M. Le Grand, we find that it must have required a prolonged contact, at all times, so to speak,—a cohabitation in the same huts,—for the infection to be produced.[2] In addition, we find leprosy remains, in a way, restricted to the natives, in those places where hygiene is wanting; and those cases in which Europeans have been attacked are almost always those of outlaws who had frequent relations with the Kanakas. If we will but consider that all felons, or very nearly all, have affairs with the

[1] A. Le Grand, La lèpre en Nouvelle-Calédonie. Clermont (Oise), 1891. Leprosy in New Caledonia.

[2] It is true that certain adherents of the theory of contagion admit periods of incubation of more than thirty years for leprosy. After that . . . !

native women, the *popinées*, there is cause for surprise at the relatively small number of those who are affected. If the transmission were rapid and *unerring*, the whole penitentiary would long since have succumbed.

Yet this only refers to New Caledonia. It is probable that things do not occur in the same manner in the East; for Dr. Zambaco, who has recently published a most interesting book[1] on the same subject, does not at all appear convinced of the direct contagion. His travels in Egypt, in Palestine, and among the islands of the Archipelago, have even strengthened him in the absolutely contrary opinion. According to him, the teachings regarding the processus of leprosy must still remain open. And, until we are furnished with more ample information, we will cling to our first hypothesis,—that this frightful disease is not directly transmitted save in infrequent cases, if not exceptional ones, as a result of living intimately for several months or years, under conditions of receptivity of a special nature, and that it develops only in a marked way in a soil good for its growth.

Besides, Dr. Le Grand himself confirms us in this view, for he concludes by saying:—

> Leprosy is caught neither by the air nor by water, let it be well understood; and a focus of lepers, were it even in the centre of a city, if it were well isolated, would never become (all idea of relations or of contact with the diseased being put aside) a centre or focus of infection. The example of lazarettoes at the gates of cities in the Middle Ages and the example of leprous Mussulmans freely circulating in their quarters are there to prove this, and *there never was more of an epidemic of leprosy than there has been an epidemic of syphilis or of phthisis.*

This is exactly our opinion.

[1] Zambaco-Pacha, Voyages chez les lépreux. Paris, 1891. Travels Among Lepers.

Dr. Zambaco does not absolutely deny the contagiousness of leprosy, but he is of the opinion that it is to be considered as most rare. He mentions a number of cases of healthy persons living among lepers without contracting leprosy, and that for twenty, thirty, and even forty years. Households are constantly seen in which one of the couple is a leper,—dying finally at the end of five, ten, fifteen, or twenty years; whereas the other one remains unaffected. The wives of lepers become pregnant, are delivered of a child which may or may not be diseased, without ever becoming subject to the trouble; and not one of the healthy persons so exposed has ever taken the most simple precautions to avoid any possible contagion. There have even been negative inoculations, the most remarkable case of the kind having been seen by Dr. Zambaco in the island of Samos. The case, which is as follows, is taken from the important work of our eminent *confrère*, published in 1891:—

> A very pretty young lady, and of good family, fell desperately in love with a commencing leper, whom she married in spite of everything, the marriage with or between lepers not being interdicted in Samos. She lived eight years with her husband, who, through jealousy and egotism, tried to communicate the disease to her by all possible means. He did not wish her to survive him. For instance, he would kiss her on the mouth continually; and he gave her his tongue to hold in her mouth for a quarter of an hour at a time, when he was affected with extensive ulcers of the palate. . . . He even inoculated her upon several occasions. No results followed. The woman is still living and healthy.[1]

The learned dermatologist admits that certain meteorological and telluric conditions are not without force in the production of the predilection to leprosy in those countries where it is found in an endemic form. Poverty, bad hygiene, and filth are also important factors whose

[1] Zambaco-Pacha, Voyages chez les lépreux.

influence must not be lost sight of. Leprosy increases in Turkey during famines, according to official reports. "To extirpate leprosy," says Zambaco, "is synonymous with suppressing misery." On the other hand, the author is, as we have already said, a strong partisan of heredity, which is admitted by the majority of dermatologists. He recites an enormous number of cases which prove the existence of hereditary antecedents in individuals who never came in contact with lepers, and in whom leprosy manifested itself at various ages. In each one a leprous ascendant was found,—the father or grandfather; for this disease may skip one or even two generations.

Our eminent and sympathetic colleague, Dr. L. Brocq, who declares himself a contagionist, recognizes, in his excellent work, that leprosy is only transmissible under very exceptional circumstances; and, despite the discovery of the bacillus of Hansen, he does not hesitate to admit, like Zambaco, the influence of the factors we have just enumerated. "In order that this transmission may occur," he says, in his article on leprosy, "there must exist conditions of receptivity and of soil, as yet badly understood, but which, perhaps, depend on race, bad hygiene, poverty, overcrowding, defective food, and heredity."[1] It would be safe to wager that the discovery of the existence of the bacillus of leprosy has brought a certain number of recruits to the camp of the contagionists, for that micro-organism has troubled—theoretically, at least—the convictions of those who uphold the contrary opinion. It is certain that, if clinical observations only were adhered to, one would be tempted to join those who are arrayed under the banner of the

[1] L. Brocq, Traité des maladies de la peau. Paris, 1892. 2d edition, page 416. Treatise on Skin Diseases.

anticontagionists. Perhaps the author indulged in the same thought, for a little farther on we find the following sentence, in which a slight doubt seems manifest: "It is certain that if leprosy is transmissible from the affected to the healthy individual, it is only so under certain conditions, as yet not well known, which make it in reality but *slightly contagious*."[1] In truth, it is hardly possible to conceive of the contagiousness of the lepra's bacillus in any other way than in these narrow limits.

Nor must it be forgotten—which explains many of the premature opinions from the point of view of contagion—that leprosy and syphilis are confounded at every moment, according to the testimony of Greek, Turkish, and Egyptian physicians. Zambaco has been able to verify this in his own case. Besides, these two diseases co-exist at times, and through that very fact aggravate each other.

What is to be concluded from these divers opinions, from these accumulated proofs, as many in number by the contagionists as by the non-contagionists, and defended with the same ardor, if not the same success even? We have read without any preconceived ideas the works of the ones and of the others, not in the hope of confirming a previous impression, but with the expectation of forming a definite opinion. Well, we believe, with Dr. Zambaco, that the question is not yet completely elucidated. If it be true that leprosy can be communicated by one human being to another, outside of procreation, are we to admit to contagion one per thousand of the cases seen? It is, perhaps, much; at all events, we would not undertake to prove it!

In the thirteenth century medical works, properly

[1] *Loc. cit.*, page 420.

so called, were not always written by practitioners, or by physicians no longer practicing medicine. Learned men—but how rare!—touch upon all scientific subjects. It is thus that in 1250 we see one Theodoric, a religious of the order of St. Dominic and bishop of Cervia (an Italian city in Romagna), write a treatise on surgery. It is true that he made a compilation of the work of Brunnus, and profited a great deal from the remarks of Hugh de Lucanes, with whom he had lived. However this may be, Chapter XLIX of Book III, which treats of the *dead disease* [mal mort] (de malo mortuo), is particularly interesting to us, for the description of it by the author is that of the principal symptoms of syphilis; he concludes by advising, for its treatment, *mercurial frictions and sweating.* Let us not forget that the manuscript dates from the thirteenth century; nevertheless, the therapeutic measures employed would not be much out of place in 1893.

Then, a little farther on, he adds this sentence, which is for us a very valuable piece of information, "I believe that this disease is a *species of leprosy.*" In another place, he states, textually, that "whosoever hath intimate relations with a woman who has formerly had to do with a *leper*, contracts a *bad disease.*" Lepers could, by direct contagion, transmit a disease *other than current leprosy*, and this disease was especially contracted by coitus. It would not require a great stretch of the imagination to find the following explanation: Theodoric, who called *leprous* the women in whom he found the plain presence of pustulo-crustaceous syphilides, without suspecting the vulvar lesions,—and especially the correlation of these latter with the cutaneous manifestations,—saw with surprise these women communicate chancres of the penis. He accordingly gave the name of *bad disease* to the *nodosities* either of the vulva or of the penis, according to the sex of the victim, which appeared to him absolutely outside of classical leprosy.

When it was observed later on that dermatic troubles in general, which primarily received the name of "leprosy" and genital sores, were almost always acquired under the same circumstances, the same word was indiscriminately applied to all affections—sexual and otherwise—in which the ancient Venus appeared to be put forward as a cause. The adjective *leprous*, as we shall have occasion to verify, was then a term which served currently in the Middle Ages to designate a *venereal* individual.

Guillaume de Salicel, professor at Verona, where he wrote in 1270, is the first physician who employed the expressions *impure*, *unhealthy*, *infected* (fœda, fœtida), *foul* (immunda), as applied to any woman or to the courtesan, the sources of venereal sores. All of these adjectives are found at every step in the writings of the authors who followed him in the thirteenth and fourteenth centuries. In his surgery,[1] he speaks "of *pustules* which are white or *red*, of small *pimples* large as millet-seeds, of erosions and of *corruptions* which show themselves on the penis and around the prepuce," and he states positively that these lesions recognize as their principal cause "*coitus* with an *impure* woman, or a prostitute."

. . . de pustulis albis vel rubeis et de millio et de scissuris et de corruptionibus quæ fiunt in virga vel circa præputium, propter coïtum cum fœtidâ muliere, aut cum meretrice, aut ab aliâ causâ.

He knew that figs grew at the anus and vulva, for one of his chapters is entitled "*De ficis et condylomatis in ano et vulvâ.*" Farther on he advises ablutions with

[1] Cyrurgia, lib. i, cap. 48.

vinegar-water to those who, "following coitus with an *infected* woman, should see some disquieting *sign* from the point of view of a former *contamination.*"

. . . dum incipit post coïtum cum fœdâ muliere aliquod corruptionis futuræ vestigium.

This passage leads to the belief that the physician of Verona had perfectly observed that a certain length of time elapsed between the suspicious coitus, or even the primary lesion (*vestigium*) contracted upon a former occasion, and the general infection of the organism (*corruptio*). In Chapter XLIX he says, speaking of the *nodosity* of the penis (*nodo in virgâ*), "I have cured many in my time." Finally, in Chapter LIII, which treats of *crusts* and *ulcers* on the legs ("*De crustis et cancrænis in cruribus*"), he describes the venereal disease and advises *frictions* by means of *mercury* quenched with saliva. At the present time mercury is quenched in lard, which is more cleanly and infinitely more practical; apart from this, the therapeutics is the same. It must not be forgotten that Guillaume de Salicet wrote in 1270; that is to say, more than two hundred years before the siege of Naples.

Muratori, in his work on the "Antiquity of Italy," reports that Guillaume Piacentino, in Chapter XLVIII of Book I of his medico-chirurgical works, written in 1275, has given a description of venereal diseases, distinguishing the lesions of the genital organs having a *specific* character from those which do not present any.

Petrus Hispanus, who later became pope under the name of John XXI (1276), after having mentioned the *fig* and ulcers of the penis, speaks of the chancre (*cancrum*), which may be found on the penis and in other places, and which is cured simply by the application of olive-tree leaves triturated with honey. "But," he adds, "centaury cures it in a few days, and more completely."

Cancrum in virgâ et alibi folia olivæ trita cum melle curant. Centaurea in paucos dies sanat cancrum perfectius.

We can see from this that the expressions *cancrum*, *cancrosum*, applied to an ulcer of the genitals, did not signify, in the minds of the authors of the Middle Ages, an ulcerated, cancerous tumor; for, in spite of the hand-bills of certain industrious individuals who cannot be recommended, cancer is not curable.

A manuscript of the thirteenth century, *small micrologue* (parvus micrologus), as it was called by its author,[1] contains a passage which also testifies to the existence of venereal ulcerations.

Ulcerantur utraque, virga scilicet et testiculi, tempore menstruorum ex coïtu ex salsis humoribus et acutis et incensis, quod satisex colore cutis et pustularum vel saniei ex pruritu et punctura et ardore perpenditur.[2]

These two organs—that is to say, the penis and testicles—become the seat of *ulcers* after a coitus at the menstrual period, by reason of the acrid humors, which are heated and corrosive, as is abundantly proven by the color of the skin and *pustules* or bad blood, as also the itching, the stinging, and the burning which is felt.

At that time, as to-day, in fact, menstrual blood had a good broad back.

Another physician of the thirteenth century, a certain Géraud, Gerarder Geraldus, who wrote about the same time as Guillaume de Salicet, is still more explicit. In a passage of Book VII of his "Explanations"[3] may be

[1] Ricardus Senior, Richard the Englishman, the Parisian, the Salernitan are among the various appellations under which he is known.

[2] MSS. No. 7056. Biblioth. Nat. Paris.

[3] Glossulæ Gerandi, *Cf.* Hist. littér. de la France, t. xxi. Literary History of France.

found a sentence which proves that the author was acquainted with the general infection which follows local lesions.

Virga patitur a coïtu cum mulieribus immundis ex spermate corrupto, vel ex humore venenoso in collo matricis recepto; nam virga inficitur et aliquando totum corpus.	The penis is diseased in consequence of coitus indulged in with *foul* women; is it due to the corruption of the sperm or to the presence of a *virulent liquid* deposited in the neck of the womb[1] in which it has sojourned? We know not. Nevertheless, the *penis is infected*, and sometimes the *whole body*.

We do not know how the partisans of the American origin will be able to interpret this sentence; but, in so far as *general infection* is concerned, it appears sufficiently clear to us. However, although we are no longer arguing, we have by no means exhausted our proofs; and, if these latter do not all have the same intrinsic value, they may, when taken altogether, have a certain weight in the balance.

The authors who follow say the same as Guillaume de Salicet, and almost in the same words. We will quote a few belonging to the end of the thirteenth and beginning of the fourteenth centuries.

Simon Januensis (1288) gives a description of *figs*. "We call *figs*," says he, "hard *pimples*, which are ulcerated and show granulations like the seeds of the fig."

Ficus vocantur durities ulcerosæ, habentes in se grana, sicut grana ficuum.

We read, in Lanfranc of Milan[2]:—

[1] That is to say, in the posterior *cul-de-sac*. The Latin word *recepto* (received) implies the idea of an external source of derivation for the contagious virus.

[2] Practica; doctr. tertia, cap. 2. Milan, 1290.

De ficu et cancero et ulcere in virga virili. Ficus est quædam excrescentia quæ nascitur super præputium virgæ et aliquando super caput; . . . quæ si corrumpitur, transit in cancrum. Ulcera veniunt ex pustulis calidis virgæ supervenientibus, vel ex commixtione cum muliere fœda quæ cum ægro talem habente morbum de novo coïerat.

Of the fig, of the chancre, and of the ulcer of the penis. The fig is an excrescence of a peculiar nature which grows on the prepuce and sometimes on the head of the penis. If it corrupt, it degenerates into a *chancre.* Ulcers originate from hot *pustules* which grow on the penis, or from a coitus with a *diseased* woman having recently had sexual relations with a *diseased man* attacked with the SAME *affection.*

The contagiousness seems to us to be pointed out clearly enough. The author then advises washing after a coitus which might give rise to fears for the future.

Bernard Gordon (1305), in speaking of diseases of the penis,[1] recognizes, amongst the external causes of *ulcers* and of *chancres*, the fact "of having had relations with a woman whose vagina is *diseased*, full of sanious matter, of virulence, of flatulence, or of analogous corruptions."

. . . jacere cum muliere cujus matrix est immunda, plena sanie aut virulentiâ, aut ventositate et similibus et corruptis.

That is to say, the entire collection of venereal contagia, which the author designates by the expressions of his epoch. In studying Avicenna, he adds, it may be seen that "every ulcerating and corrosive pustule may be called *Persian fire*,[2] *chancre*, or *chancroid*" [chancrelle, literally small chancre].

. . . omnis pustula ulcerans et corrodens . . . potest vocari ignis persicus seu carbo, seu carbunculus.

[1] Lilium medicinæ. Particula vii, cap. 2. Montpellier, 1305.

[2] In a book published in Calcutta by a society of learned men, under the title "Asiatic Researches," and quoted by Swediaur, may be seen the statement (vol. ii) that the *venereal disease* is known in Hindustan since time *immemorial* under the name of *Persian fire* (bâo), and that mercury is employed for it.

Farther on, a passage written in a peculiar manner testifies to the uncertainty of the physicians of the Middle Ages in regard to the nature and etiology of certain diseases; but it is interesting in the sense that it proves the *malum mortuum*, described by Theodoric fifty years before, to have been syphilis.

Malum mortuum est quædam species scabiei quæ oritur ex melancolia naturali adusta et ex adustione phlegmati falsi; cum livore et negredine, et pustulis crustosis, magnis, fœtidis, sine sanie, cum œrugine, et cum quædam insensibilitate, et cum turpi aspectu, et in coxis et in tibii frequentius ter eveniens.	The *dead disease* is a sort of rottenness which is caused by inflammation of the natural melancholic matter and of the false phlegm. This affection is characterized by a livid, black color; by large *pustules*, which are *scabby*, fetid, not sanious, like rust, almost insensitive, and of a repellent aspect; this disease is seen thrice as frequently upon the hips and the *tibiæ* as anywhere else.

Already Roger Bacon had said, in the twelfth century, that the *dead disease* was a sort of rotting (*scabiei genus*), causing *pustules* around the legs and shins (*circa crura et tibias facit pustulas*), and which was so called because the limb attacked by it seemed to be struck with the gangrene (*mortificari*). Lanfranc says about the same thing.

Silvaticus (1317) states that the *bothor* of the Arabians was an excrescence of flesh or a pustule (*bothor, id est eminentia carnis vel pustula*); for him, as for Theodoric (1250), *formica* is a small projecting pustule (*pustula parva quæ egreditur*). John of Gaddesden says, at about the same epoch, in regard to *ulcers* of the penis,[1] that they are derived from having coitus with a woman having her courses; and he advises, like Guillaume de Salicet and Lanfranc, to wash well the organ after each

[1] Rosa Anglica. Oxford, 1320.

suspicious intercourse, and he repeats almost verbatim the phraseology of the last :—

Si quis vult membrum ab omni corruptione servare, cum a muliere recedit, quum forte habet suspectam de immunditie, lavet illud cum aqua frigida cum aceto mixta, vel de urina. . . .

If you wish to preserve your organ from all *virus*, in case you should have reason to suspect your companion of being *infected*, wash yourself, as soon as you retire, with cold water to which vinegar has been added, or with urine. . . .

To this may be compared an analogous sentence from a manuscript of the fourteenth century by an unknown author,[1] who had certainly read the works either of Guillaume de Salicet or of Lanfranc.

Ablutio cum aqua frigida et continua abstersio cum eâdem post coïtum cum fœtidâ muliere, vel meretrice, perfecte defendit virgam a corruptione illâ ex causâ, et maxime si post ablutionem cum frigidâ aquâ fiat roratio loci abluti cum aceto.

An ablution and a continuous sprinkling with cold water after coitus with a *diseased* woman or a courtesan guarantees the penis well against *infection* by itself, and especially if, after washing with cold water, vinegar is poured over the washed part.

We also find, in the "English Rose" of Gaddesden, a very curious passage, which proves that the term *leprosy* was applied, in the minds of the physicians of the fourteenth century, to local venereal affections acquired during coitus. The paragraph has this title: *Of the contamination consecutive to intercourse with a leper* [male or female]. (De infectione ex concubitu cum leproso vel leprosâ.) The author is assured that the woman who has had sexual relations with a *leper* may protect herself against all infection if, immediately after the act, "she jumps, runs down the stairs backward, and brings on sneezing by snuffing powdered pepper and by tickling the nasal mucous membrane with a feather dipped in

[1] Fonds St. Victor, No. 218. (National Library, Paris.)

vinegar, in such manner causing the seed she has just received to flow out. Then she must be careful to make ablutions with a decoction of roses and plantain boiled in vinegar with bran." The method is of a *naïveté* which is refreshing; still, the most primitive irrigator is yet preferable to this demoniacal choregraphy.

Gordon,[1] whom we have already quoted, reports a case which confirms our view of the matter regarding the nature of leprosy during the feudal period:—

> A certain countess, who had leprosy, went to Montpellier, and I treated her toward the end. A bachelor of medicine, whom I had placed by her, shared her bed and made her big with child; but he became *leprous* himself.

Philip Shepff[2] relates a similar story relating to a carpenter who, having had to do with a leprous woman, was infected with *leprosy* a short time after.

This mode of contamination is that of syphilis, for it is only diseases of a gallant origin which can be communicated in such a manner. With what Dr. Zambaco has acquainted us in regard to true leprosy—that is, that married men and women, perfectly healthy, may live with their consorts, who are *notoriously leprous*, without ever contracting the slightest trouble—we are forced to the conclusion once more that the word *leprosy*, in the Middle Ages, was most often the synonym of *venereal disease*.

Gui de Chauliac (1360) says, in his second "Traité Doctr.," ii, cap. 3,[3] that *formica* is nothing else than *herpes* of a malign nature (*malus*), and he defines this last: *ulcerated, virulent pustules, and of bad color*. They are of two kinds: small and large. These latter

[1] Lilium medicinæ (Lily of Medicine). Montpellier, 1305. Partic. i, cap. 2.

[2] Liber de lepra. Book on Leprosy.

[3] Cyrurgia. Montpellier, 1360.

show themselves "under the appearance of the *pustules* of *ficus* and of *bothos*, some of whose characteristics they present."

. . . Videntur esse pustulæ ficales et bothorales, quia ad modum ficus et bothores sunt apparentes.

Formica is longer to disappear (*tardioris resolutionis*) than ordinary herpes, and forms no eschar, in spite of its *virulence* (virulentia). Gui de Chauliac repeats very nearly what his predecessors have said. We shall see later on a physician,[1] who lived before and after the epidemic of Naples, state, in the year 1500, that *formica* and the disease which then prevailed (the French disease) were one and the same.

A physician of the fourteenth century but little known, Magninus,[2] says that the corrupt sperm (the vehicle of the contagium) "not only *infects* the natural passages of the woman, but also her *entire organism.*"

. . . non solum feminaria vasa, sed etiam totum corpus corrumpitur.

As a matter of fact, adds he, the putrid sperm spreads itself throughout the body in the manner of a poison (*ad modum veneni*). Let us leave aside the sperm accused here in an entirely gratuitous manner; let us translate *veneni* by the word *virus*, which the author could not know, and the manner of propagation of syphilis will come out very clearly.

Valescus, of Tarentum (1400),[3] gives us some very precise information on the seat and mode of transmission of venereal ulcers and pustules. Up to that time every one was forced to perceive contagion in the

[1] Jean Salicet.

[2] Regimen sanitatis. Lugduni. (Règles pour la santé. Lyon). Rules of Health. Published in 1517.

[3] Philonium. Montpellier, 1400. Lib. vi, cap. 6.

quotations we have made from the authors of the Middle Ages, but the word was not mentioned; whence arose matter for contention. Now we shall see written out in full the word *contagiousness*, which cuts short all discussion:—

Ulcera et pustulæ fiunt in virgâ. . . . Causæ possunt esse vulnus, vel attritio et coitus cum fœtidâ vel immundâ vel cancrosâ muliere. . . . Juvenibus frequentius accidunt quod aliquando cœunt cum fœminâ habente ulcus in matrice; cum sua contagiositate inficiunt virgam, et in eâ fit ulcus.

Ulcers and *pustules* may occur upon the penis. . . . The causes thereof must be sought either in some traumatism or in the *contact* and *coitus* with an *unhealthy*, *infected*, *chancrous* woman. . . . These diseases are most often found in *young persons*, because they sometimes have relations with women having *ulcers of their genital organs*. On account of the CONTAGIOUS nature of the disease, their penis becomes *infected*, and becomes the seat of an *ulcer* of a like nature.

Astruc, who could not pass this by silently, thought that he escaped a difficulty by translating the word *cancrosa* as *cancerous*, and by saying that the terms *fœda* and *immonda* were simply applied to filthy women; for him, these ulcers of the penis were erosions without any importance. We are astonished that no physician of the eighteenth century did not call to the attention of this illustrious, stubborn man that cancer is a rare thing in young persons,—which would contradict the text of Valescus,—and has never been contagious. Poor Astruc, a little confused in the midst of his authentic writings, which all give him the lie in the most formal manner, concludes by quibbling. He recognized that, as a matter of fact, there existed in antiquity genital diseases presenting *manifestations analogous to those of syphilis*, contagious,—my God, yes! (he could not deny it!),—but, at all events, having disappeared in our days. Is this childish enough? Why take so much trouble to prove that Paris and Lutetia[1] are two different cities which have certain analogies to each other, but nothing in common, under the pretext that Lutetia disappeared with the Roman dominion, and that Paris dates from the Middle Ages?[2] As Schellig[3] says, "What matter names, as long as the thing itself is known?" But to yield to evidence is a much greater sacrifice than is generally supposed; this is why the American origin numbers so many partisans to-day.

Farther on, Valescus claims to have seen persons whose penis was the seat of a *chancrous* and *indurated* ulcer which surrounded it, which made it round like a turnip.

Virga erat circundata toto ulcere cancroso cum duritie et erat rotunda, sicut unus napus. . . .

Leonard Bertapalia (1404) speaks of a disease which he calls *morus* (by way of comparison with the fruit of the mulberry-tree); it is, he says, a sort of soft growth which is found about the anus and vulva.

Hugues Bence edited, about 1440, several reports of

[1] Lutetia was the name of Paris when it was under Roman dominion.

[2] When Cæsar, after the conquest of Gaul (about 52 B.C.), made of Lutetia a Roman city and transferred to it the seat of his military government, it was restricted to the island of *la cité*, situated in Parisis; that is to say, in that portion of the department of Seine-et-Oise (at present) comprised between the rivers Oise and Marne. It received the name of Lutetia Parisiorum (Lutetia of the Parisians). Toward the end of the sixth century, Childeric, son of Merovius, the father of Clovis, drove the Romans from it for good and all; the city was first called Parisius (a corruption of the word) from the name of the country of which it was the centre, and finally that of Paris. (*Cf.* "Paris," par A. Vitu.)

[3] "De nominibus non est curandum, cum res ipsa sit nota." Malum de Francia. Heidelberg, 1500. The French disease.

cases which were published later on by one Gozadini.[1] That which bears the number 72 is extremely interesting; the following is a condensation after Astruc and Richond des Brus.[2] The case was that of a young man of quality, 20 years old, who presented, as will be seen, symptoms of constitutional syphilis. The author relates that his patient experienced increasing pains in the head for six weeks; then there appeared, on the back, "hard *pimples* of the size of a split pea or hazel-nut. Finally, at the end of a month, there had come on a *hard tumor* on the back of the leg, near the foot." The following summer the fever recurred accompanied by *red spots over the whole body*, with pains in the mouth and over the shoulders. The spots disappeared, as well as the pains, under the influence of baths. At the end of a month new pains and a new crop of "red, rough, and furfuraceous" spots, with *pimples in the face*, which also terminated in disappearing. Some sciatic pains.

We find in "Peter of Argeletus" (1470) the following passage[3]:—

De pustulis quæ adveniunt virgæ, propter conversationem cum fœdâ muliere. Ex materiâ venenosâ quæ retinetur inter præputium et pellem virgæ istæ pustulæ tales per hunc modum . . . ex actione viri cum fœdâ muliere. . . .

Of the pustules which appear upon the penis in consequence of connections with a diseased woman. These *pustules* of diseased nature are produced by the sojourn of a *virulent* material between the prepuce and the mucous membrane of the glans . . . after a coitus with a *diseased* woman. . . .

A very valuable piece of information, and which emanates from an authoritative source, demonstrates to

[1] Consultations de médecine. Bologne, 1482. Medical Consultations.

[2] De la non-existence du virus vénéréen. Paris, 1826. On the Non-existence of the Venereal Virus.

[3] Chirurgia, lib. ii, traité 30, ch. iii. Surgery, book ii, treatise 30, ch. iii.

us that the cutaneous manifestations of syphilis were already treated under the name of *scabies*, and by *mercurial frictions*, many years before the siege of Naples. To tell the truth, the manuscript does not exist, but it is quoted by the illustrious Fracastor, who, besides his celebrated poem on syphilis, has written a treatise on contagious diseases.[1] In this little work the author searches for the causes of the French disease, and quotes the following case reported by Renault,[2] Dupuy,[3] and two or three others. We reproduce the passage from Fracastor *in extenso*:—

A barber friend of mine possessed a manuscript of quite a respectable age, a sort of formulary. One of the receipts bore this title: "*For the* SCABBY ITCH *accompanied with pain in the joints.*" The barber, when the new disease (syphilis) broke out, remembered a remedy mentioned in his manuscript, and consulted several physicians to know if the remedy might not be employed against the new disease, which *he* believed to be *nothing else than the scabby itch* mentioned therein. But the doctors, after having examined the remedy, proscribed it with violence, because it had a base of *quicksilver* and sulphur.

This contemporary of the epidemic had been able to compare the symptoms presented by the patients with those described in his book; it is on this account that he had the idea, most naturally, of applying the remedy which was counseled. But, unfortunately for him, he addressed himself to obtuse and routine minds.

Without this unfortunate idea, adds Fracastor, he would have made an incredible fortune! At all events, he did not dare to go farther, and did not decide until later on to try his remedy, when it was recognized that it was the best therapeutical agent. He then bitterly repented not having done so before, and to have let others draw from this well profits which he could have kept all to himself.[4]

[1] De morbis contagiosis (Apud Aloysium Luisinum). Venetiis, 1566.

[2] La syphilis au XVe siècle. Paris, 1868. Syphilis in the Fifteenth Century.

[3] Le Moyen-âge médical. Paris, 1888. The Medical Middle Ages.

[4] To facilitate comparison, we give the text of Fracastor with the orthography of the time: "Tonsor quidam amicus noster libellum habebat

But it was too late: the secret had fallen in the public domain. "This fact," concludes the author, "proves to us most conclusively that the disease *had already been observed* at anterior epochs."

Ex quo videre perfecto possumus alijs etiam ætatibus visum cum morbum fuisse.

Fracastor had not the slightest doubt, in all probability, that this *thick scabies* was syphilis, as he had seen the disease break out, and, like the majority of his contemporaries, he designated the *French disease*, in his writings, under the name of *scabies*.[1]

A testimony from Widman,[2] another contemporary of the epidemic (for he writes in the year 1500), proves that the word *saphati* or *asafati* (leprosy), employed by the Arabian physicians in the sense of a venereal disease, was applied to syphilis thirty-seven years before the great nosological event. Widman himself had been enabled to observe demonstrative cases long before the siege of Naples, since, six years after, he had arrived at an age sufficiently advanced to publish a work on medicine. This is the documentary evidence: "Pestilential

experimentorum quorundum antiquum satis, inter quæ unum inter alia scriptum erat cui titulas erat: *Ad scabiem crassam*, quæ *cû doloribus juncturam accidit.* Is ergo quum primum recentissimus esset morbus, memor medicaminis consuluit medicos quosdam num uti eo medicamento deberet in novâ illâ contagione, quam per scabiem crassam significari existimabat. Medici autem, inspecto medicamine, acritur prohibuere, quod ex argento vivo constaret et sulphare. Felix nisi medicos illos consulinisset incredibili quæstu dives futurus! Paruit autem nec ausus est experiri medicamêtû quod demum expectus, atque optimum agnoscens, valde indoluit quod sero usus eo fuisset, quæstu jam per alios sibi arrepto" (Lib. ii, cap. 2).

[1] This is to be compared with the epigram of the Latin poet, Ausonius, in which the word *scabies* is also taken in the sense of syphilitic ulcers. (*Cf.* La syph. chez les anciens, p. 229. Syphilis in Ancient and Prehistoric Times, p. 202.)

[2] Widman, a physician of Tübingen (Würtemberg), is also known under the names of Jean Salicet and of Meichinger.

diseases manifest themselves sometimes under the form of fevers, either by means of chancrous ulcers or by morbillous[1] or variolous eruptions; or they are cutaneous affections, such as the pustules of *formica* or those of *asafati;* also called the *French disease*, which disease has spread itself from country to country with the most grave symptoms *since the year 1457* up to the present time,—year 1500."

Morbi pestilentiales, aliquando febres interdum carbunculi, nonnunquam morbilli et variolæ; vel aliæ cutis infectiones, quales etiam sunt vel pustulæ formicales; vel asafaticæ dictæ malum Franciæ quæ nunc ab anno 1457 usque ad præsentem annum 1500 de regione in regionem dilatatæ sunt, cum sævis accidentibus.

This text demonstrates to us, besides, that the *formica* of the authors of the Galenic school (μυρμήκιον) and the *asafati* of the Arabians were forms of the pox which, for a certain time, was called the *French disease.*

To have an end with the information emanating from purely medical works, we will give an extract from a communication made by Broca[2] to the Société d'Anthropologie, March 16, 1876:—

During all the Middle Ages, patients suffering from syphilitic dermatoses of a grave nature were confounded with lepers. I have found a large number of *syphilitic lesions on bones derived from an ancient leper-asylum* whose cemetery was dug up about fifteen years ago (about 1860), rue de Bruxelles, Paris.[3]

M. Lancereaux having gone to the catacombs of Paris, a few years later, examined closely the bones coming from cemeteries which remained *in situ* at the crossing of the streets de Douai and de Bruxelles, upon the site of an old leper-asylum. Like Broca, our learned master recognized that these bones, notably the skulls

[1] Measles.

[2] *Cf.* Bull. de la Soc. d'Anthropol., 1876.

[3] Upon the site of this cemetery (Place de Vintimille) ther is at present a square, in the middle of which is the statue of Berlioz.

and femurs, were profoundly altered, and, for the most part, in the same manner. These alterations not answering at all to the description of the lesions of leprosy in bones as given by Danielssen and Bœck in their treatise, and different too much in other respects from the drawing furnished by Steudener[1] in connection with a case of lepra mutilans, it was more natural to attribute them to syphilis, as they were types of specific exostoses.

M. Lancereaux caused the two most remarkable skulls to be drawn for his excellent "Traité d'Anatomie Pathologique,"[2] in which he gives the following description:—

> The different bones which go to make up the base of these skulls have undergone no appreciable change; on the other hand, those of the calvarium are profoundly altered. These last bones have a thickness of about one centimetre; moreover, they show upon their convexity elevations circumscribed by feeble depressions or even by losses of substance, and, as a result, marked irregularities of the surface of the cranial bones, which resemble, so to speak, plowed ground. As to the femurs, they are very long and plainly thickened, as may be seen on section, but not deformed. Their unequal surface indicates that they are affected with hyperostoses, and besides small exostoses exist in the neighborhood of the articular surfaces. . . . The radii, the clavicles, and the humeri presented similar alterations, but not so marked.

M. Lancereaux adds that there exists, in the anatomopathological museum of Geneva, bones which are considered syphilitic, and which have the most perfect resemblance in alteration and origin with those he has just described, seeing that, like them, they are derived from an old cemetery. The same holds with a skeleton sent from Australia to the museum of Freiburg, in which the bones show alterations identical, so to speak, with those

[1] J. Steudener, Beiträge zur Pathologie der Lepra Mutilans. Contribution to the Pathology of Lepra Mutilans. Erlangen, 1867.

[2] Treatise on Pathological Anatomy. Paris, 1885. Vol. iii, pages 69 *et seq.*

of the finds of the Place de Vintimille. From the description of this skeleton, given by Œffinger, the two femurs, the left radius, the right clavicle, the two humeri, and the flat bones of the head are simultaneously affected.

The long bones, says M. Lancereaux, changed in almost their entire extent, are dotted with asperities and irregular depressions; the skull is, here and there, on its convexity, the seat of depressions and elevations which have a great similarity to the skulls we have met with in the catacombs. There seems to be a reason to connect these different alterations; and if it be admitted, which is true, that the syphilis of former times was more severe and more acute than that of our days, and could give rise to more extensive lesions of the bony system, we can *without hesitation* attribute them to this disease.

These material proofs, perforce not to be discussed, step in to corroborate the opinion which we have advanced, that three-fourths of the lepers of the Middle Ages were syphilitics. Besides, this manner of looking at the matter is shared by a number of authors; among others Vercelloni,[1] who wrote in Latin verse in 1701, and was translated by Devaux. "When I read the books of the Ancients on leprosy," says the Italian author, "it seems to me that I am reading works on the pox, and the titles alone of these books persuade me that they are treatises on this disease."

So much for the purely scientific works; we will now examine the historical and literary documents.

[1] J. Vercelloni (transl. by Devaux): Traité des malad. q. arriv. aux part. génit. des 2 sexes. Paris, 1730. Treatise on the Diseases which Come on the Genital Parts of the Two Sexes.

CHAPTER II.

Historical and Literary Documents.

Incredible manners of the Middle Ages.—Latin inscriptions discussed in the ruins of Pompeii; expression found on the walls of a brothel of the first century.—Curious anecdotes; free poems and historical notes relating to venereal diseases.—*Ex-votos* found in the Côte-d'Or.—The "burning" in the twelfth century; the *bite of the geese of Winchester;* the *fig;* the *disease of St. Giles;* the *Mal Boubil* and the *Mal Malan.*—Thirteenth century: the *inguinal plague.*—Fourteenth century: the *vermocane;* the disease of lecherousness.—Beginning of the fifteenth century: the *spits (broches);* *fix;* the *big evil;* *impurity.*

In order that our readers may understand the expressions—at times obscure—of the writers of the Middle Ages, we will begin by giving a short sketch of the manners of that period. Alas! it will necessitate our stirring up of much muck, the spreading out of many shameless things; but it is indispensable. It is certain that we shall thereby awaken much ill-feeling and many angers which are, fortunately, impotent. It is not our fault that the *auto da fé* no longer exists except as a memory, and that mourning must be assumed for the privileges of past years! But there will always remain for the discontented the privilege of continuing to say that our writings contain "nothing scientific." Aside from this we are unconcerned; we shall not see any more than previously—and for a good reason—the shadow of a reputation.

During the feudal epoch, debauchery, which seemed to slumber somewhat, or at least limited itself to certain points during more or less protracted periods, would at times awaken with an unusual frenzy. From this arose epidemics known under the names of the *inguinal plague,* the *sacred disease*, the *burning disease*, that of *St. Main*, of *St. Giles*, of *St. Marcellus*, *St. Anthony's fire*, *hell's fire*, etc., which we will investigate later on. The debauched of all classes took their risks in the Cour des miracles (Paris), or in certain streets in the neighborhood of the ramparts; these streets were the resorts of cut-throats and of prostitutes (*ribaudes*). These highways have almost all disappeared in our days. There is, however, one whose present name, which signifies nothing, recalls only by its phonetic resemblance its primitive appellation. This corruption occurred through the lapse of time, the names of streets and places having undergone a series of transformations in passing from mouth to mouth during centuries. It is not very long since, as a matter of fact, that the names of the streets were for the first time written at the angles of streets, upon the houses. The street to which we have alluded is the rue Petit-Meuse, which runs from the Quai des Célestins to the rue St. Antoine, and whose original name was *rue Pute-y-musse*, which meant *strumpet there hides* (*catin s'y cache*).

In convents, where everything was thought permissible, the monstrous occurrences caused the Roman debauches of the Merovingian times to pale.[1] If we are to believe Dufour,[2] all the varieties of bestiality (hogs, mares, geese, bitches, etc.) were indulged in. The greater part of the Templars perished in torture on account of their awful habits, which gave rise to a far-

[1] A Catholic historian thus describes the depravity of the priests and monks of the fourteenth century: "Alas! alas! how many religious and priests in their convents and retreats, especially in Italy, have established, publicly in a certain way, a sort of infamous gymnasium and race-course where they exercise in the most abominable debauches; the most distinguished young men are consecrated to these places of prostitution." (Alvar Pelag., De Planctus Ecclesiæ, lib. ii, cap. 2.)

[2] *Loc. cit.*

sounding trial. It may be permissible to ask what, in the beginning, were the causes of the habits of sodomy. "They are found," says Dufour, "in the long sojourn of the Templars in the Orient, where the vice against nature is almost endemic, and where the fear of *leprosy*, of the *disease of fire*, and of different cutaneous and organic diseases, is always connected with commerce with women. The Templars, fearful of becoming leprous and *measly*,[1] had soiled their soul and body in accepting, in approving the most shameful of all prostitutions." Certain nunneries were also places of debauchery against nature. "The women, even the religious," says the author, "indulged amongst themselves in orgies in which the art of the *fellator* had forgotten nothing of the obscene lessons of antiquity. And the laity, authorized by example, abandoned itself equally to debauchery."

It was this general depravity which led to the belief of the end of the world and the arrival of Antichrist: a new deluge was awaited for the year 1000. But, says Dufour again, "The end of the world and Antichrist having failed their appointment for the year 1000, those who survived that fatal date believed themselves authorized to fear no celestial vengeance, and plunged deeper in the dung-heap of their unholy license." . . . A passage of Nicolas de Clémenges, archdeacon of Bayeux about the year 1400,—and whom on that very account one cannot suspect of partiality in regard to religious establishments,[2]—gives us the exact status of the mo-

[1] This measly condition (*la mêsellerie*) was the venereal disease. In the Norman patois, it is still said to-day, in speaking of a woman who has had some scuffles with Venus, that she is *meselle*.

[2] Jean Gerson, priest of St. Jean-en-Gréve, canon of Notre Dame and chancellor of the Church of Paris, who died in 1429, gives out the same sentiment on the convents which covered France at the close of the fourteenth century: "Open your eyes, and see if these convents of female monks do not resemble the haunts of prostitution." (Declaratio defectuum virorum ecclesiast.)

rality of convents toward the end of the fourteenth century. "In regard to the virgins consecrated to the Lord," says this Christian philosopher, "it would be necessary to retrace all the infamous doings of the haunts of prostitution; all the arts and the impudence of courtesans; all the execrable methods of fornication and of incest. What, as a matter of fact, are the monasteries of women of our times, if not sanctuaries consecrated not to the worship of the true God, but to that of Venus? Impure receptacles where a youth which no longer knows a check abandons itself to all the tumults of luxury in such a manner that *now it is the same, either to cause a young girl to take the veil or to expose her publicly in a place of debauchery!*"[1]

Evidently the good abbe imagines himself in the pulpit, and he fulminates; and when a preacher fulminates, he always has a tendency to exaggerate. Nevertheless, without losing sight of the hyperbole, one cannot help concluding that the *fin de siécle* subjects ruled by poor Charles VI—more than twenty years before his mental breakdown—did not particularly shine for their chastity.

During all these perturbations syphilis was emerging from some shallow place where it was incubating, and burst forth with such violence that patients and physicians alike believed in a fire from above. As each epidemic was separated from the preceding one by several centuries, there was always a belief in the novelty of the disease, which each time was consecrated with a new name. Let us not lose sight of the fact either, that numerous viruses which were non-syphilitic—that of the phagedenic chancre, not to go any farther—were

[1] Extract from the work of Nicolas de Clémenges, entitled "De corruptio statu ecclesiæ." On the Corrupt State of the Church.

included in the affair, and were not always the least frightful.

Before entering upon the purely literary domain of the subject, we will examine a few curious documents connected almost with antiquity, and which consist of inscriptions and ex-votos discovered during the past few years.

First, let us cite two Latin inscriptions found in the ruins of Pompeii, a city buried, as is well known, by an eruption of Vesuvius in the year 79 of our era: hence it may be affirmed that the sentences which have been gathered are not subsequent in origin to that date. It is even probable that the young Pompeians, who experienced the necessity of engraving upon stone the subject of their disappointment, lived in the time of Martial (reign of Nero, about A.D. 65). Without wishing to pretend that this documentary evidence—necessarily vague—is conclusive, we believe that it possesses a certain value, and comes as a useful re-inforcement of the proofs which we have extracted from the Priapidæ. The analogy presented to the latter is quite marked.

Discovered accidentally in 1755, Herculaneum and Pompeii offered to the archæologist and to the historian the most valuable evidences of a civilization which no longer exists to-day. As might be expected after reading the authors contemporaneous with the fall of Rome, the paintings, the frescoes, the sculptures, the statues, the pottery, and even jewelry testify to the most loose manners. The Italian government, to prevent thievery and acts of vandalism which had taken place for a long number of years, finally took charge of the excavations and caused the most valuable objects to be placed in the museum of Naples. There are there finds of inestimable value, and every day new ones are discovered.

As to the obscene paintings and statues, as well as the bäs-reliefs and mosaics representing lascivious scenes, they were relegated to a special room, which has received the name of *Secret Museum.* If we are to judge by the reproductions given by Barré in his work,[1] there is very little there for the syphilographer to glean from a retrospective point of view. The dominant note in all these drawings is the phallus, which is found everywhere, under all circumstances,—on the walls, vases, statues of fawns and satyrs, etc. In gold or silver it serves as jewelry, as an amulet; in bronze, it constitutes the wick-holder of lamps and the attachments for the chains; in wood or marble, it is the fantastic appendage of the celebrated god Priapus, whom the Romans placed everywhere,—in gardens and at the four corners of their fields.

One single fresco is instructive from a medical point of view. It concerns the special offering which was made to the God of Gardens—or, rather, to his appendage—by young virgins, or those supposedly so before marriage. In our first volume[2] we advanced the opinion that this custom among the Romans must have been—outside of libertinage—one of the most frequent causes of the propagation of venereal diseases. We could no longer doubt this, now that we have before our eyes a reproduction of the realistic scene preserved in the Secret Museum of Naples. This drawing proves to us that the numerous statues of Priapus, with their attributes, were left to the free use of the public,—a fact which was pregnant with consequences. As a matter of fact, the woman whom the artist represents clinging to the horns of the god with one hand, and with the other

[1] Barré, Herculaneum et Pompéi. Paris, 1837–40. The Musée Sécret is contained in the last volume.

[2] Chapter xi, pp. 172 and 173.

preparing the passage for the projecting object situated lower down, seems to us to be more anxious to make a complete offering than a mere simulation.

But entire houses cannot be transported into a museum; it would certainly be interesting to be able to examine closely the structures rid of the masses of ashes and scoriæ under which they have remained embalmed for upward of sixteen centuries. We are persuaded that there would be found evidence of the greatest value relative to the history of syphilis.

This remark is suggested to us by a sentence of Dr. Galligo, of Florence, who visited the ruins of Herculaneum and Pompeii nearly thirty years ago. As a matter of fact, this author says, in Book VIII of his work,[1] respecting the prophylaxis of syphilis, that he saw in the ruins of Pompeii several brothels, on the walls of which were found, on the outside as well as inside, "not only erotic paintings, but also obscene inscriptions, which were plainly making allusions to the *venereal disease.*" The author then gives a reference to a note in which are reproduced a few inscriptions which were given to him by a colleague and by the director of the excavations at Pompeii. These are the texts which we propose to study.

The first inscription, engraved on a stone, emanates from a prowler in luck, desirous no doubt of informing his contemporaries that, in matters of gallantry, appearances must not always be trusted, and that the handsomest creature is sometimes the most tainted. He is proud of his victory, but that which he discovered—when it was too late—spoiled his pleasure. "Even here," he writes in very raw terms, "I have just had a beautiful

[1] I. Galligo, Trattato teorico pratico sulle malattie veneree. Firenze, 1864. Theoretical and Practical Treatise on Venereal Diseases. Florence, 1864.

girl, having a remarkable and much-praised external form." . . . He should have stopped at a general view, and not gone into details: he would have spared himself a disillusion; for he adds that, "within, it was nothing but a *dung-heap.*"

HIC EGO NUNC FUTUI FORMOSAM FORMÆ PUELLAM. LAUDATAM A MULTIS: SED LUTUS INTUS ERAT.

Laudatam a multis corresponds to the latter-day expression "way up." The gallant Pompeian takes good care to call attention to the fact that he did not address himself to the first-comer; and yet this woman, although one of the most in fashion, was contaminated. The young innocent seems to be ignorant of the fact that, the more a gallant woman is sought the more chances she has of being syphilitic by the very reason of the extent of her patronage. This dung-heap (*lutus*) of which the author speaks was no doubt very palpable for him, a man ignorant of medicine, to have perceived: and we can scarcely see anything but confluent ano-vulvar syphilides, and having a fetid ichor, to justify the expression employed. Soft chancres, phagedenic chancres, on account of the pain they occasion upon the least contact, would certainly have proven an absolute obstacle to an accidental walk in the gardens of Priapus. The diagnosis of *vegetations* could, if strictly necessary, be defended; but these rarely—outside of pregnancy—attain the size and confluence necessary to merit the name of *dung-heap.* And, to conclude, the demonstrative documents which we have drawn from ancient literature relieve us in advance from answering the objections which have already been refuted. As we stated at the beginning of this volume, we will now restrict ourself to presenting the proofs such as they exist: it is for the reader who is not yet entirely convinced to base his opinion, by a due consideration of the entire matter taken as a whole.

The second inscription was engraved on the wall of a brothel in Pompeii. Although it is incomplete and several letters have been obliterated during the course of time, it is readily understood that it concerns a disease contracted with one of the boarders of the place. It is probable that the customer, enraged at having been deceived concerning the *quality of the goods*, felt a malign pleasure in informing passers-by—possible purchasers at some future time—that the most beautiful woman of that establishment had "the disease capable of producing eating ulcers."

HIC FUTUI FORMOSAM FO . . . Æ PUELLAM: MORBUS QU . . SANGUINI . . . AM FACIT . . . NOME . . .

It is easy to restore the incomplete words FORMÆ and QUI, especially when given the tenor of the first inscription, whose beginning is identical with that of the second; but the remainder escapes us. It may be asked what part does blood play in this sentence. Was the woman in question at her menstrual period? Did the author look upon this blood as a vehicle capable of transmitting the disease, or even of originating it? Or did he mean to imply that the disease passed into the blood before producing ulcers? We know not; but the thinly-veiled words which can be read plainly state that there were sexual relations; then there is immediate mention made of a disease characterized by venereal ulcers (*nome*). Accordingly, one can hardly avoid seeing relations of cause to effect in the group of words which have remained intact.

On the whole, everything leads to the belief that the young Pompeian was himself contaminated, for his inscription, engraved on the wall itself of the brothel,

—with the evident design of injuring the prosperity of the business carried on inside,—shows clearly a spirit of revenge. And revenge—how sweet may be this "pleasure of the gods"!—is only wreaked against those who are reproached, right or wrong, with having caused some injury. Here the injury is written out in full, and the word *nome*,[1] which expresses it, has resisted the ravages of time for nearly twenty centuries.

So far as *ex-votos* are concerned, they have been discovered in France, as we are informed by a scientific report published in *l'Union médicale* of December 22, 1852. At its meeting of October 17th of the same year, Becquerel had reported to the Société Médicale des Hôpitaux de Paris "the inferences of an antiquary of the Côte-d'Or who, at the ruins of a temple near the Seine, where baths were taken, had found numerous *ex-votos* attesting cures of different diseases of the genito-urinary organs by the use of those waters. These *ex-votos* were lithographed, and there are seen examples of *tumors* of the scrotum, of *buboes*, of destruction of the penis, and of other *changes* which might, perhaps, be referred to *syphilis*. In such a case the circumstance would be very curious, for it would establish the existence of that disease in the *thirtieth year of the Christian era*." Evidently this is very vague, and this proof would be very weak did we not possess others to support it; but, with what we know concerning antiquity, the conclusions of Becquerel can only be approved.

A legend reported by Rollet demonstrates that syphilis existed in Mexico from time immemorial. It deals with the apotheosis of Manahuath, who was trans-

[1] An archaism for *nomæ*,—an expression which Pliny the naturalist frequently employs in his works in the sense of *eating ulcers;* it is derived from the Greek word *νομαί*, which has exactly the same meaning.

formed into a sun (" Annales anciènnes des peuples de l'Anahuac ").[1]

> The pyre is lit; he who has the courage to cast himself upon it will merit the honors of apotheosis, for from his ashes will be renewed the god which will illumine the universe. Manahuath is there with the others, but he suffers from *a disease which is terrible, incurable.* . . . " It is for you," the others tell him, " to keep the heaven and earth."

Manahuath, determined by his disease, springs in the flames. All the traditions recall the memory of this disease which the Mexican aborigine divined, so to speak; for the word *buboso*, which was applied to it, still means *syphilitic.* The word *puz*, in the Tzendal and Zotzil dialects, designates the ill-swelling and corrupt matter which characterizes the sores of the *buboso* patient.

Hœser[2] quotes a letter written by a bishop named Basil, who lived in the tenth century. This prelate speaks of a deacon who had his lips *polluted* by a venereal affection (*diaconus qui pollutus est in labiis*), and he calls attention to the conduct to be followed in reference to clerks who were affected with a similar trouble.

In the chronicles of Conrad of Ausperg, the following passage is found : " The bishop Jean de Spire contracted an *ulcer* on the shameful parts; he was ill for a long time, and died in the year 1104."

W. Beckett[3] reports that in the " Constitutions " of 1162, relative to furnished lodgings, there is found, among other things, the prohibition: " No stew-holder

[1] Annals of the Ancient Peoples of Anahuac.

[2] Lehrbuch der Geschichte der Medizin, Jena, 1882. Hand-book of the History of Medicine.

[3] Philosophical Transactions. London, 1720.

to keep any woman that hath the periculous infirmity of burning" (*arsure*).[1]

A manuscript dated 1430 repeats this ordinance with more details; here we see that those who violated it were subjected to a fine. In the prison of the Bishop of Winchester, this manuscript states, could be found a book in which the same police regulation could be found bearing this title: "*Concerning those who conceal girls having the detestable disease.*"

De his qui custodiunt mulieres habentes nephandam infirmitatem.

Beckett gives this at length in Middle-Age English and with the orthography of the time: "That no Stewholder Keep noo Woman within his hous that hath any Sycknesse of *Brenning*, but that she be putte out upon the peyne of make it a fyne unto the Lord of a hundred schylyngs."[2]

The expressions *brenning* and *burning* were applied, in the twelfth century, to venereal disease in general. That which proves it in an irrefutable manner are two documents of the sixteenth century in which the *corroding* action of syphilis, which was then known, is designated by the verbs *burn* and *brenn.* The same words employed for four hundred years must certainly have served to specify the same affections.

In the first place, if we are to believe history, we see Simon Fish presenting to Henry VIII, in 1530, a report in which he makes complaint of the licentiousness of the Romish priests "that corrupt the whole generation of

1 *Arsure* is an old French word which is found in several authors of the Middle Ages, and notably in Villon (fifteenth century), with the meaning *conflagration* or *burn*, and, by extension of the sense, of *venereal disease.* [As will be seen above, the English term is identically the same, being doubtless derived from the sensation experienced more especially in gonorrhœa.—O-D.]

2 At the time this ordinance was in force one hundred shillings were considered comparatively an enormous sum of money.

mankind in your Realm, that catch the Pockes of one Woman and bear them to another; that be *Burnt* with one Woman and bear it to another," etc.

The second proof emanates from a manuscript of which we have already spoken in Chapter V of our first volume, and in which it is stated that the Dean of Windsor, Weston, was the most debauched canon of the time (1556), and much skilled in the art of treating *Burning.* He was himself the subject of it, for Cardinal Bernard Polus, who deposed him, says, in his order: "He not long ago *brent* a Beggar in St. Botolph's Parish."[1] . . .

To express the fact that this same Weston had been heavily touched by venereal disease, the author employs a circumlocution which has long since become a proverb: "He had been sore *Bitten by a Winchester Goose*, and was not healed thereof."

We are told by Beckett that at that time this was the "common Phrase for the Pox," because the stews were under the jurisdiction of the Bishop of Winchester. The manuscript of 1430, which we quoted above, shows that this jurisdiction existed quite some time before the siege of Naples. It is evident from all these documents that there existed in England, in the Middle

[1] The word *beggar* here signifies not a mendicant, but an unfortunate individual in the same sense in which it is used to-day by the English. Dr. Buret translates the expression as a *female beggar*, but he is evidently at fault. That a female is meant is probable, for, as he justly observes, if Weston had been a sodomite the author would not have failed to lay stress upon the fact. As the word appears in the original English text there can be no doubt unless it would be an error in the manuscript itself, for by the simple change of a letter it would make the word appear "bugger." So far as the word *burn* is concerned as applied to venereal disease, it is one which is still current in the English language. Among the lower classes it is the ordinary word employed to express venereal infection. An individual will refer to the matter by saying that he has been *burnt.* The origin is probably due to the fact that the most common venereal diseases among the lower classes are chancroid and gonorrhœa, both of which transmit a decided burning sensation to their possessors.—O-D.

Ages, a sexual disease, which was contagious, which was contracted from girls leading a bad life (*whores*), and which it was not easy to cure. Samuel Cooper, in his "Elements of Surgery," completes our knowledge in regard to this matter. In that quarter of London known as Southwork there were, it appears, in the Middle Ages, special places in which sick prostitutes were kept to be treated, "so as to prevent," so the rules state, "the rest of the inhabitants from *contracting their disease*."[1]

The collection of poems of the Middle Ages, collated by Leyser, and published at Magdeburg[2] in 1721, offers us, here and there, a few verses which prove that, in the twelfth and thirteenth centuries, attention was drawn to sexual affections of a gallant origin. It was known that the worship of Venus brought on not only social inconveniences, but that in addition the *virus* of the goddess was to be feared,—that is to say, *pimples, hidden tumors*, the *filthy things* which are not seen externally; the venereal *dung-heap*, on the whole, and the *ulcers* which might cover the *entire body*.

In an elegy "on the caprices of fortune," in book i, the poet Henricus Septimellensis wrote, in 1192, the attributes of the principal divinities of paganism. The "formidable virulence" which he places in the hands of the Goddess of Cythera seems to us to be very difficult to interpret in a purely moral sense. "Saturn holds a scythe; Jupiter, a thunderbolt; Mars, arms; the sun, heat; Venus, *terrible poisons*."

> Saturnus falcem; fulmen Jupiter; Arma
> Mars; Sol Fervorem; Dira venena Venus.

[1] Samuel Cooper, First Lines of Surgery.

[2] Polycarpe Leyser, Historia poetarum et poematum medii ævi. Halæ Magdeb., MDCCXXI.

Alain de l'Isle (1294), whose works are also included as a part of the collection of Leyser, has written numerous loose poems in satirical and especially erotic style. In Chapter V of the "Book of Parables" we see him cruelly jesting at a certain Drusus who must certainly have become acquainted with the *dira venena* of the Goddess of Paphos. From the very nature of the conflict between the poet and his "Turk's head," it is permissible to suppose that Alain de l'Isle had himself been slightly scratched by little Eros.

Drusus, he tells us, shaves himself with care, shampoos his head, washes his face and hands; all this is very well, but there are other parts which deserve a good cleansing. "So much for the outside; but, so far as concerns the *filthy things which grow upon his body* in places which are not seen, he takes care not to scrape them."

Hoc facit externis, sed sordes colligit intus
Nec sibi crescentes radere curat eas.

And he has the audacity to wipe the sacred vessels! True, he has washed his hands: a great thing, indeed! But it suffices for the cloth which he uses to touch the "dung-heap" which he has on him, and the former will bring back the "shameful soils," and then the vessels are filthier than before.

Tacta tuto turpes subito trahit instita sordes.

We see the case of this so-called Drusus very plainly defined. The poet adds: "It is in poor taste to reproach me for my *pimples*, when it comes from this man who is so lenient for the *tumors* which he carries on his body. Let him first cure himself of the *ulcers with which he is covered:* then he may make sport of my *pimples*."

Non me verrucas juste reprehendit habentem
  Qui sibi portanti tubera parcit homo
Ulceribus plenum primo se liberet ipsum
  Postea verrucas rideat ille meas.

Even if those who contradict our position can only see in the word "sordes" a repelling filth due to neglect of the intimate toilet,—something rather strange in a man who takes so much care of his face and hands,[1]—we will humbly call attention to the fact that filth has never engendered either *tumors* or *ulcers*, and as much cannot be said of syphilis.

Littré has drawn attention[2] to a very curious little book of the thirteenth century which was published about 1833, and bore the title of "The XXII Kinds of Villains" (*Des XXII manières de Vilains*). There are noted a few verses in which are mentioned, among other diseases, figs, gonorrhœa, and syphilis in general, under the name of the "disease of St. Giles." We will give the translation and the original text, which is in old French, and not easily interpreted: "May God send them sore unhappiness, and disease of heart, and disease of head, disease of mouth and also of the teeth, and disease without and disease within, gutta rosea and *figs* on *figs!*—in manner such that the clergy will of it say 'Fi—the wolf,[3] the wandering gout, scrofula, and madness!' May the male and female villains all have the *disease of St. Giles*, the stationary gout and the

[1] Without desiring to impugn the observation of the author, we would like to call attention to the fact that instances are occasionally encountered in which individuals who are scrupulously careful of their hands and faces will not bathe their bodies. A marked case of this kind was that of Hugh Mottram Brooks, alias Maxwell, who was always scrupulously neat about his face and hands. After his execution his body was found to be horribly filthy.—O-D.

[2] Gazette médicale de Paris, 1846.

[3] Lupus (which also signifies *wolf* in Latin) is here meant, and most probably that form which is rapidly destructive in its character.—O-D.

gout of joints, and the disease called hectic, the itch, small-pox, abscesses; and that they be full of scales, of fever, and of jaundice; and that they may have the clap, and disease which causes groans, and sores which cannot heal."

Que Diex leur envoit grant mischief,
Et mal au cueur et mal au chief,
Mal es bouche et pis es dens,
Et mal dehors et mal dedens,
Goutte rose, et fi pour fi !
Si en dirai li clergiés fi,
Le leu[1] et la goutte volage,
Les escrœles et la rage !
Toutes vilaines et vilain
Aient tout le mal Saint-Gillain
Et goutte feske et goutte arthique,
Et le mal ke on dist étique,
Rogne, vairole et apostume !
Et si aient plenté[2] de grume
Plenté de fièvre et de jaunisse !
Et si aient la chade-pisse,
Mal ki les faiche rechaner,
Et plaie ki ne puist saner.

What would Astruc—who, in common with many others of the time, believed in the syphilitic nature of gonorrhœa—have said if he had known of the existence of this document? He might perhaps—on finding, in a manuscript of the thirteenth century, the word *chade-pisse* (gonorrhœa)—have said :—

[1] This expression will not be easily understood even by students of old French. It has remained in the patois of Picardy, and signifies *wolf.* It may be found in a quotation from La Fontaine, book iv, table 16; but there it refers to the animal. For those who may be interested we give the quotation referred to :—

Biaux chires *leups*, n'écontez mie
Mère tenchent chen fieux qui crie.

[2] The analogy of this word to our English *plenty* is not confined to the sound, for the meaning is identical. The last word of the first line (mischief) is identical in orthography and meaning with the English word.—O-D.

Plenty of fever and of jaundice!
[Plenté de fièvre et de jaunisse!]

About the same epoch—that is to say, at the beginning of the thirteenth century—we see Gauthier de Coinci, Prior of the Abbey of St. Médard, near Soissons, advising the monks placed under his orders to be careful not to touch the *mal boubil* or *mal malan*,—a contagious affection situated about the ano-genital region.[1] "The monks, the clerks, and the priest should not at all or, at least, be careful to touch in a *bad place* all those who elevate and replace the image of God, who must handle the body of God; they must not touch, either with the hand or with the finger, the *mal boubil* or the *mal malan*, which attacks so many persons."

Li moines, li clercs, et li prestre
Ne doivent être à tout le mains
Moult doivent bien garder leur mains
Qu'en vilain lieu ne les attouchent
Tuit cil Diu levent et couchent,
Qui le cors Diu manoier doit,
Ne doit toucher ne main ne doit
Au mal boubil, au mal malan[2]
Qui tantes genz met en mal an.[3]

"As early as the twelfth century," says Dupouy,[4] "there already existed, in France, discussion of the mal malan or mal boubil, which was characterized by sores and ulcers of the anus and on the genital parts."

We find, as a result of our personal researches in regard to the Middle Ages, that by the *mal boubil* or *bubuis*,

[1] It is impossible to find English equivalents for these expressions which would at all be adequate. The *mal boubil* is the bubonic disease, or bubo; whereas the *mal malan* would seem to signify the virulent disease, and refers to the chancre, as will be seen farther on. These phrases are not even susceptible of synonyms in the French.—O-D.

[2] Certain editions have *mal bubuis* and *mal malen* or *malon*.

[3] Gauthier de Coinci, Mir., lib. i, ch. xxxiii, manuscript.

[4] Le moyen-âge médical. Paris, 1888. Medicine of the Middle Ages.

or yet the *bube*, is designated more especially the bubo; the *mal malan*, *malen*, *malem*, or *malon* aimed at the chancre and secondary lesions of an ulcerative nature. "Taken as an adjective," says Godefroy,[1] the word *malan* qualified every disease which manifested itself by an eruption,—leprosy, the itch, etc.; taken as a noun, it is the disease itself,—chancre, bubo, or ulcer." Here are a few quotations, derived from divers manuscripts of the Middle Ages, which leave no doubt as to the venereal nature of the disease aimed at by the trouvères of that period:—

It concerns, in the first place, a woman remarkable for her physical perfection: the author very clearly makes it understood that she is free of all venereal poison. "The flesh more soft than wool, having neither *bubos* nor *contagious ulcers;* even as far as Jerusalem no woman could be found the possessor of a more beautiful throat."

> La char plus sœf que toison,
> Si n'i ot bube ne malem,
> N'avoit jusqu'en Jerusalem
> Fame qui plus bel col portast.[2]

Per contra, the author of another poem, entitled "*le Cheval de bois*" ("The Wooden Horse"), speaks of a woman who has the *malan*, and in whom the mouth is the part which is most abused. The remainder is nothing in comparison with the state of her buccal mucous membrane. "But if you had seen her *mouth!* Never was there one found so ugly, so large, so hideous, so *diseased;* for the interior was lined with enormous *venereal ulcers.*"

[1] Dictionaire de l'ancienne langue française. Paris, 1889. Dictionary of the Ancient French Language.

[2] Rose, manuscript 1573, fo. 5c.

Mais si sa bouche veissiez,
Ainz si laide ne fu trouvee,
Granz fu, hideuse et decrevee,
De granz malanz pleine dedenz.[1]

Now, it is St. Genevieve who appears to a young nunlet and ironically offers her to remove, by a " twist of the wrist," the small *venereal ulcer* which she has somewhere *under her petticoat.* The latter, very much surprised, protests, saying that she is perfectly *healthy,* and that she has nothing which could justify such an accusation. Perhaps an indurated chancre was involved in the matter; we know that this erosion, being indolent, frequently remains ignored, more especially in women.

SAINTE-GENEVIÈVE:

Or souffrez que je vous oste
. I . malon qu'avez sous la coste;
Mez vous doubtez . . .

LA NONNAIN:

Dame, je me sens toute saine,
Pourquoy parlez-vous de tel chose ?[2]

In whatever manner these texts are interpreted, it cannot be denied that there existed, in the thirteenth century, a contagious disease located sometimes in the mouth, at other times on the sexual organs, and again at the anus, and found most often in easy women. To name these different localities in connection with the same disease which owes its origin to sexual indulgences is to simply designate the disease, for it is only syphilis which can answer to such a description.

In the " Annales des Frères Mineurs "[3] (" Annals of the Minor Brothers "), in the year 1265, the first of the

[1] Du Cheval de fust. Rom. V, p. 112.
[2] Le mir. Mme St. Genev., Jub. myst., vol. i, p. 218.
[3] Annales minorum, vol. iv, p. 254.

pontificate of Clement IV, it is related that a contagious disease, most probably of genital origin, reigned in Venice in an epidemic form, and that the inhabitants were rid of it only by the force of prayers and ex-votos. "The Venetians had to suffer much from the *inguinal disease*, a sort of pestilential affection. In order to be freed of it and at the same time escape the danger, they erected in the church itself a remarkable chapel with an inscription extolling the virtues of the Blessed Virgin. Their prayer was fulfilled."

Venetentes lue inguinaria, morbove pestifero graviter oppressi ut liberarentur, periculumque evaderent, Sacellum titulo Dominæ nostræ de virtutibus insignitum, in eadem Ecclesia extruxerunt, sicque votorum compotes sunt effecti.

We shall see later on that the epidemic of the fifteenth century was also designated by some authors under the name of *lues inguinaria.* Besides, an epitaph which may be seen on a tomb-stone in the church of Santa Maria del Popolo, in Rome, proves, in a very clear manner, that this disease has not been an isolated epidemic, but a current affection, since it was noted in the thirteenth and fifteenth centuries. In addition, if certain authors contemporaneous with the epidemic of Naples have given it the appellation of a scourge which was still making victims nine years previously, it must be concluded that they did not find any great differences between the symptoms which they observed in both cases. The following is the epitaph in question: "To Marcus, son of Antony the Roman Knight, of the noble family of the Albertons, endowed with a lofty soul and a remarkable body, who died of the *inguinal pest*, in his thirtieth year, July 22d, in the year 1485 of the Christian era," etc.

MARCO ANTONII EQUITIS ROMANI
FILIO, EX NOBILI ALBERTONUM FAMILIA
CORPORE ANIMOQ. INSIGNI
QUI, ANNUM AGENS XXX
PESTE INGUINARIA INTERIT
ANNO SALUTIS CHRISTIANÆ
MCCCCLXXXV. DIE XXII JULII.
HEREDES B. M. P.

Dufour even says that the *inguinal disease* appeared in France about the middle of the sixth century (546). Dom Ruinart[1] explains the origin of this appellation: "It was called *inguinal pest* because, arising at first either in the groin or in the armpit, it killed by means of an *ulcer*, after the fashion of the serpent."

. . . Lues inguinaria sic dicebatur, quod, nascente in inguine vel in axilla, ulcere in modum serpentis inteficeret.

A certain Master Vulgerius wrote a pamphlet against Boniface VIII, elected pope in 1294, in which he represented that pontiff as a man addicted to all forms of debauchery. There are to be found a few verses in which the author reproaches him of being attacked by a virulent disease which is seen on the *face;* now, as Vulgerius has said, immediately before, that the sovereign pontiff was an amateur of the fair sex, a gutter-rake,— in one word, a mighty hunter before the Eternal . . . Venus,—it is impossible to cavil upon the nature of the morbid principle garnered by his saintship. The virus mentioned can be nothing else than the *venereal virus.* The pamphleteer, making a play of words on the expressions *vir* and *virus*, perpetrates a pun which we have attempted to reprc luce in our translation. "Unceasingly in search of a new amorous prey, he makes the rounds of the places of prostitution. . . . This man

[1] Hist. de Gregoire de Tours. History of Gregory of Tours.

is a Dean; he has a masculine appearance, but he is not *virile;* with his *diseased* face, he is *virus* itself."[1] . . .

> Qui loca circuit Venator Veneris,
>
> . . . .
>
> Hic Vir Decanus est, qui viri specie
> Non Vir; sed Virus est, virosa facie.[2]

March 16, 1876, at a meeting of the Société d'Anthropologie, Broca, in a discussion on the antiquity of syphilis, mentioned a map of Copenhagen, dating from the fourteenth century, in which the *French disease* is already spoken of as a contagious affection of the genital organs. Besides, in a document relating to the foundation of St. Victor, in Maintz, having the date of the year 1472, it may be seen that the services of a chorister are dispensed with because he suffers from the disease called *Mala Franzos.* J. Meursius has reproduced two Greek verses written by an anonymous author, in which is found the Greek word barbarous,—φραντζάζειν (to have the French disease): the poem was composed in the Middle Ages, and most probably before the epidemic of Naples. The texts quoted and the declaration of Widman, which we have given in the preceding chapter, prove that the expression *French disease* was current a number of years before the expedition of Charles VIII. From this it seems conclusive that the letter of P. Martyr, of 1488, was in no manner antedated.

According to Doglioni,[3] it was ordered by the Senate,

[1] It is impossible to render this in English in a manner at all satisfactory; in French it may be done. Dr. Buret very cleverly renders it as follows: "Il a l'aspect masculin, mais ce n'est pas un mâle: avec sa face *malsaine*, c'est le *mal* lui-même." . . .

[2] Eccard, Corpus historicum medii ævi (History of the Middle Ages). Leipzig, 1723, vol. ii, p. 1854. [Versus in Bonifacium VIII, papam et mores cleri. Magister Vulgerius (Poem against pope Boniface VIII and the manners of the clergy).]

[3] Cose notabili di Venetia. Remarkable Things of Venice.

in 1302, that "he who should communicate to another the *vermocane* (a species of disease) should each time pay a fine of twenty cents."

L'anno 1302, fu proveduto chi mandova a qualch'uno il vermocane (ch'e è specie di malatia) pagavi ogni volta xx soldi.

If we are to believe Plisson,[1] Reynaud,[2] and others, this disease was caught in public houses (*lupanaria*).

We read in the "Chronique d'Ottakar"[3]: "King Wencelaus of Bohemia (at the beginning of the fourteenth century) acquired from a concubine a *disease* which caused him to die as soon as the *rottenness* attacked those parts which a man is ashamed of letting others see." This occurrence is confirmed in the "Chronique d'Hornek"[4]: "The King of Bohemia died of a *love-gift* from his well-beloved Agnes."

According to P. Paul Verger,[5] Ubertin VII, third prince of the city, died at Padua, March 29, 1345, "of a *disease* which he had contracted on his *shameful parts* by his excesses of *libertinage* with women."

We now arrive, by following a chronological order, to the statutes of Jeanne I, Queen of the Two Sicilys and Countess of Provence. These statutes were intended to regulate, in the fourteenth century, the brothel of Avignon; they have been quoted by the majority of syphilographers who followed Astruc: but they have given rise to so much controversy that we will limit ourself to reproducing them without committing ourself respecting their authenticity, which is of quite a

[1] Syphilographie. Paris, 1825. Syphilography.

[2] Traité pratique des malad. vénér. Toulon, 1845. Practical Treatise on Venereal Diseases.

[3] Chronicle of Ottakar.

[4] Chronicle of Hornek.

[5] Hist. de la famille des Carrares. Padua, 1395. History of the Family of the Carraras.

secondary importance. However, we will state that certain authors look upon them as apocryphal because an anonymous note, written on a copy of the "Cacomonade" of Linguet, relates a supposed mystification of which Astruc was the victim. Unfortunately, as is said by Dufour, who made a serious inquiry in this regard, there is noted among the accomplices an individual from Avignon, by name Commin, who was born ten years after the publication of Astruc's work in which the celebrated statutes appeared for the first time. And, adds the author, if such a colossal joke had been involved, being given the fame of Astruc, "the whole of Europe would have resounded with an immense burst of laughter." Undoubtedly the author would have been apprised of this, and he would not have failed to suppress the fantastic statutes in the second edition of his "De morbis venereis." Besides, this work having been translated in French and several other languages, how is it that not one translator has mentioned the supposed joke in his notes? Such is, in a few words, the argument of Dufour; it must be admitted that his objections have a certain weight.

These regulations, written in old Provençal, have for title *Statuts pour le lieu public de débauche d'Avignon*,[1] and date from August 8, 1347. Article IV, the only one which interests us, is thus conceived: "The Queen wishes that every Saturday the bailiff's wife (the go-between) and a barber (surgeon) delegated by the consuls shall examine all debauched girls who may be in the brothel; and, if there be found any one having *disease acquired in lechery*, that such girl be separated from the others and lodged apart, so that no intercourse shall be held with her, in order to avoid the *disease which youth might contract.*"

[1] Statutes for the Public Place of Debauchery of Avignon.

L'an mil très cent quaranto set, au hueit dan mès d'avous . . . La Reino vol que toudès lous samdès la baylouns et un barbier deputat des Consouls visitoun todos las fillios debauchados que seran au Bourdeou ; et se sen trobo qualcuno qu'abia mal vengut de paillardiso, que talos fillios sian separados et longeados à part, afin que non las connougoun ; per evita lou mal que la jouinesso pourrié prenré.

Astruc also expresses a slight doubt concerning the authenticity of these statutes, but assuming a point of view which excludes all suspicion of mystification. He is surprised at this action being taken "by a queen of 23,"[1] seeming to forget that a queen signs, but does not draw up, laws. Then he concludes by saying that, after all, she did nothing but follow the custom of the times. The principal cities of Italy, he relates, had possessed houses of prostitution for many years ; they were found even in Rome, particularly in the close vicinity of the palace of the popes ; and, as an edifying detail, there was one of these brothels from which the Marshal of the Court of Rome drew *a sort of tribute.* The scandal was such that Guillaume Durand[2] demanded, from the Council of Vienna, the abolition of this privilege.

A Florentine chronicler, Donatio Velluti (fourteenth century), speaking of his own son, relates that the child, at first confided to a nurse but *little sound*, became covered with *pimples* (pruzza) and *wasted ;* and then that a second nurse, who was younger, took the place of the other in the suckling of the child, and did not delay in contracting the *same disease.* Corradi, who notes this

[1] She was only 19 years old in reality, and was the widow of Andrew of Hungary, the first one of her four husbands, and he whom Prince Louis of Tarentum caused to be assassinated. Jeanne not only passed this by, but even married the murderer as soon as a year had elapsed after the deed. This is hardly in accord with candor. Astruc should have been more careful.

[2] De modo celebrandi Consilii generali, p. 2, titul. 10. Proceedings of the General Council.

fact, sees in it infantile syphilis. It would really be rather difficult to see anything else in it.

A document quoted by Friedberg deals with a disease of which a certain Nicolas Kurnik, Bishop of Posen, died in 1382.

"As he employed two of his organs for the purpose of giving himself up without shame to illicit deeds, he was, in *those same parts*, punished by Divine wrath . . . for he was attacked with the *chancrous disease* and suffered from *ulcerations of the tongue and throat* to such a degree that, before his death, he could scarcely speak, swallow his food, and close his mouth."

Comme il se servait de deux de ses membres pour se livrer sans pudeur à des actes illicites, il fut, dans ces mêmes parties, puni par la vengeance divine . . . car il fut atteint du mal chancreux et souffrit d'ulcerations de la langue et de la gorge, à ce point qu'avant sa mort il pouvait à peine parler, avaler ses aliments et fermer la bouche.

Raynaldus, quoted by Hœser, states that "Ladislaus, King of Poland (1414), contracted on his *genital parts* a *disease* which was attributed to a *poison* deposited by a *courtesan* of Perouse, and of which he died."

Rabelais, who wrote in the sixteenth century, tells us of a teacher of Gargantua, Maistre Thubal Holoferne (Master Tubal Holofernes), whom he causes to die of syphilis in 1420.

'Twas fourteen hundred and a score,
That pox did come to him full sore.

Et fut l'an mil quatre cents vingt,
De la vérole qui lui vint.[1]

If this sally do not demonstrate that syphilis was known at the beginning of the fifteenth century, it

[1] Gargantua, bk. i, ch. xiv.

tends, at all events, to prove that Rabelais considered it anterior to the siege of Naples.[1]

Beckett, of whom we have already spoken, quotes a manuscript of the fifteenth century, which was found in Lincoln's College at Oxford. The author, one Thomas Gascoigne, doctor of theology, states that he has known "several individuals who died as a result of a *rotting* of their genital organs and of their bodies; and that this *corruption*, this *putrefaction*, had for its cause, from their own admission, *carnal relations* with women."

. . . diversos viros qui mortui fuerunt ex putrefactione membrorum genitalium et corporis sui; qua corruptio et putrefactio, ut ipsi dixerunt, causata fuit per exercitium copulæ carnalis cum mulieribus.

As an instance he reports the case of a gentleman of high position, John of Gaunt, Duke of Lancaster, called Plantagenet,[2] who died in this fashion. It would appear that this prince was a great lecher (*magnus fornicator*), in the sight and knowledge of the whole English nation. "Before his death, whilst he was lying on his bed of torture, he showed his *rottenness* to the King of England, Richard II, who had come to visit him in the course of his disease; and this was told to me by one who knew,—a faithful Bachelor of Sacred Theology."

. . . ante mortem suam jacens sic infirmus in lecto, eamdem putrefactionem regi Angliæ Ricardo II ostendit, cum idem rex eumdem ducem in sua infirmitate visitavit; et dixit mihi qui ista novit unus fidelis sacræ Theologiæ Baccalaureus.

Kitchen Latin, which must have made Cicero's ashes tremble in their urn! The author also speaks of a cer-

[1] Not only this, but in another part of Rabelais (Pantagruel, bk. ii, ch. xxx) we find Pope Sixtus spoken of as "an anointer (of mercurial ointment) of those who have the pox," showing that the treatment of the disease was also known, as well as the affection itself.—O-D.

[2] He was the fourth son of Edward III; he died in the reign of his brother, Richard II.

tain Will, a man of ripe age, who lived in London, and who was also carried away by a *sexual disease distributed all over his body* and acquired in commerce with women. "He acknowledged it to me several times before his death, when he distributed alms with his own hand; it was then that I came to know him, in the year of our Lord 1430."

Willus etiam longe vir maturæ ætatis et de civitat. Londonii, mortuus est ex tali putrefactione membrorum suorum genitalium et corporis sui, causata per copulam carnalem cum mulieribus, ut ipsemet pluries confessus est ante mortem suam, quum manus sua propria eleemosynas distribuit ut ego novi anno Dni 1430.

A document of 1456 informs us that venereal disease was sometimes denominated, at that time, under the name of *spits* (*broches*). In that year the Dauphin—who became Louis XI later on—had an estrangement with his august father, Charles VII. He left the court of France and for five years he received a most generous hospitality in the fortress of Genappe, removed a few miles from Brussels. It was nothing but feasting and merriment ("*nopces et festins*"), and many shady stories were told: the young prince was much pleased especially, after drinking, in relating and hearing the relation of gallant stories. These subjects were gathered by the chroniclers of the times, and these latter have transmitted them to us, considerably augmented, under the title "Les cent nouvelles nouvelles" ("The Hundred New Stories") of Louis XI. In the second story, entitled "The Gray-Friar Physician" ("Le Cordelier médecin"), are to be found several passages which are extremely interesting from the point of view of the history of medicine.

It concerns a very pretty girl of London, aged 15 years, much sought after, who had probably had weaknesses and, without doubt, misfortunes of an entirely special sort. If the disease with which this little girl with a tender heart had acquired had only consisted of ordinary hæmorrhoids,—the interpretation of the word *broches* given by certain authors,—the event would not have been sufficiently important to arouse all the neighborhood and necessitate the arrival of a large number of physicians. The author brings out prominently this circumstance as a proof of the grave nature of the disease; besides, it is quite certain that an insignificant trouble would not have been mentioned in the chronicles of the time, and more especially with such circumstantial details. However, the reader can readily appreciate the matter.

"She fell ill of a *dangerous* and unpleasant malady, which was commonly known as *broches* (spits)." . . .

Elle chéut, en une *dangereuse* et desplaisante maladie que communément on appelle broches. . . .

It is certain that the lesion was located upon an organ which is delicate, fragile,—which can be guessed, however,—and was of an ulcerative nature and most likely contagious, for the text says that the disease "attacked its prey in a *dangerous* and damagable place."

"The poor girl, frenzied by this *great disease*, could not hold her countenance but to weep and sigh. . . . The physicians could scarcely see the *great mischief* which tormented her so much."

La povre fille, de ce grant mal toute affolée, ne sçait sa contenance que de plourer et souspirer. . . . Les médecins virent apertement le grant meschief qui fort la tourmentoit.

It was evidently a disease which was out of the ordinary, since the "relatives, friends, and neighbors of this house of woe" came to visit and comfort "the company."

A beginning was made by administering old women's remedies; but the disease became worse despite the drugs of the "matron" who was consulted, or, rather, on account of them. Then recourse was had to men of the art.

"There came master Peter, master John, master this and master that,—as many physicians as you will,—who were willing to see the patient together and the portions of the body uncovered in which this *accursed disease* of the spits had—alas!—long ambushed itself."

Or sont venus maistre Pierre, maistre Jehan, maistre cy, maistre là, tant de physiciens que vous vouldrez; qui veulent bien veoir la paciente ensemble et les parties du corps à descouvert où ce mauldit mal de broches s'estoit hélas! longuement embusché.

But from the very beginning the girl did not wish to show her trouble; it was necessary to point out to her that she might die of it; then she yielded.

"She took and did all that was desired in order to recover her health. But it all availed not, for there is neither feat nor machine with which the said physicians were acquainted to allay in ever so small a degree this *distressing disease;* nor in their books could they find it, nor in their experience."

Elle print et fit tout ce que on voulut pour recouvrer santé. Mais tout rien n'y vault, car il n'est tour ne engin que les dictz médicins saichent pour allegier quelque peu de ce destresseux mal, ne en leurs livres n'ont véu ni acoustumé.

As a result, surprise of the physicians,—just like in 1495, after the siege of Naples,—which, to say the least, would be very odd in reference to simple rectal varices. Let us also remember that it concerns a very young girl, almost a child; besides, we believe that we may contend that hæmorrhoids were known before the reign of Charles VII.

At length, in despair, the family had recourse to the science of an old gray friar, blind of one eye, who, after having examined the *corpus delicti* and well measured his distances, prepared himself to insufflate,—*in loco dolenti*,—by the aid of a quill, an astringent and even caustic powder. This procedure, taking the times into consideration, was not so artless. But young Agnes, who was slily watching him, burst out laughing at the critical moment; there resulted on the part of the patient a sudden movement, with an escape of gas, which sent the powder into the only sound eye of the friar. He lost his eye in consequence; "for in a few days the powder, which was corrosive, spoilt and ate up the entire eye, and by this token, the other being already lost, he became blind, and thus remained the said gray friar."

. . . car en peu de jours la pouldre qui corrosive estoit, luy gasta et mangea trestout l'œil, et par ce point l'aultre qui ja estoit perdu, advengle fut, et ainsi demoura ledict cordelier.

At all events the remedy was a good one, for the young girl recovered, and this adventure even made her the fashion.

. . . "she became known to everybody by this accursed disease of the spits, of which, in the end, she was healed."

. . . devint notoire à tout le monde par ce mauldit mal de broches, dont en la fin fut garie.[1]

The diagnosis "ano-vulvar syphilides" seems to us infinitely more rational here than that of *hæmorrhoids.* The popular expressions *broches* (spits) or *brokes*, in use in the fifteenth century, must, like the *marisca* of the Romans, have served to designate, in a general way, the

[1] Louis XI. Cent. novelles, 2.

morbid products of the ano-genital region; especially those of a gallant origin, and that by reason of the primitive meaning (a point, dart) of the word (spit).

This entire chapter was written in 1889; now, two manuscripts of the Middle Ages, which we have recently consulted, demonstrate in the clearest manner that the spits, as we stated in studying the preceding text, were not simple hæmorrhoids.

In the first one the author enumerates some of the disagreeable diseases with which the patient is affected: "suffocations, *spits*, diarrhœa, hæmorrhoids, lancinating pains," etc.

Aratelles, broches, menoisons,
Amorrhoïdes, aguillons.[1] . . .

The words *spits* and *hæmorrhoids* both occur in a description of very different symptoms, and could not designate one and the same thing.

The second text is still more conclusive, for it demonstrates that the "spits," analogues of the *figs* (fici) of which Martial speaks so often, could be observed in other places besides the anal region. Now, hæmorrhoids, deriving their name from the veins of the rectum called *hæmorrhoidal*, of which they are simply the varices, can be found nowhere else, in spite of all the argumentation of this world. The *physicist*, author of the manuscript, recommends a topical remedy good for several cases, and which cures *spits*, employed as a lotion, when that disease affects the anus. "This same is good to wash the *spits*, when they are at the seat, and also cures them."

Ce mesme est bon à laver les broches, quant ou les a au siége, si garist on.[2]

[1] E. Desch, Poés., mss. 840, fol. 211a.

[2] Liv. de fisiq. Book on Physics. Mss. Turin, lxxxvi, k. iv, 37, fol. 15r.

We will once more establish that in the Middle Ages, as among the Greeks and Romans, the different symptoms of syphilis had been perfectly noted and described under as many names, which varied according to the location of these manifestations. At one time it is the buccal syphilides (*malanz dedenz la bouche*); at another vulvar lesions (*mal malan en vilain lieu*, *malon sous la coste*); farther on, syphilides of the anus (*broches*). At other times it is simply *arsure*, the *malem*, the *big disease*, the *fix*, *fig*, or *fi*, *leprosy*, etc.,—general terms which became, according to epochs, at one time, the *burning disease;* at another the *sacred disease*, the *fire disease*, the *fire of St. Anthony*, the *inguinal plague*, etc., each time that the disease assumed its epidemic character or, rather, occupied the most prominent place in an epidemic.

In the "Grand Testament" of Villon, a French poet who wrote about 1460, may be found a few more or less vague allusions to venereal disease. In one place it is a courtesan at the turn of life who laments at being obliged to be content with the gallants whom she can find. "The glutton, *tainted with disease*, was kissing me."

> Le glouton, de *mal entaché*,
> M'embrassoit.[1] . . .

When she was young there was no man of high birth who would not have stripped himself for her on account of her beauty, providing that she would have granted him the favors which the dregs of the people now refuse for nothing. She is old! And yet the gallants of former days did not hesitate, not even before the pathological consequences of those amours of which

[1] Les regrets de la belle heaulmière jà parvenue à vieillesse. The laments of the beautiful free lance already arrived at old age.

they often had to *repent.* "Then there was not man born who all of his would not have given to me, not if he *repented*, even providing that I abandoned to him what now is refused by beggars."

> . . . alors n'etait homme né
> Qui tout le sien ne m'eust donné,
> Quoy qu'il en fust des repentailles
> Mais que luy eusse abandonné
> Ce que reffusent truandailles.

Farther on it is a rather obscure picture of what was encountered in brothels of the fifteenth century. First of all, *sublimate*, a poisonous substance which was not to be handled carelessly; then the "quick flow" (coulette vive) of the navel. Was this an allusion to gonorrhœa? It is possible, for the green flow is mentioned. Next, the cloths stained with black blood which are placed to dry every month by the stove (hygiene and perfume!); *chancres*, *figs*, and the filthy tubs in which the nurses wash their linen stained with blood; in conclusion, the water which has served for the secret washing of the prostitutes.

The author calls attention to the fact that those who have not frequented the bawdy-houses of that time will catch the meaning of these allusions with much difficulty; it is still less easy for readers of the nineteenth century to do so.

He concludes by consigning to the flames the bad tongues, which he would be pleased to see sizzling with all the nice ingredients he has just enumerated. "In sublimate, dangerous to touch, and at the navel of a quick flow; in blood, which is put by stoves to dry on cloths when the moon comes full, of which one is black, the other greener than chives; in chancre and fix and in those filthy tubs in which the nurses exsanguinate their (flags) cloths;[1] in the small baths of amorous girls (who does not understand me has never been in brothels) may those venomous tongues be fried."

En sublimé, dangereux à toucher
Et au nombril d'une coulette vive,
En sang, qu'on mect en poylettes sécher
Chez ces barbiers, quand plaine lune arrive,
Dont l'ung est noir, l'autre plus vert que cive;
En chancre et fix et en ces ords cuveaulx,
Où nourrices essanguent leurs drappeaulx;
En petits baings de filles amoureuses
(Qui ne m'entend n'a suivy les bordeaulx)
Soient frittes ces langues venimeuses.[2]

Daremberg, in ransacking some legal documents preserved in the archives of Dijon,[3] found several dating from the Middle Ages, and very valuable for the history of venereal diseases.

The first, which bears date of *June 13, 1430*, relates to the case of a wet-nurse of the name of Jeannotte, who was turned over to a debauched sergeant by one widow Bigot. The poor nurse, having acquired a venereal disease as a result of this act of ravishing, the mayor caused her to be examined by two barbers and two matrons; these, after having been sworn, declared that the deed had been consummated and that the patient was threatened with infection, for the parts were inflamed and could not delay, according to them, in becoming chancrous if remedies were not applied in the shortest time. "They state by their oaths that the said Jean-

[1] *Drappeaux* in Old French means either cloths (whence the English word *drapery*) or flags. A query which naturally arises is as to whether the English expression of "having the red flag out" traces its origin to this French word.—O-D.

[2] Ballade cxxxi.

[3] Archives de la ville de Dijon. Série C. Jurisprudence municipale. Procès criminels. Archives of the City of Dijon. Municipal Jurisprudence. Criminal trials.

notte has been ravished and carnally corrupted, as it appeared to them, and, what no one can deny, the said Joanne is on the road to *perdition;* they consider that she is already *heated within*, and already commences to *take the chancre*, unless remedy and provision be made in a very brief time."

Ilz dient par leurs sermens que ladicte Jehanotte a esté vyolee et corrompue charnelment comme il leur a apparu et, qui n'y pourverra, ladicte Jehanotte est en voye de perdicion ; considere de desja elle est eschauffée par dedans et se encommence ja à prendre le chancre se remede et provision n'y est mis bien brief.

The real meaning of the word *chancre*—which we have also seen in the ballade of Villon—was certainly known at that time; indeed, we again find this same word in another place relating to an œdema of the penis whose cause is not specified. This new document is dated *August 5, 1445.* It begins thus: " The case is such for about a month that by heating of the yard or virile member of Jacot du Mex, a baker living in Dijon, it swelled and had neither *chancre* nor other disease except the swelling." . . .

Le cas est tel à environ ung mois que par eschauffoison de la verge ou le membre virile de Jacot du Mex, boulangier demeurant à Dijon, luy estoit enflee et ny avoit ne *chancre* ne aultre maladie que tant seulement enfleure. . . .

It was then known that there could be something else involving the genital organs besides swelling. We will find the proof of this in a third text, emanating from the same source, and in which it is shown that, long before the voyages of Columbus, there existed a *great* disease, of sexual origin, and which no one cared to acquire. The document in question is dated *July 25, 1463.*

"In the year one thousand four hundred and sixty-three, Tuesday the twenty-fifth day of July, Jehan Jehannin, a varlet serving in the inn of Vergy, at Dijon, aged about thirty-three years, held a prisoner in the prison at the request of the prosecutor of the city and commune for a rape by him made and committed on the person of Jacote, daughter of Alexandre de Chateauvilain, deceased, is interrogated by his worship the mayor."

L'an mil cccclxiii, le mardy xxve jour du mois de juillet, Jehan Jehannin, varlet servant en l'ostel de Vergy, à Dijon, eagié d'environ xxxiii ans, détenu prisonnier ez prisons à la requeste du procureur de la ville et commune pour le ravissement par luy faict et commis en la personne de Jacote, fille de feu Alexandre de Chauteauvilain, est interrogé par M. le Mayeur.

This inn-waiter relates, in his examination, that, in a conversation with a priest of the name of Guillaume Clerget, he learns that there is in town a girl who is not a virgin, and who has "rubbed" (*reverchié*) against the ecclesiastics of Dijon: this bit of news immediately gives him the idea of possessing this girl in his turn. He then comes to an understanding with a procuress, who, that very evening, brings the ex-virgin to his room under some pretext. The latter wishes to leave; but he forces her, by his threats, to share his bed. However, the enterprising young man is not at the end of his trouble, for, as soon as he wishes to show himself gallant, a Homeric struggle begins. The Lovelace is fighting at a pure loss, for, being strongly excited, he . . . comes to a conclusion in the environs of the promised land without being able to enter it.

. . . "by the heat in which he was . . . he spilled his seed without ever knowing her, notwithstanding that his intention was such."

. . . par la chaleur en le quelle il estoit . . . fist semence sans aulcunement la cognoistre, conbien que son intencion feust telle. . . .

Nevertheless, the jade became angry and, during the forced respite accorded to her by her partner, she burst into reproaches; the other answered that he was posted on her ways, and that, for a runner of vestries, she put on a great deal of style.

"The said girl told him, after he had come down, she would make a complaint against dame Simonne, who had sold her thus. To which he answered and remonstrated, asking why she should complain, for the latter had not sold her, and, besides, she had served the mistress of the brothel and had been with priests."

La dicte fille luy deist, après ce qu'il feust descendu, qu'elle se plaindrist de dame Symonne qui ainsi l'avoit vendue. A quoy il depposant luy respondit et remonstra pourquoy elle se plaindroit, car elle ne l'avoit pas vendue, et, d'aultre part, elle avoit servit la maistresse du bourdeaul et avoit esté avec des prebstres.

Finally, he once more came to the assault, in such a manner that the girl, seeing that she would have to yield, took an heroic course and confessed that she had the greatest sort of *great* affections in the line of venereal diseases.

"And since the said deponent held her in his embrace and also did the said girl, and, after a certain time, for the second time, and in getting on her with the intention of knowing her carnally, the said girl told him that she had the GREAT DISEASE, on which account he, all dismayed and having horror of the *disease*, no longer labored to know her carnally, and they remained until morning." . . .

Et depuis ledict depposant la tint embrassée et aussi fit ladicte fille et, après certain espace de tems pour la seconde fois et en montant sur elle en intencion de la cognoistre charnelement, ladicte fille luy deist qu'elle avait le gros mal, pourquoy luy, tout espardu et ayant horreur du mal, ne se travaille plus avant de la cognoistre charnelement, et illeques demeurerent jusques le matin. . . .

This avowal had the power of immediately cooling the ardent young man; accordingly he abandoned the attack and remained quiet until the next morning as soon as he had reasons to make him believe that his companion was dangerous. The reason given must have been the true one; otherwise such resistance could not be explained on the part of a *professional.*

Daremberg draws certain conclusions in reference to the matter which we regard as our duty to reproduce:—

What can this GREAT DISEASE (*gros mal*) which I print in large letters be,—this disease whose name affrights the gallant, steals from him all valor, and puts him to flight; this disease which *is caught*,—if it is not the *big pox?* For my part, I have but small doubt in its identity, and I hold that the girl Jacote was convicted of having acquired the pox probably in a "brothel" ("bourdeaul"); but, at the same time, I would almost grant her absolution for having shown herself less ignorant than the physicians of her time, and having without pretexts recognized the fact that she had a contagious disease acquired in the pursuit of her duties.[1]

These remarks are quite just. Certainly, the gibberish of the erudites of the feudal epoch and the inflated dithyrambics of the troubadours are not, as a general thing, booked in a manner to enlighten us in a satisfactory manner. Fortunately, we come across, from time to time, a brutal and little-veiled report of some registrar of the times; this enables us to place proofs under the eyes of the incredulous; for, if the orthography appear fantastic, at all events the points are plain enough.

The story of the honest Jacote—this style of probity

[1] Union Médicale, 1868.

is rare—has some points of resemblance with that of the martyr of Palladius,[1] which we related in Chapter X of our first volume.[2] It is probable that the *fetid ulcer* of the Greeks of the first century and the *great disease* of the Burgundians of the fifteenth century had close ties of relationship, since, at an interval of fourteen centuries, in calling up one of these two different names, each one of those interested immediately obtained the same result under analogous circumstances. The text of the Dijon parchment sufficiently demonstrates of itself that the *great disease* of feudal times and the only *pox* which has come down the ages are one and the same thing.

We will now speak of the letter,[3] so often quoted by Peter Martyrus, of Milan, addressed to a certain Aryas, a Portuguese by nativity and professor of Greek in the University of Salamanca. This letter does not prove the antiquity of syphilis; but it shows that the invasion of the disease in Europe was anterior to the return of Christopher Columbus and to the siege of Naples. "Thou writest to me freely concerning a peculiar affection of our times which the Spaniards call *las bubas;* the Italians, *French disease;* others, the *elephantiasis* of physicians, etc., and that you are attacked by it." . . .

In peculiarem te nostræ tempestatis morbum, qui appellatione hispana bubarum dicitur (ab Italis morbus gallicus, medicorum elephantiam alii, alii aliter appellant), incidisse præcipitem, libero ad me scribis pede. . . .

Then follows a description of the most marked

[1] Patrologie. Pères Grecs, tome 34. The *Patrology*, or collection of works of the Fathers of the Church, comprises no less than 384 volumes, of which 163 are in Greek and 221 in Latin.

[2] Syphilis in Ancient and Prehistoric Times, p. 152.

[3] Opus epistolarum Petri Martyris, lib. i, capist. 68. Collection of Letters of Peter Martyrus, book i, letter 68. Amsterdam, 1670.

symptoms of syphilis: pains in the joints, ulcers, fetid breath, etc.; and the author thus concludes his missive: "I sincerely pity thee, my dear Aryas, and I would gladly know thee well, but I understand nothing of the disease which overcomes thee. Adieu. Genoa, this 9th of April, 1488."[1]

. . . Misereor quidem, Ari amicissime, tui, cuperemque, te bene valere, sed minime, quod te prosternas, ignosco. Vale. Gienno, in nonis Aprilis, MCCCCLXXXVIII.

An analogous document also proves that, if syphilis were, in 1494, a public calamity officially spread throughout Europe, it had officially begun, practically in epidemic form, in many countries at a distance from each other, and at an anterior date. "*Two years before* the arrival of Charles in Italy," says J. B. Fulgose,[2] "there was a new disease discovered among men, called by different names, according to the countries."

. . . biennio antequam Carolus in Italiam veniret, nova ægretudo inter mortales detecta, varie, ut regiones erant, appellata.

It was then in 1492; Christopher Columbus had left for America, but he had not yet returned.[3] It is known besides, through the testimony of Infessura, that Pope Alexander VI, the infamous Borgia, wrote to Charles VIII in April, 1492, to dissuade him from his expedition

[1] According to certain authors, the date is a false one, and it should be "1498" that is read. Granted; as the value of this document, even if authentic, would not pay for the loss of time necessary to employ in researches, we will admit, if this is insisted upon, that it is antedated. The ample harvest of texts containing better proofs which we have gathered will readily permit us to make this slight sacrifice.

[2] Milan, 1509. Bartolomeo Sonarega, of Genoa, says the same thing in his "Commentaries" (1488–1514); he was ambassador to Charles VIII in 1492.

[3] Christopher Columbus, having left Palos August 3, 1492, returned in 1493, landing at Valparaiso, near Lisbon, on March 4th, remained there nine days, and arrived at Seville on the 15th.

to Naples, giving for a reason that an epidemic disease was devastating Italy; it was a *plague* (the inguinal plague) which was attributed to the presence of the Jews in that country.

A poet of the times, Pacificus Maximus, of Florence, who in 1489 composed several distichs which one might believe were extracts of the Priapridæ, makes some allusions to syphilis. In Book III is found an Ode to Priapus which presents a certain analogy to an ex-voto formula which we have given in Chapter XI of our first volume. Here, also, an unfortunate venereal addresses himself to the God of Gardens asking him to cure his penis; it is the same local disease, with this difference, that the patient knows that he is liable to general lesions, such as ophthalmias and caries of the bones of the nose. "If thou dost not hasten to cure my organ, alas! he will *drop off* by himself! . . . Do not wait until I *lose my sight*, or until my *nose*, *disappearing piecemeal*, will leave me a repulsive face. . . . Miserable being that I am! to be rotten! to carry in the mouth *putrid ulcers!* . . . Cure me; make my penis healthy as it was."

> Tuque meum, si non properas sanare Priapum,
> Decedet; heu! . . .
> Ante meis oculis orbatus priver, vel ante
> Abscissus fœdo nasus ab ore cadat!
> . . . .
> Me miserum!
> Ulcera quæ fœdo marcidus ore gerit!
> . . . .
> Fac valeat, fac sit sanus ut ante fuit.

In Book X (De matronâ) the author reproaches several individuals for giving themselves up to unnatural practices. "This is why," he exclaims, "you have the anus irritated, which induces you to excoriate yourselves with your finger-nails; this is why the *fig* and the *marisca* invade your miserable buttocks!"

> Inde calet culus, digitisque avellitur, inde
> Ficus habet miseras atque marisca nates.

An important document found among the official papers of a notary of Florence gives the proof that, several years before the expedition of Charles VIII, different forms of diseases, acquired in sexual congress with prostitutes and capable of spreading themselves in a city after the fashion of epidemics, were known. It concerns the attestation of the mayor or analogous functionary of the city—entered by a Florentine notary of the fifteenth century, by name Raphael de Cerchi. This document forms part of the legal papers and acts arranged in chronological order since the year 1400, which were found at the ministerial officer's. The document in question is found assigned to a register immediately preceding a note, without interest to us, written in 1491; it is therefore impossible that this act should have been written at a later date. The following is the substance of it: "By these presents, we, Jo. A., of Florence, . . . attest that the French *courtesan* resides for more than two months already in the said city and continually plies *her trade* there; that the said city since that time has not had to suffer from any epidemic or *disease* of whatever nature it may be, as well the men who inhabit it as," etc.

Præsentium tenore, nos Jo. A., de Flor., . . . attestamur, Francischetam meretricem iam per duos menses et ultra continue in dicta civitate stetit et commoravit artem suam continue faciendo; et dicta civitas a nulla peste seu morbo gravatur, seu homines in ea habitentes. . . .

This attestation, in its general nature, presents a close analogy to an ordinance adopted at about the same time by the municipality of Venice. This new document, which we will bring up, is much more explicit than the preceding one. Here it is no more a simple allusion to the disease which might be transmitted by courtesans; there have been victims. The number without doubt was increasing to alarming proportions, since the magistrates of the city saw themselves obliged to pursue clandestine prostitutes and to force them to live in specified houses, where it would be easier to watch over their . . . health. The text positively states that they were the foci of infection, because they accepted the first-comer as a customer and then transmitted the contagium to those who had nothing. Moreover, they hid their pathological state,—just like the loose women of our times. However, the following are the principal conclusions of the ordinance, which bears the date of March 21, 1490. "In view of the fact that it is brought to the attention of our administration, from various sides, that the public girls who live in the different quarters of this city are a *large source of infection*, on account of the relations they hold, as much with *contaminated* people as with others; for not only do they receive at their places *men affected with the contagious virus*, but, if there be contagion, they say nothing of it, so as not to be expelled from the houses in which they lodge," etc.

Cum ex variis personis officio nostro denunciatum sit quod meretrices in variis huius urbis locis habitantes, sunt maxima causa infectionis propter conversationem quam ibi faciunt tam infecti quam alii, quia non solum infestores domi recipiunt, verum si aliquid est domi clam retinent ne domibus expellantur. . . .

Finally, in a satire of the Middle Ages, given by Jourdan,[1] it is said that dissolute manners expose one

[1] Traité complet des malad. vénér. Paris, 1826. Complete Treatise on Venereal Diseases.

to an unhealthy state and to a contagious disease. This satire, which was found in Switzerland in an old manuscript, was written a long time before the Reformation. The title suggests that it is anterior to the year 1000, a date which was then thought to be that of the end of the world. The following is a translation of this curious piece:—

"*On the General Corruption and the Imminent Ruin of the World.*—Shamelessness is connected with three followers with which it has spread itself through the world with a stupefying rapidity. Of these three consequences, scarcely is there one which does not leave behind it some *disgusting stigmata.* I wish to speak of adultery; next comes *impurity*, and finally the *contagious leprosy of sodomites.*"

De Corruptionne Omnium Statuum et Imminente Interitu Mundi.

Ternis est libido fœda
Conjuncta pedissequis,
Per quas totum replet mundum
Vaga petulantia.
Quarum trium vix est ullus
Non fœdatus macula;
Scilicet adulterorum;
Post hunc immundicia;
Et leprosa sodomorum
Tertiant contagiosa.

This *impurity*, according to the testimony of the authors of those times, was a morbid state of a peculiar sort, into which one fell as a result of frequenting cour tesans. Guillaume de Salicet and his successors (Gérard, Gordon, Valois de Tarante) have taught us that the chancres of the penis were taken, at that time, from *impure* women (fœda immunda). As to the "contagium of leprous nature" which was acquired, as the text states, in unnatural practices, it is infinitely more rational to see in them the *ficus* of the Roman Cinedi than anything else; in default of which one would inevitably derive fantastic conclusions. The work of Astruc is the best proof of this.

Such are the documents which bear testimony to syphilitic lesions before the epidemic of Naples, so celebrated and yet so badly known. For this reason, and in order to enlighten ourselves on the nature of this great medical event, we will once more interrogate history.

CHAPTER III.

Syphilis and the Epidemics.

The great epidemics of the Middle Ages compared with those of antiquity.—The disease of the god Siva; curious therapeutics.—The *inguinal disease*; the *sacred fire*; the church of Notre Dame transformed into a hospital for venereal patients.—The worship of Venus in the monasteries of the tenth century.—The death of Hugues Capet.—The *disease of the burning* (mal des ardens); the *disease of fire*; the *disease of St. Main*; the *fire of the Blessed Mary*, the *sacred disease*, and *St. Anthony's fire*.—*Measliness* (mésellerie) or *Oriental leprosy*.—The part played by syphilis.

The history of epidemics is founded, for primitive ages, on legends whose origin is lost in the obscurity of time. All epidemic diseases presupposing a certain agglomeration of individuals, these scourges must have had their birth in places where there was overcrowding, or in which hygiene was wanting, and under the influence of certain telluric or animal miasms. The accounts are, from the very force of circumstances, very vague, for the morbid principles did not wait, before showing themselves, for the advent of physicians to study them or even for historians to describe their effects. Nevertheless, these events have at times manifested themselves with such brutality, and in a manner so fearful and at the same time so murderous, that primitive peoples have retained the remembrance thereof and transmitted the account to their descendants. Having passed from mouth to mouth for centuries up to the time that writing was invented, these recitals took on an allegorical form bearing an analogy with the poetry peculiar to each people.

Man having been, from all time, avid of the marvelous, the unusual diseases which attacked an entire nation were always looked upon as the effects of divine wrath; this explains why those medical events are so intimately bound up with fable; that is to say, the *sacred history* of the pagan nations of antiquity. For this reason, it is to mythology that we must first address ourselves to give the history of the great epidemics which attacked the human race.

We have seen, in studying the documents relative to the sexual diseases of the ancient Hindoos,[1] that a great epidemic of a venereal nature raged in India at a time which it would be impossible to determine within a thousand years. At all events, it is permissible to suppose that this event dates back to the origin of men and closely followed the first attempts at civilization; for it is known that India is the cradle of the human race. Those who have read our preceding volume will remember the legend in which the three persons of the Hindoo Trinity play the principal part. The god Siva, just like the Jupiter of the Greeks and Romans, allows himself gallantries very little to the taste of the husbands of the time. These latter, less easy to indoctrinate than a certain Jewish carpenter,—long since canonized,—had recourse to cabalistic science. Poor Siva was punished where he had sinned; but he concealed his case and continued to have the same success, in such a way that the trouble ended by falling upon its authors. Great consternation upon earth; great uneasiness in the Hindoo paradise. Finally, Brahma and Vishnu, the colleagues of Siva, came to a grand determination; they had recourse to homœopathy in the etymological sense of the word. Accordingly, after having assumed the form of

[1] Syphilis in Ancient and Prehistoric Times, chap. ix, pp. 107 *et seq.*

the genital apparatus of woman, they received the diseased organ of the libidinous god and, say the Vedas, "the burning was stopped." According to one of these Vedas, venereal diseases have for their origin the debaucheries of the wife of Brahma; but that is not the question. The interesting fact which develops itself out of this religious fable is that there certainly was, at a very remote period, an epidemic of venereal nature, and in which syphilis no doubt shone in the front rank.

We have also shown that an analogous condition occurred among the Greeks. Priapus, the son of Venus, driven from Lampsacus by the husbands whose wives he had seduced, revenged himself by sending to them a venereal disease having an epidemic character. The Athenians were punished in the same manner by Bacchus, the father of Priapus, because they did not receive the images of the god with all the honors which were due to them.

In taking up the documents written by eye-witnesses of the memorable events of antiquity, we especially note the *Sixth Plague of Egypt* (about 1410 B.C.), which was characterized by certain pustules which could very well be of venereal nature, and the *plague of Baal-Peor* (1451 B.C.), whose syphilitic character we have already demonstrated in another place.[1] Next come the *plague of Athens*[2] (fifth century B.C.), concerning which Thucydides and Lucretius call attention to the terrible lesions on the side of the generative organs; then a transitory

[1] *Loc. cit.*, chap. viii, p. 88.

[2] In our first volume we quoted the passages of Thucydides and Lucretius regarding the plague of Athens, and we stated that certain descriptions could refer to tertiary lesions. It was simply an hypothesis on our part; for if a few of the patients of that time may have presented venereal lesions, syphilitic and other,—which is very probable,—it remains none the less demonstrated to-day that that plague was especially an epidemic of typhus.

epidemic related by Hippocrates, in the course of the same century, and in which similar lesions are described with more details. Still later, the epidemic,[1] evidently venereal, which followed the return of Manlius to Rome (183 B.C.), and finally an epidemic of the same kind a century later. Pliny the Elder has described the symptoms under the names of *lichen* and of *mentagra* (80 B.C.).

All these episodes have been studied in detail in our preceding volume; so that we need not stop to consider them. We shall now see that the epidemics of the Middle Ages, endowed with names of the most divers kinds, manifested themselves in the same manner, have equally astonished the people by their unusual characteristics, and have, in reality, presented the same general phenomena without differing very much in their particular symptoms.

It is necessary to come to the year 542 of our era to find a description of a venereal epidemic deserving a special name. At that time unnatural debauchery reigned throughout the empire. Then burst forth that epidemic which we have described before under the name of the *inguinal disease.*[2] We have seen that it was again noted upon several occasions, and notably in the thirteenth and the fifteenth centuries. In that epidemic, eminently venereal, the phagedenic ulcer, with its suppurating and undermining buboes, must have been the dominant note; and when syphilis—which is as nothing in comparison with these local troubles—lined itself with serpiginous chancres invading the

[1] "Pestem perniciemque," says the poet Lucilius. See chap. xi of our first volume, page 157.

[2] According to Procopius, a Greek historian born at Cæsarea in 500, it originated in Constantinople and ravaged Syria, the Gauls, and Spain. It should have originated in Ethiopia, if we are to believe Desruelles. (Traité pratiq. des malad. vénér. Paris, 1836.)

groins, we leave it to the imagination to conceive in what state the patients found themselves! There is no astonishment, then, in learning that the larger number of them succumbed. The people, absolutely stricken to the earth, noticed only the principal symptom, the adenitis, and passed over the other details.

After a calm of four centuries, the disease again appeared under the epidemic form. But it is probable that the general manifestations were of a character which overshadowed the local lesions in intensity, at that time, for the name of *sacred fire* was given to this disease. Perhaps it was also better observed. The time was after the Norman invasion, about 945; same picture as in the sixth century; the same terror; the same impotence of the physicians. As at other times the Romans did, the French of that time tried invocations to the Divinity; men pass away, religions change, but superstition remains! It is for this reason, because of the modifications which worship had undergone, that the Virgin replaced Isis, as is testified to by the following passage from Sauval: "As remedies were of no avail, recourse was had to the Virgin, in the Church of Notre Dame, which served as a hospital in that extremity."

Comme les remèdes ne servirent de rien, on eut recours à la Vierge, dans l'église Nostre-Dame, qui servit d'hospital dans cette occasion.

The great Pastoral of Notre Dame confirms this fact, for in it is found a detailed exhibit of 1248 relative to the lamps which were used for lighting, and in which it is positively stated that it was "in this church that the sick and those who were attacked by the disease called the *sacred fire* ordinarily came to find an asylum."

. . . ubi infirmi et morbo, qui ignis sacer vocatur, in acclesiâ laborantes consueverunt reponi.

This disease especially attacked the masculine sex, which is readily explained by the pederastic habits of the invading hordes of that period. Let us also add that the inhabitants of the invaded countries authorized, as we have already stated, by the example of the religious, were far from being little saints. We only require, as a proof of this, the following edifying passage from Dufour,[1] which we turn over to the meditations of our readers:—

The most shameful corruption had penetrated into convents as far back as the Merovingian epochs. In 742, St. Boniface, bishop of Mayence, wrote to Pope Zachariah: . . . "*I have found among those who are called deacons men accustomed from childhood to debauchery, to adultery, to the most infamous vices . . . ; they have all night long, in their beds, four or five concubines, and even more.*"[2] This is not the place to expose the coarse vices of church peoples,[3] who believed that everything should be permitted to them because they had the right to grant

[1] Histoire de la prostitution. History of Prostitution.

[2] For the benefit of those who, in spite of these testimonies, "prefer to doubt," as was said to me at one time by a pious person at a loss for arguments, we give the Latin text of the principal passages of the letter of Bishop Boniface: . . . "Inveni inter illos diaconos quos nominent, qui a pueritiâ semper in stupris, semper in adulteriis et in omnibus semper spurcitiis viam ducentes . . . ; concubinas quatuor, vel quinque vel plures noctu in lecto habentes . . . ." (Act. SS, ord. L Bened., vol. ii, p. 54.)

At a meeting of the Société d'Anthropologie, held December 18, 1890, M. Vinson, in an answer to M. Fauvelle during a discussion on the decreased birth-rate in France, said the following: "The clergy never shone on the side of chastity, to such a degree that at certain times it was necessary to allot it concubines to avoid graver abuses." In our humble opinion marriage would have been much more preferable and especially less scandalous.

[3] Pederasty, which had attained its height at the time of the Roman decadence, blossomed in the Middle Ages at the beginning of the year 1000 and toward the end of the fifteenth century. It came naturally from Italy, from which also came faith in *incubi* and *succubi*, imagined, as Garnier says, to suit the necessities of the case. "Princes, queens, and popes," adds this author, "filled the world with their lewdness. Sixtus IV, of a family of sodomites, went so far as to justify this ignominy by authorizing its practice, during three months of the year, in an infamous brief. Leo X also distinguished himself in this manner." Pope Sixtus IV (1471), as practical as he was debauched, also laid a tax on courtesans.

absolution to sinners placed in their hands; we will not attempt to penetrate into the archives of convents and to recover the long list of those which were reformed, excommunicated, suppressed on account of the monstrous debaucheries of their inmates; it will suffice to say that perhaps not an abbey of any celebrity could be found in which the cloistered customs did not, upon numerous occasions, suffer from the contagion of shamelessness. To quote a few examples among a thousand of this kind, the monks of Moyen Moutier and of Senones, in Lorraine, led such a frightful life, in the tenth century, that they were expelled by order of the Emperor of Germany; but their successors who were given did nothing but surpass them in the science of libertinage.

And these are the beings who caused others to be burned for a question of dogma or a chop eaten on Friday! But cupidity, at least as much as fanaticism, served to stimulate the zeal of the demoniacs of the feudal period; for it must not be forgotten that the property of the heretic subjected to torture was confiscated to the profit of the Church. The chronicles of the times acquaint us with still more horrible things. Apart from the question of religion, the victims were sometimes unfortunate women who had refused to submit to the lubricity of the debauched monks. Then these sensual brutes, weary of orgies, came, in the hope of having new sensations, to gaze upon the naked bodies of women writhing under the red-hot pincers of the tormentor!

The *sacred fire* or *sacred disease* re-appeared in 994. It had lain dormant almost fifty years to again manifest itself in an epidemic form, following upon the heels of a recrudescence in the debauchery of European peoples. It was as murderous as upon its first appearance; and the chroniclers record that the King of France, Hugues Capet, succumbed to it himself, a victim of the attentions he gave to the sick. This terrible disease, against which art could not successfully battle because vice was always disputing the field, was called the *sacred disease* by antithesis; for, says the book "De l'Excellence de Sainte Geneviève" ("The Excellence of St. Genevieve"), "in the system of the formation of names, a name is frequently given to a thing which means the contrary of that which it implies. This is why the physicians call *sacred fire* the disease of fire (*mal de feu*)."[1]

But it was hardly to medicine that recourse was had to arrest the scourge; it was rather to public prayers, fasting, and penances, which restrained the contagion by putting a curb to debauchery. For during the long crises of public health bawdy-houses were closed; women leading loose lives had to suspend the traffic in their persons under penalty of terrible punishments, or the suspected girls were either driven away or confined until the end of the epidemic.

Then the sacred disease was unchristened to call it the *disease of burning* (*mal des ardens*, from *ardere*, to burn), which the people later on called *disease of St. Main* and *St. Anthony's fire*, because, among other reasons, these two saints, well and duly invoked, should have had the honor of curing or improving some patients. Besides, a filthy imprecation of those times, preserved by the populace until the sixteenth century, proves well that the disease of burning, or St. Anthony's fire, was of venereal origin, since the seat of the disease is mentioned. The expression is found at length

[1] In a treatise on internal pathology ("Pathologie Interne") of Grisolle, there is found, as a synonym for scarlatina, *ignis sacer*. It should not be concluded from this that the two diseases are identical, for, if the "sacred fire" had been of a simple exanthematous nature, the chronicler would not have called attention to the fact that the word *sacred* was employed there in an ironical manner, so to speak. Naturally, the opposite of *blessed disease* can be nothing but *disease which one is ashamed to acknowledge;* that is to say, *venereal disease.*

. . . morbus igneus, quem physici sacrum ignem appellant eâ nominum institutione, quâ nomen unius contrarii alterius significationem sortitur.

in Rabelais:[1] "May the fire of Saint Anthony burn the *bum-gut* of the goldsmith who" . . . Let us not forget that it is in the anal region more especially that we find the syphilides known as *mucous patches.* Another phrase demonstrates that the disease manifested itself equally upon other parts of the body: . . . "passed his time and enjoyed the good will with which they sought flight, thinking that the fire of St. Anthony had them *by the legs.*"

. . . prenoit son passe-temps à voir la bonne grâce qu'ils avoient en fuyant, pensants que le feu sainct Antoine les tinst *aux jambes.*[2]

"May the fire of Saint Anthony burn them!" also says Scarron[3] at the end of the seventeenth century.

It may be objected to us that Rabelais, who speaks so easily of the *fire of St. Anthony*, was very well acquainted with the *pox*, and that, nevertheless, he never said that the two diseases were identical; he ought to have done so, will be added, or otherwise only employ but one of these two terms. We will answer that Rabelais wrote for his contemporaries, who knew well how to judge, and that the word *pox* related to the disease in general, and the *fire of St. Anthony* to certain local phenomena. It is thus that, in our days, we still say *painters' colic*, or *saturnine intoxication; gravel, gout*, etc., without forgetting the *uric-acid diathesis;*

[1] Gargantua, book i, chap. xiii.

[2] Pantagruel, book ii, chap. xvi. In the same chapter there is mentioned a practical joke played by Panurge on a gray friar who said mass at court. In helping him to put on the vestments, he had tied together the alb and the shirt of the frater. The latter, in wishing to remove the alb, after the *Ita missa est*, permitted to be seen in a state of nudity a posterior region which is generally kept hidden. Then exclaimed a courtier: "What, this nice father makes us the oblation and wishes us to kiss his a—e! May the *fire of St. Anthony* kiss it." Here again the anus is designated as the principal seat of the disease.

[3] Roman comique, chap. ii.

croup, instead of *laryngitis diphtheritica*, etc. The witty priest of Meudon may, accordingly, have gaily consigned some to the *fire of St. Anthony* at one time, if they did not think as he did, and at another time sing the praises of "the most precious poxy" (verollez trez pretieulz), without any of his contemporaries, up to and including Francis I,—and for good cause,—making any mistake concerning the medical significance of these different expressions.

There were still several recrudescences of this disease,—notably in 1043, in 1089, in 1130 (under Louis VI, called the "Bruiser"), and in 1374; it was also called the *sacred fire* or *fire of burning.* As may be seen, all these designations resembled each other, which is not at all surprising, as they served for centuries to express one and the same thing. Besides, even to-day syphilis is spoken of as the *sacred disease* (mal sacré), but by placing the adjective before the noun.[1]

Such were the informations which we had been able to find, up to 1890, upon these diseases of venereal nature, considered during the entire Middle Ages as epidemics and dubbed with the most whimsical names. For the past two years we have been unable to find, on this subject, any document of a complementary nature which was worth noticing. Nevertheless, we were destined, before giving the manuscript to the printer, to experience the double satisfaction not only of being able to add some new texts to those we have quoted, but also of seeing our conviction shared in by an extremely competent practitioner This practitioner is our distinguished *confrère*, Dr. J. Eraud, of Lyons, who has sent us his interesting study on "The Dis-

[1] This would make the expression *sacré mal*, which, in French, entirely changes the meaning, the translation being "d—d disease."—O-D.

ease Called St. Anthony's Fire," which was published recently.[1]

There we found, with valuable bibliographical points, very suggestive Greek and Latin quotations, which the author did not translate. It is true that his paper was only written for those capable of translating for themselves. But, as we have adopted the custom of explaining and of discussing all our documentary evidence, we must needs continue; our *confrères* will pardon us for having deprived them, in our work, of the pleasure of interpreting themselves the meaning of these curious texts.

Dr. Eraud informs us that there exists, in the Department of Isère, a village of the name of St. Antoine. It owes its name to the neighborhood of an old abbey whose ruins still exist, and which was founded about the year 1080. According to the tradition, the church of the place possesses the relics of St. Anthony, brought from Judea at the time of the Crusades by a certain Prince Jocelyn. There was established there an order of monks who, under the name of *Antonines*, gave for six hundred years their best attention to sick people in general and applied themselves especially to the treatment of the terrible disease known in the Middle Ages by the term *Saint Anthony's fire.*

Evidently the disease derived its name from the hospital, or, rather, from the abbey, where it was treated in a manner more empirical than medical. As a result of this the scientific men of the feudal period are perhaps the only ones who did not speak of it; at the very least, under this appellation. Accordingly, as Dr. Eraud very justly remarks, "not much dependence must be placed

[1] "La maladie dite feu Saint-Antoine," Lyon Médical, July 31 and August 7, 1892.

upon the descriptions of the writers of that distant epoch; for, either through ignorance or through lack of observation, the imagination especially helping, they devote themselves before all to express the agonies, the pains, the fears experienced by the patients, but at the same time completely neglect the local symptoms."

We see some authors call this disease *ignis occultus* (hidden fire); the descriptions are always the same, subjective, but slightly scientific; the terms *pest*, *leprosy*, *sacred fire*, and *disease of burning* constantly recur and relate to the same symptoms. A certain Jean Boucher already had, in the seventeenth century, suspected the bond of relationship which united to syphilis these morbid manifestations so diversely denominated. At least, this is what we are told by the Jesuit Théophile Raynaud, of Lyons, who wrote in 1662: "Jean Boucher, after having declared that this *sacred fire* was totally unknown to him, supposes that it was the affection called by the French *mal de Naples* (Neapolitan disease), and by the Italians *French disease*," etc.

Joannes Boucherus, hunc ignem sacrum plane sibi ignotum professus, conjectat esse quem Galli neapolitanam luem vocant, Itali Gallicam. . . .[1]

He adds farther on that there is no question of the flames of hell, but, indeed, of "that *sacred fire* whose appearance on earth is due, in most instances, to bad Angels, and it is for this reason that it is called *infernal fire*."

. . . hoc igne sacro, cujus immissio est plerumque per Angelos malos, et iduirco dicitur ignis infernalis.

Raynaud also calls it *fire of carnal concupiscence* (ignem concupiscentiæ carnalis), which decisively proves

[1] Theophilus Raynaudus, Hagiologium. Lugduni, 1662.

the gallant origin of the disease. So far as the symptoms are concerned, their serious study must not be asked for. Scarcely are a few phrases found which relate to the most marked general symptoms: the pain, losses of substance, the corruption and fetid odor of wounds (*ex putræ carnis fœtore*), at times cachexia and death, are mentioned. Then it is a diatribe against luxuriousness, the primal cause of these evils, and the work terminates without an exact detail which can bear witness to the slightest clinical observation. However, we have remarked the same thing regarding the works of Antiquity,[1] if my readers will remember, and notably in reference to the Bible.

In the Middle Ages—just as in Antiquity—every time that the chroniclers speak of the epidemic then prevailing, whatever be the name which they give it, they all agree in saying that the disease attacks every one, without distinction of age or sex, and may be seated upon the most diverse places of the body. Witness the following text, entitled "Divine Fire; Sacred Fire": "In the same year (1129) the plague of *Divine Fire* invaded in an astonishing manner Chartres, Paris, Soissons, and many other places; but what is still more astonishing is that it was extinguished by Saint Mary, Mother of God. For young people, old people and children, even tender virgins, were attacked, either on the feet, or on the hands, or on the breasts, and, what is more grave, on the cheeks: nevertheless, they were rapidly cured."

Ignis divinus, *ignis sacer*. Eodem anno plaga Ignis Divini Carnotum, Parisius, Suessionem . . . et alia multa loca mirabiliter perdavit, sed mirabilius per S. Dei genitricem Mariam extinguitur. Juvenes etenim, senes cum junioribus, virgines etiam teneræ in pedi-

[1] Syphilis in Ancient and Prehistoric Times.

bus, in manibus, in mamillis, et quod gravius est in genis exuruntur, et celeritur extinguuntur.[1]

At other times, as it is consigned in the royal archives, it is the arm which is the seat of the disease, and this is probably an ulcerated porrigo; but the treatment is quite radical: "The fire of St. Anthony and of St. Andrew fastened upon his arm, and for this it was cut off."

Le feu Sainct-Anthoyne et Saint-Andrieu se prist en son braz et pour ce lui fut copé.[2]

The title was: "The Disease of St. Andrew, which is also that of St. Anthony." Another manuscript, entitled "Mal de Sainte-Geneviève, ou Feu Sacré" ("Disease of St. Genevieve, or *Sacred Fire*"), designates the leg, and demonstrates that for Isis and Priapus were substituted, as patrons of venereals, a respectable number of male and female saints.

"The said Jeanne, who was sick in her leg of the disease which is called of St. Genevieve and of St. Anthony," etc.

Icelle Jehanne qui estoit malade en sa jambe du mal que l'on dict de Saincte-Geneviève et de Sainct-Anthoine, etc.[3]

It always concerns the same virus, whatever may have been the name which fancy or circumstances may have given it.

Then the centres of election are designated in a more precise fashion. Thus, one may read, in the same archives: "*Fire of the Blessed Mary, a sort of disease which raged with violence in the reign of John, King of*

[1] Chronicon Andrense, vol. ix. Spiceleg. Acher.

[2] Morbus S. Andreæ qui et S. Antonii. Lit. remiss., ann. 1346, in reg. 75, chartoph. reg., ch. 423.

[3] Morbus S. Genevofæ, Sacer ignis. Lit. remiss., ann. 1411, in reg. 166, chartoph. reg., ch. 85.

France. The said Persil had the *Fire of the Blessed Mary* in his *tongue* and in his *throat* . . ; he died of the above-named *fire.*"

Ignis B. Mariæ. Morbi genus qui sub Joanne Franc. rege desæviit. Dictus Persil habebat Ignem Beatæ Mariæ in linguâ suâ et gutture suo . . . ; ex igne predicto expiravit.[1]

Now come ulcers of the nose and lips; the patient was rid of it for a candle to the Virgin; however, the scar persisted: "A woman who was attacked by the *sacred fire* on the *nose* and *lips* went to the Church of the Blessed Mary of Soissons and offered a wax taper very devoutly: the *fire* was extinguished, but she retained a *shameful* deformity, which she hid under a moist rag."

Cûm quedam mulier, habens in naso et labiis ignem sacrum venisset ad ecclesiam Beata Mariæ Suessionensis, offerens devote candelam, extinctus est ignis ille, sed remansit deformitatis verecundia, que sub panno humido occultabatur.[2]

It is self-evident that our opponents will be able to say that in that case it was one of lupus or of cancer; but why not a precocious tertiary syphilis? Was it ever seen that shame (*verecundia*) was attached to the lesions of lupus vorax or of ulcerated carcinoma? Do luxuriousness (*concupiscentia carnalis*), sodomy, etc., play any part in the genesis of scrofulides, epitheliomata, or lupous ulcers? Without taking into consideration that cicatrization, in these different morbid processes, seldom takes place spontaneously; whereas the miraculous cure quoted above took place in the reign of John II, surnamed the Good (1350–1364), and, as related

[1] Registrum cartophylacii regii. Register of the Royal Archives, No. 81, sign. 13.

[2] Et. de Bourbon, Anecdotes, histoires, et apologues. Anecdotes, stories, and apologues.

by the chroniclers, is rather in conformity with the general method of evolution of syphilitic lesions.

In the same measure as the texts succeed each other, the points which can be preferably referred to syphilis are seen to be more and more distinctly described. After the tongue, the throat, the hands and the feet, the nostrils and the buccal orifice, it is the genital organs and especially the anal region which are mentioned. In Du Cange, in speaking of this "fire," at each moment there recur the words *infernum* (infernal, from an inferior region), *anus*, *podex* (fundament), etc.; and in a very ancient manuscript the following sentence is found: "This is why the Lord often smites the sodomite in his genital organs, and sends to him that *fire* which is called *infernal* or of *St. Anthony*, and whose cure takes place by a miracle."

Quare hac . . . sodomiticum percutit Dominus sepe in membris genitalibus illo igne qui dicitur inferni vel santi antonii cujus cura miraculosa est.[1]

In conclusion we will quote a passage of the *Chroniques* of Monstrelet, in which it is stated that King Henry V, of England, the victor of Agincourt, died in 1422 of a disease localized in the margin of the *anus*, and that this conflagration, arsure, sacred disease, disease of burning, or whatever one may wish, was *St. Anthony's fire*, according to the current expression of that time. "And as it was pretty truly known, the chief disease of the said king went from life to death, came to him by *fire* which took him from under *at the fundament*, very similar to that which is said to be the disease of Saint Anthony."

[1] Et. de Bourbon, De septum donis spiritus sancti. Of the Seven Gifts of the Holy Ghost, f. 518. Mss. fonds latin, No. 15, 970.

Et comme il fut assez véritablement sceu, la principalle maladie don le dict roy alla de vie à mort, luy vint par feu qui lui print par dessoubs au fondement assez semblable à ce l'on dict estre la maladie de Sainct-Anthoine.[1]

Dr. Eraud devotes one-half of his monograph,—that is to say, seven pages—to demonstrate that the inseparable companion of St. Anthony, the small *mascot*, is nothing else than a picture of the famous temptation of which the saint was the object. The *pig*, as a sequel, was also to recall the idea of the disease treated by the *Antonines*, since that animal was the symbol of the organ which tempts, of which the Supreme Being, by one of those ironies whose object escapes us, made a focus of infection at the same time as a focus of voluptuousness. One focus can produce but one *fire*, moral or physical: as we have seen, it was most frequently the two, the one following the other.

The researches of our colleague, in regard to the legendary small grunter, are very curious, but they teach us nothing more in regard to the history of syphilis. Therefore, we will limit ourselves to saying that, among the Greeks and among the Romans, the words χοῖρος and *porcus* signified both *pig* and the *external genital parts of a woman;* sometimes, and by extension of meaning, *virginity*.

To sum up, the vulva, or seat of lasciviousness, was represented among the ancients by the animal which today constitutes the stock-in-trade of the pork-seller. The Greeks had even the verb χοιροπωλεῖν, which meant, at the same time, *to sell hogs* and *to prostitute one's self*. It may be readily imagined to what jokes, more or less refined, the double meaning of these words

[1] Enguerrand de Monstrelet, Chroniques, Paris, 1595, vol. i, chap. lxv, fol. 325

could give rise; we find, for instance, in certain pieces of Aristophanes,[1] a few puns of which the word χοῖρος naturally forms the foundation. In the Church of Neuvage, if we are to believe M. Gingue,[2] lasciviousness is represented by a woman mounted on a hog and half-lying down. In the Church of Notre Dame du Bourg, at Digne, is to be found another fresco which shows us a woman astraddle on a sow; beneath may be read an inscription in Provençal, whose meaning it is easy to catch: "Because I gave myself up to lasciviousness, the sow carries me off to hell."

Quar a luxurie me soy donea
En infer me porta la troya.[3]

Thus continually pictures, but nothing precise. As our *confrère* Eraud says, "The therapeutic methods of that time can furnish no explanatory sign; it was too uniform and too frequently of no value to enable one to derive from it any serious explanation. After all, at St. Antoine as everywhere else, lepers, the plague-stricken, and others were found congregated pell-mell and huddled together, the empiric medicine of the time being powerless most of the time, either through ignorance or through material impotence." Nevertheless, like the intervention of *Satan*, *concupiscence*, the invocations to the *Virgin*, to *Anthony* and other saints, are continually found connected with different lesions, more especially those localized in the mouth, at the anus, and in the sexual regions; and these lesions have names, numerous

[1] *Cf.* Aristophanes, The Acharnians, v. 781 *et seq.*

[2] Ch. Gingue, Légende du grand Saint-Antoine. Legend of the Great St. Anthony. Introduction, 1889.

[3] J. Roman, Tableau des vertus et des vices; mémoires des antiquaires de France, vol. xli, p. 25. Picture of Virtues and of Vices; Memoirs of the Antiquarians of France.

it is true, but always implying the idea of ulcer, of virulent sore, of gnawing chancre (devouring fire, infernal fire, disease of burning, sacred fire); so that it appears to us not to be too bold to see in this the ancient and eternal *pox.*

Indeed, a curious painting of the Museum of Colmar (Alsace) produces testimony in favor of this hypothesis. It is a canvas dating from the end of the fifteenth century, and from the brush of Mathias Grünewald; the author, having wished to represent the famous temptation of St. Anthony, has, above all, figured the classic scene of the nightmare, in which the agents of hell persecute the poor saint. Now, one of the characters, we have been assured by our excellent colleague Dr. Larger,—a native of Colmar and at present in Maisons-Laffitte,—is the bearer of syphilitic gummata in every phase of their evolution, and *so typical that we would believe them painted from nature.* Grünewald must certainly have had for a model a patient afflicted with *St. Anthony's fire;* for our part, we have not the shadow of a doubt about it.

The eleventh century was marked by a medical event of importance, the appearance of *leprosy* [1] in an epidemic form.

On the return of the Crusaders, all the undisciplined hordes of *hangers on*, who wallowed in the camps with their *queans*, had not failed, in Palestine, to give themselves up to excesses of all kinds. So that all the Crusaders—all, with very few exceptions—brought back

[1] To tell the truth, leprosy had existed in Europe for a long time in an endemic form; the law of Rotharis, King of the Lombards, proves this. This law, published in 630, the same as the statute due to Charlemagne (789), prohibited lepers from associating with healthy persons. In the same century (eighth) Nicolais, Abbot of Corbie, caused a leprosery (lazar-house) to be constructed, which clearly demonstrates that lepers were already numerous at that time.

Oriental leprosy or *measliness.*[1] Immediately the most severe measures were adopted to prevent lepers from living with healthy persons or among them. Then Europe was seen to become covered with *leproseries*, in which the sick who were most affected were placed. As soon as a leper was discovered, say the chronicles, he was brought to the church, where the service of the dead was read. The patient was then declared dead in law; he was no longer to communicate with healthy persons. His *line* (hut or cell) was designated, and he could not go beyond it without shaking his wooden rattle, so that all might take flight upon his approach.[2] For leprosy had its degrees, and was even not always apparent. Certain lepers were married, but their gangrened race did not delay in becoming extinct from want of care. Some of the less contaminated, especially those in whom the disease was not externally visible, propagated the morbid principle.

From this information it is easy to see that the leprosy of the Middle Ages differed in a marked degree from that which we are enabled to study in our days. The former was contagious in the first degree; the precautions taken show this; whereas it is still a matter of discussion as to whether the latter is transmissible by contact. We have already examined this disputed point, and we will not recur to it. But we repeat that everything justifies us in holding that the word *leprosy*

[1] Leprosy was also called *ladrerie*, *maladrerie*, *éléphantie*, *léphantie*, etc. [Like *mésellerie*, ladrerie and maladrerie have no definite English equivalents, being translated leprosy, sordid, scabby, etc.—O-D.]

[2] However, the warning signal varied according to the locality. Thus, at Lille, they had to blow a horn twenty times; at Caen, they carried a bell "made of bronze, and struck it ten times every hundred paces" (faicte d'airain et en frappoient dix fois chaque cent pas); at Arles, "they sang in a loud voice the psalm *De Profundis*" (ils chantoient en haulte gueule le psaulme *De Profundis*).

served to designate, in the Middle Ages, a host of diseases, among which true leprosy was certainly one, but principally the contagious affections of the sexual organs. The proof of this is furnished by the works of the physicians of the time,—those, for example, of Roger Bacon (twelfth century), of Theodoric (1250), of Gordon (1300), and of John of Gaddesden (1320), etc. We have related, in our first chapter, the occurrence of a passage in the "English Rose," which leaves no doubt in this respect; and when we come to study the authors of the fifteenth and sixteenth centuries we shall also see that, among those who were contemporaries of the epidemic of Naples, the term *leprosy* was employed to designate venereal diseases.

Then this word fell into desuetude for a very simple reason,—the almost complete disappearance of the so-called lepers. After the epidemic, venereal disease having been studied and classified, the immediate result was a great event which could not fail to strike all observers,—the NINETEEN THOUSAND leper-asylums of Europe fell in ruins *for the want of patients*, and . . . the syphilitics ran over the world!

CHAPTER IV.

The Epidemic of Naples.

The great epidemic of the fifteenth century, or the "ninety-three of the pox."—Sanitary state or medical constitution of Europe at that time.—The exact date of the scourge according to the physicians and historians of the time.—Manifest identity of the leprosy of the Middle Ages with syphilis.—The true nature of the epidemic of Naples; why it received that name; its march and direction.—Height and end of the epidemic; syphilis frees itself from the pathological chaos.—A word from Ricord.

When the greater number of the epidemics of antiquity have been reviewed in the same manner as we have done, it is permissible to ask one's self if venereal diseases have always shown themselves under the same appearances. It may be readily admitted, it seems to us, without being accused of heresy for that, that those affections may have undergone a large number of metamorphoses,—at all events, more apparent than real,—and this on account of the divers local atmospheric conditions which have produced themselves in the course of centuries. The syphilitic disease, so far as being a general affection such as we know it to-day, with its three periods, has always been the same; but the successive manifestations, especially the genital sores, must have presented variations in intensity, appearance, form, etc., according to the temperaments, the medical constitutions of nations and of epochs, or to the redhibitory vices of each one. "This hideous scourge," says Dufour, "which science, after three and a half centuries of profound study, still looks upon as a Proteus which cannot be seized, did not possess, before the year 1493 or 1496, the fearful characteristics, and especially the propagating virus, which are observed for the first time at that epoch, when the exceptional cases became general ones."

In other words, the horrible genital sores, which are the rarest in our days, were then very frequent. There would not have been any more uneasiness about syphilis than about any other disease of slow evolution if a host of unforeseen circumstances had not come up, at that very time, to aid in its propagation; for it is quite certain that venereal disease had always existed in a chronic state in isolated individuals. Prostitution being its most active focus, the debauched were about the only ones contaminated, in the Middle Ages; so that the scourge remained perforce circumscribed. However, at certain periods, as we have just seen, it became irritated under different influences, passed beyond its ordinary bounds, and associated itself with other epidemic or contagious diseases.

Everything would lead to the belief that the historic plagues of antiquity were nothing else than a blending of infectious diseases, one complicating the other, and that there were, among the victims, persons suffering as well from typhus, cholera, scurvy, gangrene, and hospital rot, as from phagedenic ulcers with dissecting buboes, and from syphilitic lesions. We know, besides, that syphilis does not protect from other infections of the organism, and the cumulation—excuse the word—must have been one of the greatest causes of error, if not the only one. But it was written that the syphilitic virus, so long unrecognized or confounded, was not to be freed from this chaos and receive its baptismal name in a final manner before the end of the fifteenth century!

It must not be forgotten that mixed chancres are only known since yesterday, thanks to Ricord. who, adopting the way of seeing of Bassereau, has well separated the non-infecting chancre from the primary lesion of syphilis. It is, therefore, not surprising that the latter should have been considered a terrible disease in those cases in which the unfortunate patients, attacked by horrible, eating ulcers, found themselves attacked by the pox at the same time, and died from the consequences of their *non-infecting* chancres at the very time of the appearance of the general symptoms of syphilis.

It may be objected that similar cases must have presented themselves before the taking of Naples and outside of the epidemics, and that, notwithstanding this, no one ever separated the syphilitic virus from this mingling of diseases. We will answer that this morbid entity had several names then, or, rather, that these different symptoms each had one; but that, on the other hand, the nosological bond which inclosed within it these manifestations was still in the darkness. In addition, from the beginning of the twelfth century, venereal diseases were left in the shadow, being eclipsed by *leprosy*,—a generic term which included all cutaneous affections, whatever their origin might be. That which proves it is that it has been applied, by extension of meaning, to venereal diseases in general: we have seen that, in certain authors of the Middle Ages, this word designates exclusively diseases of the genital organs, even *gonorrhœa*. The words *elephantiasis* and *leontiasis* were attached to very marked dermatoses, but not necessarily of genital origin. And, as we have already stated in one of our papers,[1] we remained convinced that the leper-asylums contained all the varieties of diseases of the

[1] F. Buret, Les mesures répressives à l'égard des vénériens. Autrefois, aujourd'hui. Clermont (Oise), 1890. Repressive Measures in Regard to Venereal Persons. Formerly and To-day.

skin, notably common itch, with this difference, that we cure them to-day, whereas then they knew no better than to take flight upon seeing the diseased. Our present Hôpital St. Louis was represented in Europe by nineteen thousand leper-asylums,—of which there were five thousand for France alone,—in which poor treatment or none at all was given.

When venereal disease went out beyond its ordinary limits the greater part of the cases seen was malignant syphilis, such as is so rarely seen in our days. The scourge multiplied itself with the most terrible symptoms, and threatened to invade the entire population. Sanitary measures were immediately adopted; but, as soon as the danger had passed, the regulations fell into neglect and manners became relaxed more than ever, until a new epidemic appeared. Let us add to this that hygiene was reduced to its most simple expression, especially in the quarters of prostitutes. When we state that, before the sixteenth century, a *leech* or *physician* (medical practitioners of the period) had never penetrated into the Cour des Miracles,[1] an idea may be formed of the sanitary state which reigned during the Middle Ages in this celebrated corner of old Paris.

Nevertheless, toward the end of the fifteenth century, the *great leprosy*, or elephantiasis, had about disappeared, thanks to the precautions taken and especially on account of the deaths of those affected with it. They hardly succeeded, as a matter of fact, in perpetuating themselves beyond the third or fourth generations. As to the *little leprosy*, which included venereal diseases of external benign appearance, it also became weaker, as we have already said, by reason of continence. Fear

[1] A low quarter of Paris, the abiding-place of thieves, rag-pickers, etc., destroyed by Baron Haussman when he built the Boulevards.

alone placed a restraint upon licentiousness; for the finest sermons of preachers upon seraphic joys, which beget chastity, had but a moderate success during this period of general debauchery. And naturally, as soon as the first respite came, the libertines took heart and commenced to frequent more than ever the quarters reserved for prostitution. This is exactly what occurred toward the end of the fifteenth century: venereal diseases broke forth anew from the foci in which they had continued to brood silently. This time they were to declare themselves in a terrible manner, and give rise to the most celebrated epidemic which has ever been known in the history of peoples.

It should not be thought, however, that this event burst forth suddenly, like a stroke of lightning. Quite the contrary; the epidemic hung fire for a long time. The proof lies in the lack of agreement of the dates assigned by different authors—historians or physicians —who undertook to write an account. Although it has been generally agreed upon for the years 1493 or 1494, it is more true to say that venereal lesions, which had always existed in an endemic form, increased in a marked degree for several years, and assumed the appearances of a scourge of general character from 1492 to 1496. We have quoted a passage from an author of the time, J. B. Fulgose, who assigns the beginning of the epidemic to 1492 (*two years before Charles came to Italy*). We have also observed that Pope Alexander VI (the famous Borgia), warned of the expedition contemplated by the King of France, wrote to him to dissuade him, urging as a reason the epidemic of inguinal plague then prevailing in Italy. Jean Salicet makes the origin of the disease date back to 1457, and confirms (being a contemporary of the epidemic of

Naples) the opinion of the authors of the preceding three centuries, who then called *leprosy* what was called, later on, the *French disease* (mal Français). Wendelin Hock, of Brackenaw, who had completed his studies at the University of Bologna, begins, in his work, by repeating what he had heard said in Italy on the origin of syphilis: "Since the year 1494 up to the present year, 1502, a certain contagious disease, the *French disease*, has made considerable ravages" . . .; then, in the course of the same volume, he restores the truth—then known to all his German colleagues—by saying: "This disease, which had begun, to speak more exactly, *ever since the year 1483* of Our Lord." . . . This is something which abundantly proves that the famous epidemic evolved itself with remarkable sloth.

The symptoms of syphilis varying in an infinite number of ways and not always manifesting themselves by cutaneous lesions, the physicians of the time must have inevitably made continual mistakes by confounding classic leprosy and the new disease. We have seen that, already in the thirteenth century, Theodorus called attention to the fact that leprous women were capable of giving a *bad disease*. Well, three centuries later—that is to say, thirty years *after the epidemic*—Jean Manard, of Ferrara, says about the same thing in his "Letters on Medicine." This shows very well that they had not yet emerged from the chaos in which, for more than a thousand years, leprosy and venereal affections remained plunged. The leper-asylums were deserted, it is true; but men of science had not yet been struck with the fact that common leprosy disappeared in proportion as syphilitic lesions, better known and more studied, were classified under their appropriate names.

However, here is the text of Manard, whose analogy

to that of Theodoric is absolutely striking: "Those who have carnal relations with a woman coming from the arms of a *leper* (it is thus that the elephantiasic is called)—that is to say, whilst the seed is still in the vagina—sometimes catch leprosy *and at times other diseases* more or less considerable, according to the circumstances in which they are placed, like the leper who *infected* the woman."

Qui mulieri coierint, quæ parùm anteà cum leproso (sic enim Elephantiacum vocant) rem habuerit, semine quidem adhuc in utero manente, elephantiasim quandoque incurrere, quandoque non, sed alias ablæsiones, majores minoresve, prout et ipsi affecti et Elephantiosus ille qui mulierem infecit.[1]

Replace the word *leprous* by that of *venereal*, and all the obscurity in the quotation disappears.

It will be summed up in that axiom which is to-day a truth of la Palisse[2]: "The sexual act accomplished with the mistress of a venereal individual renders liable to the same lesions as those with which the latter is affected." Astruc himself furnishes us with a document more and more favorable to the opinion which we have been defending. Respecting the expressions *impure*, *spoiled*, and *chancrous*, employed by the authors of the Middle Ages, he maintains that they referred to *leprous* women, and he supports himself by several passages of Arabian physicians of the same period in which it is stated that "there ordinarily come on *ulcers of the penis* in those who have intercourse with women infected by *leprosy*." It required the monumental blindness of the celebrated syphilographer of the eighteenth century not to have been struck by these palpable proofs.

When we come to study the authors of the sixteenth

[1] Jean Manard, Epistolæ medicinales, 1525.

[2] La Palisse is a fictitious character who is always stating self-evident truths.—O-D.

century we shall see that the term "leprosy" is employed less and less; we shall also see that it finally disappears completely from works on venereal diseases to give way to the words *pox* or *disease*. These words summed up, at that time, and included the venereal trinity officially recognized as a morbid entity; but the three elements which compose it were not to be classified as distinct and independent viruses until toward the middle of the nineteenth century.

The undeniable fact which is deduced from the documents of the time is that the epidemic, whose nature we are going to study, had been preparing itself during at least two years, was going at a *crescendo* gait, and arrived at its maximum of intensity at the time of the siege of Naples by the French. The movements of troops, which were the consequence of the expedition of Charles VIII, contributed, in a large measure, to the dissemination of the contagium everywhere, in a small quantity. This explains how an epidemic, which was, in a certain measure, limited to the peninsula of Italy for two years, could in a few months spread itself to the four corners of Europe and sow its murderous elements. It is not unimportant, either, to add that the flooding rains which fell that year may have complicated the epidemic by disengaging telluric miasms, which came to add themselves to the animal micro-organisms.

It should not be supposed, as Dufour most judiciously remarks, in calling attention to the point, that this horrible disease, which was at first regarded as incurable, had at its beginning the same appearance as at the time of its decrease and of its stationary period. What certainly proves that the epidemic was composed of several grave diseases, among which is syphilis, is that the latter, observed in its true light after the first panic, which lasted for years, was reduced to a few only of the more or less serious symptoms which had been observed at the beginning. From the year 1540, according to the testimony of Guicchardin, the disease "had become much milder and had changed itself into several varieties differing from the first one."

Thus, that which had struck observers when the scourge was at its height was the mortal symptoms appertaining either to pernicious fever, or to scurvy, or to "black" small-pox, or to typhus,—perhaps to farcy? —or even to so-called malignant syphilis, and showing, in a very short time, frightful tertiary symptoms; or to that virus, not yet named, but a stranger to syphilis, which engenders phagedenic ulcers, dissecting buboes, and the enormous losses of substance. The signs properly appertaining to ordinary classic syphilis, such as it must have existed among the Romans as well as among the French of the Middle Ages,—that is to say, the symptoms which we observe to-day in current pathology, —had certainly not attracted much attention. At all events, they must have appeared quite pale in comparison with the frightful picture which the unfortunate victims of the epidemic presented.

It would become tiresome to accumulate the proofs and pile documents on documents to prove that syphilis and the disease designated during all the Middle Ages under the names of sacred fire, St. Anthony's fire, leprosy, etc., have never been anything but one and the same thing. The complete rout of the body medical at the moment of the epidemic of Naples has contributed not a little to make this false idea, which consists in carrying back the dates of the origin of syphilis to the year 1494, deeply rooted. There reigns in all the writings of this period such a confusion that the reader is quite confounded in seeing there an insurmountable barrier beyond which no description relating to syphilitic lesions may be found. So far as we are concerned, who have permitted ourselves to go to the bottom of things, and who have pushed our investigations as far as it was humanly possible to do so, we will make the following *résumé* of our opinion on the evolution of syphilis from ancient times up to the end of the fifteenth century, and upon the great medical event of that epoch :—

1. It follows from secular documents that syphilis is contemporaneous with remote ages.

2. During the period of about one thousand years, which received the name of *Middle Ages*, syphilis always existed in an endemic state, especially limited in places of debauchery, where it was treated by empirical methods.

3. From time to time it emerged from the domain of libertinage to disseminate itself over the frightened populations, by reason of a concatenation of circumstances, of which debauchery and bad hygiene were the principal factors; then it received a name which varied according to the impressions formed at the time.

4. Current *leprosy* referred itself to all skin diseases,—syphilitic and otherwise,—and it ended by designating exclusively venereal diseases in their sexual manifestations up to and including the gonorrhœal discharge. [All authors agree in saying that, in the fifteenth century, the leprosy of that time was communicated by coitus.]

5. Popular common sense took it upon itself to demonstrate this by attributing the origin of venereal disease to the intercourse of healthy persons with leprous ones, which proves very well that the symptoms, in both cases, did not differ in any material degree.

6. The epidemic of Naples was represented by a group of grave diseases which mingled themselves with cases of malignant syphilis and masked the current pox,—that is to say, benign cases.

7. Finally, the use of quicksilver, which the physicians, forced to the wall, were obliged to accept from the hands of empirics, constitutes the tangible proof of the identity of the leprosy of the Middle Ages with the syphilis of to-day. The lewd and licentious who treated the lepers thus,—that is to say, venereal patients,—and had transmitted the secret from century to century, had for many years the monopoly of the treatment of specific diseases in which physicians were too uninterested at the beginning. It results in this, that, even to-day, the mountebanks still retain the better portion of venereal patronage; and, although four centuries separate us from the siege of Naples, the bass-drum, cymbals, and the cap and bells are far from being out of fashion!

Now that we know what to understand in regard to the so-called novelty of the syphilitic disease in 1494, let us study the epidemic in regard to its nature, its course, and its duration.

Let us say, first of all, for the edification of the reader, that the French troops arrived at Naples, February 22, 1495, according to the Gregorian calendar, then adopted by the inhabitants of Italy. The French year commencing, under Charles VIII, on the feast of Easter, the first day of the year fell on the 19th of April; so that the siege of Naples, noted down by the French under date of 1494, really occurred in 1495, if the new year be taken as occurring January 1. And the Italian authors, who were the first to attribute the cause of the epidemic to this expedition, have given evidence of preconceived notions, if not of bad faith. The siege of

Naples was certainly one of the great causes of the diffusion of the contagium, but the French soldiers could not have imported into that country a disease which had already reigned there for two years in an epidemic state, seen and known by the entire Italian population.

Philippe Albert[1] reproduces a letter written by a contemporary of the expedition which leaves no room for doubt on this point. It emanates from an Italian of the name of Delphini, and bears the date of February 20, 1494. "It is to be feared, on the occasion of the arrival of the French," he writes to Cardinal de Gienne, "that such great passages of troops will spread still farther the disease in Italy, *which is not yet freed of this scourge*." This is at least one point firmly established.

Now, it is, perhaps, not useless to condense in a few lines the history of that disastrous expedition of Naples, of which the only apparent result was, as happens but too often in similar cases, a great loss of men and money.

In 1493 Charles VIII, King of France, badly inspired or, rather, badly counseled, desired to establish the claims of the House of Anjou—whose heir he claimed to be—to the throne of Naples, occupied by Ferdinand II. As a result of this he raised a considerable army and equipped a fleet at Genoa. August 20, 1494, he took the road to Italy, but an illness delayed him a month at Asti. As soon as recovered he traversed Lombardy and Tuscany and arrived at Rome December 31, 1494. February 21, 1495 (1494 according to the French calendar of the time, whose year began at Easter), he was beneath the walls of Naples, where he was crowned May 20th. Then he returned to France,

[1] Ph. Albert, Mémoire sur les malad. vénér. Bordeaux, 1836. Memoir on Venereal Diseases.

leaving an army of occupation under the command of Gilles de Montpensier,—a prince of the royal blood. The King of Spain, fearing that Charles VIII, emboldened by success, might wish to seize Sicily, dispatched Gonzalves de Cordona to Italy (1495). This latter drove off the troops of occupation which Charles VIII had left and restored Ferdinand II to the throne.

As a matter of fact, the disease did not exist in the State of Naples alone; it was observed in other localities long before the expedition of the King of France. A Spanish physician, Gaspard Torella, bishop of St. Juste (Sardinia) and physician of the Borgias, relates, indeed, that "this infectious disease began *in Auvergne* in 1493, and that the contagium spread itself in Spain, in the islands," etc.

Incepit hæc maligna ægretudo anno MCCCCXCIII in Alverniâ, et sic contagionem in Hispaniam, ad insulas, etc.[1]

The disease, then, did not burst in a sudden manner, since there are such diverse opinions in regard to the place of its origin!

We have seen that syphilis had always produced the same ravages up to the fifteenth century without attracting the attention of the men of learning of the feudal epoch. The physicists described its numerous symptoms as so many distinct diseases, and very little did they suspect the bonds of relationship which held together so closely those manifestations. Scarcely did the most clear-sighted insist on the fact that, in certain cases of infecting coitus, with contagion (*contagiositate*) several different lesions could arise in the same individual without inevitably having their seat in the genito-anal region. Certain authors of the thirteenth century have well said

[1] G. Torella, Dialogus de dolore in pudendagrâ, 1500 (Ap. Luisinum). Dialogue on the Disease of the Affected Genitals.

—as we have seen in Chapter I—that the *contaminated* woman transmitted local lesions and that the virus (*venenum*) sometimes spread throughout the body; but they sought no farther. One more step, nevertheless, and the nosological thread which binds together the three periods of syphilis was discovered.

But the symptoms which the authors of the Middle Ages describe have nothing very frightful about them. To sum up: they are those of current venereal pathology, those which we know at present. "The lesions which we observe to day," said Ricord,[1] "resemble infinitely more those described at all times than the epidemic of the fifteenth century." And he was perfectly right.

We are, as a matter of fact, far from—and fortunately—the terrifying descriptions which have been transmitted to us, by common consent, by the authors of the end of the fifteenth century, in regard to the epidemic of Naples. Why? The reason for this is very simple. This epidemic, like nearly all destructive epidemics, presented—it cannot be repeated too often—a crowd of symptoms peculiar to several grave diseases combined, and in the midst of which syphilis was submerged, in a manner. Comparatively speaking, the manifestations of the latter were really but an accessory affair, and, so to say, easily overlooked. On the other hand, we will not insist upon a refusal to admit that many of the patients, affected either with horrible ulcers, consequent upon gummata, or to losses of substance with necrosis of the bones or other grave tertiary lesions, may not have contributed, to a certain degree, in making still darker a sufficiently gloomy picture. We will even add that, in many patients, their condition of being syphilitics, or *lepers*, whichever is preferred, must have been

[1] Lettres sur la Syphilis, Paris, 1851.

a serious addition to the gravity of the epidemic disease to which they might not otherwise have succumbed. Do we not see, in our own days, syphilis sometimes awaken a latent tuberculosis or even throw wide open the doors to the comma bacillus in subjects free of all hereditary taint?

Now, what was the nature of this famous epidemic? It is difficult to know it exactly, but it may easily be surmised, in reading the accounts of authors of the time, that it was extremely complex. According to Rosenbaum, it was, above all, a typhoid condition. We have seen that, in the plagues of antiquity, and notably in that of Athens, it was typhus which especially produced its ravages. Many other pernicious elements came on to aggravate the state of the sick, in such a manner that, at the beginning,—as the rule holds in all epidemics,—almost all succumbed. The same Rosenbaum calls attention to the fact that gangrenous erysipelas,[1] which was a frequent symptom in this condition, was especially deplorable when it attacked the *pubic region* and the *genital parts;* "so that," he adds, "a multitude of patients found themselves affected with ulcerations of the sexual organs,—ulcerations which, under the influence of the reigning typhoid condition, were rapidly seized with an erysipelatous inflammation terminating in moist gangrene.[2] The localization in the genital organs of these gangrenous ulcers, which were almost always mortal, must certainly have made them attributed to syphilis.

[1] It must not be forgotten that hygiene was very much neglected at that time, and that rye came in for a large proportion in the popular food. The ergot of rye, whose toxic or hæmostatic properties were not then known, may possibly have played a part in some of the cases of gangrene observed; or, is this an improbable assumption?

[2] Rosenbaum, Geschichte der Lustseuche im Alterthume. Halle, 1845. History of Lasciviousness in Antiquity.

Then, it will be understood to what a degree modern physicians, when they ignore these details, may find themselves puzzled in comparing the descriptions regarding the epidemic of Naples with the symptoms of classic syphilis. "But it is not at all the same thing!" they involuntarily cry out; and they are right. Besides, each one can account for it to himself by studying contemporaneous authors, and especially Fracastor,[1] whose work on *contagious diseases* is yet one of the most complete for the time.[2]

We know that certain cases of malignant syphilis may, even to-day,—but how rarely!—present a gangrenous character and even bring on losses of substance.[3] These abnormal cases, absolutely exceptional, *even in the fifteenth century*, whatever may be said to the contrary, came and added themselves to the reigning epidemic and contributed in no slight degree in increasing the causes of error for all those who have endeavored to decipher the great pathological enigma. As a matter of fact, the expressions "*infectious*" and "*venereal*" must not be confounded. The infectious principle, the soul of an epidemic, is like a leaven which rises and then sinks low down on the same place; "in a given time all is said: nothing remains but to count the dead."

[1] De morbis contagiosis. Venetiis, 1546.

[2] The descriptions of authors of the fifteenth century and even of the beginning of the sixteenth are almost all identical; it must be said that they copied each other a great deal, especially at the beginning.

[3] At its meeting of February 11, 1892, M. E. Besnier presented to the Société de Dermatologie et de Syphiligraphie a patient affected with abnormal syphilis of a gangrenous nature. This man was covered with ulcers which had in places brought on considerable losses of tissue. He was an *alcoholic;* that is to say, an excellent soil for the cultivation of the syphilitic virus. M. Besnier concluded from this that the disease may sometimes show itself with the grave characteristics observed at the time of occurrence of the epidemic of the fifteenth century. This is possible, but it does not prove that all the frightful cases of that epoch were from the domain of syphilis.

Venereal diseases, essentially chronic, develop according to an unchangeable type and with varied symptoms, but always identical: the soil, alone, creates the differences in intensity in the manifestations; and the word "horrible" never could have been nor ever can be applied to the generality. There always have been, in current venereal pathology, benign cases and grave cases; but these latter, by reason of progress made, as much in individual hygiene as in therapeutics, will become more and more exceptional.

We have stated that the descriptions given by the historians of the epidemic of Naples rarely referred to syphilis. It will suffice, to prove this, for us to quote a few extracts from the contemporaneous authors. Here, for example, is a passage from Fracastor applicable only to soft chancres unceasingly inoculable, as we know, upon the same individual. It is true that, during more than three centuries, the expressions *lues venerea*, *venereal disease*, *pox*, and *syphilis* designated indifferently every contagious disease of sexual origin:—

> There came on most often small ulcers (*ulcuscula*) on the shameful parts; these ulcers were stubborn. When they had been cured in one place they appeared in another, and it was always a matter of beginning again.

This is certainly neither the appearance nor the progress of the infecting chancre, which, on account of its insensibility and its small importance, must have more than once—like to-day—been taken for an insignificant abrasion.

Farther on Fracastor describes the corroding ulcers which are not frequently met, with their characteristics, in classic syphilis. The author makes an evident mistake between ulcers of malignant tertiary syphilis and the terrible non-infecting, but undermining, chancres; he mixes the symptomatology of the two viruses :—

> They were true phagedenic ulcers which consumed not only the flesh, but the bones. . . . In the upper portions, the palate, the uvula, and the pharynx were sometimes destroyed. A few lost the lips, the nose, or the eyes ; in others the shameful parts were entirely eaten.

Were these ulcers the result of the gangrenous erysipelas of which Rosenbaum speaks, or of that local virus not yet named, but the generator of the chancres which we call to-day by the adjectives "phagedenic" and "serpiginous"? Were there also included, in these descriptions, cases of *lupus vorax* or even of ulcerated cancer? These are conjectures of which it is not easy to furnish the proof.

At all events, the virulent sores so described certainly did not arise from ulcerated gummata, for Fracastor describes these latter a few lines farther on :—

> In many patients there appeared, on the limbs, *gummy tumors*, which disfigured them and which were often of the size of an egg or of a roll. When they opened a white liquid, which was *mucilaginous*, escaped. They attacked chiefly the arms and legs ; at one time they ulcerated, at another they persisted until death without any apparent change.

This is something which leads us to think that all these swellings were of specific origin, since certain ones brought on death without there being any visible sore.

Now we enter into the domain of classic syphilis. Here comes, for example, a description of the different pustulo-crustaceous, papular, and psoriatiform syphilides :—

> Then there arose upon the skin pustules with crusts (*crustulosæ pustulæ*), which began upon the hairy scalp (this was most frequently the case) or in other parts of the body. To begin with, they were small ; then they gradually increased in size until they had attained

the dimensions of the cup of an acorn, very much in appearance like to the milk-crust of infants. In some these pustules were small and dry, in others large and moist; at times livid, at other times white, or else hard and reddish.

Then the author describes the terrible pains in the limbs coincident, at times, with the pustules, the nocturnal headache, the syphilitic cachexia, and fever.

A slight fever sometimes occurred, but rarely.

On the other hand, here is something which is not connected with syphilis:—

The face and the legs swelled.

Was not this swelling of the face rather symptomatic of true leprosy? This is what seems to appear from a passage of Sebastianus Aquilanus,[1] in which this author, contemporaneous with the epidemic, says about the same thing as Fracastor, in the barbarous Latin of the period:—

This disease causes the limbs to swell (*ingrossantur membra per hunc morbu*); the skin becomes covered with pustules of such a size that, in many places, it looks like the skin of an elephant. The face is also tumefied in such a manner that it takes on the satiric mask. Galen has described these same symptoms in connection with elephantiasis (*quæ omnia tribuit Galen, elephantiasi morbo*).

We are very far from the lesions—even the rarest—of classic syphilis; one would more readily think of the tubercular form of leprosy. It is true that the work of Aquilanus is devoted almost entirely to a demonstration of the identity of the syphilis of the fifteenth century with the elephantiasis of the Greeks. It is nothing but a long list of quotations, taken from the works of Hippocrates and of Galen, and discussed by the author.

Leoniceno[2] states that the prevailing disease is

[1] De morbo gallico, 1498. Aquilanus was Bishop of Mantua.

[2] Nicolas Leoniceno, De epidemiâ quam Itali morbum Gallicum, galli vero Neapolitanum vocant. Vicence, 1497. Of the Epidemic which the Italians call *French Disease* and the French *Neapolitan Disease.*

nothing else but ancient leprosy, that it cannot be a new disease, and he adds a thought which has its own value:—

> Men having always been constituted in the same fashion, having always been born under the same sky, and have grown under the same stars, I am forced to conclude therefrom that they must have always had the same diseases.

Jean Manard, whom we have already quoted, did not believe in the antiquity of syphilis; but he attributed the birth of the virus to the sexual relations at Valencia (Spain) of a *leper* and a courtesan. This latter, then, had, probably, subsequently contaminated a few of the future soldiers of Charles VIII. According to Matthiole, these same soldiers should have been the first infected with the new disease in Italy, after carnal relations with leprous women. According to Paracelsus, a public woman, who was affected with venereal buboes, had intercourse with a French *leper;* all those who subsequently visited her acquired syphilis. For Cæsalpinus, the French troops having drank wine contaminated by Spaniards with the blood of *lepers*, presented the first symptoms of syphilis known.

When Bishop Torella, of Valencia (Spain), a contemporary of the epidemic of Naples, himself contracted, at that time, the *French disease*, he at first believed himself "lost beyond all hope," because he was told that he had "leprosy."

Let us once more quote Peter Martyrus, who hesitated in 1488—six years before the siege of Naples—about the name he should give to the disease of his friend Aryas, and who calls it, without hesitation, *elephantiasis* in his three hundred and seventy-fifth and last letter sent from Burgos to another professor in

1507.[1] Now, he had, in the time intervening between his two letters, made the voyage to America with Columbus; and he would, doubtless, have been greatly astonished if it had been advanced before him that the disease identical with the leprosy of the Middle Ages, and recognized as such at that moment, must be a product of the New Continent. The important fact to bear in mind is that, the disease already called in 1488 *las bubas*, the *French disease*, by the greater part of the people, was, for the physicians of the time, *elephantiasis* (elephantia medicorum); that is to say, the disease known as *leprosy* during the entire feudal period.

As has been easy to see, each time that there was a question, either of naming venereal lesions or of explaining the origin of the disease which was believed to be new, leprosy was almost always placed in the foreground. And assuredly the confusion between the two diseases must also have arisen in antiquity. There is even reason to believe that the physicians who lived at the beginning of the Christian era must have, upon occasions, observed and described, under the name of leprosy, true cases of constitutional syphilis. The proof of this is in the following narrative from a contemporary of Celsus (first century), Aretæus, of Cappadocia,[2] who had studied leprosy in Asia Minor. This passage can be profitably compared with any descriptions of the symptoms of classic syphilis; certain details agree even perfectly with modern denominations:—

No alteration, no blemish, first attacks the organism, nor shows itself upon the body, nor reveals the existence of a growing fire; but

[1] Opus epistolarum Petri Martyris annegleri mediolanensis. Amsterodami, 1670.

[2] De causis et signis diuturnorum morborum, lib. ii, chap. 13. On the Causes and Signs of Daily Diseases.

this latent fire, after having remained a long time enshrouded in the viscera, finally bursts forth and spreads without, only after having invaded all the interior parts of the body (*incubation*). This deleterious fire commences in some through the face, in others at the elbows, the knees, the joints of the hands and of the feet. . . . The disease increases; the breath of the patient (*ἀναπνοὴ βρομώδης*) is fetid (*specific angina*). . . . *The abdomen* (*τὴν κατω κοιλίαν*) *is the centre of the disease;* tuberosities (*ὄχθοι*) grow out one after the other; they are thick and rough (*papulo-hypertrophic syphilides*). . . . The disease does not delay in showing itself; similar tuberosities appear all over the body. Already the hair withers and falls; the head (*τρίχες προτεθνήσκουσι καί επὶ τῆ κεφαλῆ κόμαι*) becomes bare (*alopecia*).[1] . . . The tongue becomes covered with tubercles (*γλῶσσα χαλαζώδεσι ἰόνθουσι τρηχεῖα*) when the disease manifests itself by a violent eruption (*generalized roseola*), pimples (*λειχῆνες*) involving the fingers, the knees, and the chin.

The author also speaks of the palmar and plantar syphilides; the interdigital mucous patches may be equally recognized in his description, but it would take too long to quote them.

Without seeking to justify our way of interpreting the text of the Greek writer, we will reproduce a para-

[1] It is known—and the majority of dermatologists are agreed on this point—that classic leprosy does not count alopecia as among its ordinary symptoms, the hairy scalp being only attacked in very exceptional cases. We had this note read by Dr. Zambaco Pacha, who quite recently honored us with a visit. "I approve of it without reservation," he declared to us, "for, *in all my life*, I have never been able to see but one case of alopecia in a leper; it is even so abnormal that I still ask myself if that falling out of the hair was due to leprosy itself. The patients, on the contrary, are remarkable for the abundance and beauty of their hair, even in those cases in which the face is smooth; that is to say, when the beard, the eyelashes, and eyebrows have completely disappeared." But the ability of the learned dermatologist is known, and he is competent to speak on the above subject, having for fifteen years studied *in loco* the lepers of the whole world.

It is also due to the indefatigable activity of our *confrère* that we are indebted for the knowledge that the famous Morvan's disease, by which so many neuropathologists have been taken in,—and not the least among them,—is nothing else than mutilating leprosy; the photographs which Dr. Zambaco has brought back with him from Finistère (Brittany) leave no doubt on the point.

graph from Jourdan de Pellerin, who summarizes exactly our view of the matter:—

In a word, so soon as I shall find an individual infected with a disease which will involve the entire body; which will corrupt the fluids in the viscera; which will also taint the flesh, the bones, the cartilages, the nerves, and the entire nervous portion: that buboes will show themselves in the groins, that the genital parts will be ulcerated, the skin loaded with pustules, and other symptoms of that kind, there may be given to that disease such an appellation and such a name as may be desired; as for me, I cannot help saying that it is the pox.[1]

Again, how can we explain, otherwise than by syphilis, the case of that religious monk of whom John Moschus,[2] a Father of the Church who lived at Pergamos (Asia Minor) toward the end of the sixth century, under the reign of Maurice, speaks? The Greek historian relates an occurrence which he claims to have obtained from a certain Abbé Polychronius.

A monk of the Convent of Pentucula (Πενθουκλᾶ), being no longer able to resist physiological needs too long repressed, went to Jericho to obey that law of nature which commands encouraging the propagation of the species. Spurred on by the spirit of fornication (*a spiritu fornicationis*), he went to the nearest, without taking the time to make an intelligent choice. Misfortune overtook him, for he returned to his monastery with the leprosy (*leprosus effectus est*). He then told himself that God had chastised him in order to save his soul,—which is as good a way as another of consoling one's self.

Ὡς εἰσῆλθεν εἰς τό καταγώγιον τῆς πορνείας εὐθέως ἐλεπρώθη ὅλως.	As he had entered in the temple of *prostitution*, it was not long before he was completely covered with *leprosy*.

[1] Jourdan de Pellerin, Traité sur les maladies vénériennes. Paris, 1749. Treatise on Venereal Diseases.

[2] Patrologie. Pères Grecs, tome lxxxvii. J. Moschus, Pratum, cap. 14. Patrology. The Greek Fathers, vol. lxxxvii.

Now that we know that true leprosy is not communicated between those conjoined—even after a life in common of twenty years or more—we are forced to the conclusion that the Greek verb λεπρόμαι in all gallant affairs expressed the fact of contracting a venereal disease. And as the word "leprosy" among the ancients designated more especially scaly eruptions of the skin, whatever may have been the origin of the dermatosis, we can only see syphilides in the particular case of the frater from Pentucula. Leprosy, such as we know it, does not lie within the domain of prostitution; and, were one even an anchorite, an escapade in the neighboring city would not suffice to bring on the disease.

An author of the time, Ulrich von Hutten,[1] was himself affected with syphilis; in the treatise which he wrote upon the solicitations of the physician, P. Ricinius, in 1519, he has given us a description from which it appears that at that time symptoms were referred to syphilis which were absolutely foreign to it,—abscesses, for instance:—

> There come on abscesses (*vomicæ*) which sometimes end in chancres or in fistulas; or else there are interminable ulcers which become putrid or denude the bones at first and subsequently cause their necrosis.

Even admitting that the German knight took gummata for abscesses, he hardly could have noted fistulas in classic syphilis. It is known how rare—and especially limited—is the denudation of bones. The symptoms which he describes are those of gangrene or of phagedenic ulcers, even taking into consideration the greater frequency of grave cases of syphilis in the fifteenth century. Besides, the author mentions so much suppu-

[1] De guaiaci medicinâ et morbo gallico. Moguntia, MDXIX. The French Disease and Medication by Guaiac. Mainz, 1519.

ration in these ulcers that they cannot be referred to any of the three periods of the venereal disease, with any semblance of probability :—

There escaped from these ulcers an ichorous pus which was so fetid (*spurcus profluens humor*) that it was believed the smell alone was capable of producing contagion.

It is to be supposed that the cruel Henry VIII, King of England, had either not read the work of Ulrich von Hutten or did not share his way of seeing the matter. In fact, the historian Hume[1] tells us that he ordered Cardinal Wolsey to be beheaded in 1530, under the pretext that the latter, affected with the pox, had whispered in his ear with the object, the monarch pretended, of communicating it by his breath. This idea of contagion by the breath or by the odor of virulent sores was especially imagined—according to the judicious remark of a philosopher of the time—to explain cases of syphilis in high-born persons and religious men and women ; that is to say, in all those whom it would not have been prudent for physicians then to have considered as debauchees.

The symptoms which we have just narrated in connection with the disease of Naples are the same which the contemporaneous authors were enabled to observe until toward 1514 or 1519 ; which means that, during a period of twenty to twenty-five years, the prevailing disease was clothed with a particular character almost unknown to-day, or, rather, that the most frightful symptoms did not all belong to syphilis. On the whole, it was the gangrenous sores which dominated in that terrible tragedy. Nor must it be forgotten that many true syphilitics saw their condition made worse by the unskillful and barbarous treatment which they were forced to submit to ; so that many of them were rendered

[1] History of England, vol. iv.

worse by reason of the treatment rather than from the manifestations of their pox. We will reserve a detailed examination of this interesting point to the time when we shall study the sixteenth century.

Then the picture becomes a little less gloomy. Physicians who had at first taken flight at the approach of patients began to study seriously. This explains the reason why exostoses with osteocopic pains and caries of the bones were mentioned only later on, in the course of a second period, which extends to about 1526. It was Jean de Vigo who first described these two new symptoms:—

> At the same time with the pustules or, at least, after their appearance the patient felt, for a month or a month and a half, sometimes in the forehead, at other times in the shoulder-blades, in the shoulders and in the arm, occasionally in the legs, in the thighs, and in the hips, pains which made him cry out aloud. Long after—that is to say, at the end of a year and sometimes longer—there came on bony tumors which greatly tortured patients, especially at night. . . . These pains always ended in the rotting and in the corruption of the bone.[1]

It is certain that the grave tertiary lesions, which are quite infrequently seen in these days, must have presented themselves at that time with comparative frequency, on account of the poorly-adapted treatment followed by patients, when they were treated at all.

Then the local manifestations commenced to be better observed, for another author, Peter Maynard,[2] describes the pustular syphilides of the sexual organs:—

> We say, agreeably with experience, that the principal sign of the French disease consists in pustules which come at the extremity of the penis in men, at the entrance of the vulva or at the neck of the womb in

[1] Jean de Vigo, Pratica Chirurgica. Genuæ, 1514, lib. v, cap. 1. Surgical Practice. Genoa, 1514.

[2] De morbo gallico. Tractatus primus. Veronæ, 1518. On the French Disease. Verona, 1518.

women, and in an itching of the parts which contain the seed. Most frequently these pustules ulcerate.

The new period extends to 1540. The scourge becomes more and more mitigated according to the testimony of Fracastor[1]:—

Since about six years the disease has again changed considerably. Pustules are no longer seen except in a very few patients, almost no pains or very light pains, but many gummy tumors. One thing which has astonished everybody is the falling out of the hair of the head and of other parts of the body,—a thing which made the patients appear almost ridiculous.

The author adds that this falling out of the hair, beard, eyebrows, etc., was at first attributed to the remedies employed against syphilis and especially to mercury;[2] "but," says he, "it did not take long to see that these lesions were due to the disease itself."

Very soon everything will limit itself to the classic phenomena which was known, and malignant cases will no longer be mentioned except here and there. Let us make a note of the fact that, in 1519 already, Ulrich von Hutten had very distinctly said: "When the disease appeared it was so disgusting (*tantâ fœtiditate*) that it is hard to believe that the present disease can be of the *same nature*." This is certainly very clear. We may be allowed to conclude that the grave diseases which came on to complicate the scourge—and *alone* gave it its epidemic character—had considerably changed for the better or had even completely disappeared, leaving standing upon their ruins SYPHILIS, which was then to receive its official consecration. There remained noth-

[1] De morbis contagiosis. Veronæ, 1530, cap. 1. On Contagious Diseases. Verona, 1530.

[2] There exist even to-day persons of that sort; but it must be said that the medical failures, who live off of human credulity, take good care not to undeceive people.

ing of all the symptoms which were so frightful and had literally mowed down patients and terrorized populations for nearly thirty years,—there remained nothing, I say,—but the ordinary manifestations of the venereal trilogy; that is to say, syphilitic lesions, the chancroid, and gonorrhœa.

Besides, Ricord, whose clear-sightedness in matters of venereology needs no demonstration, had remained cold before "the immense romance published by Astruc," in the hope of explaining the nature and origin of the scourge of the fifteenth century,—"that frightful epidemic, that veritable *ninety-three* of the pox."[1] Ricord —whom we have not been commissioned to try retrospectively, whatever may have been his whims—was of too keen an intellect not to have noticed, at the first glance, that the descriptions of the terrible disease coinciding with the siege of Naples, and the discovery of printing and that of America, in no wise fitted in with the classic symptoms of syphilis. Besides, we do not think that we can, in this chapter, do better than by giving a few extracts from Letter X,—the only profession of faith of the master relative to the origin of syphilis:—

What strikes every man who studies history without preconceived ideas is to find in the ancient authors, and especially in those who were anterior to the epidemic of the fifteenth century, perfect descriptions of all that we know to-day and which we range among the primary symptoms. Could we trace out at the present day a description more exact and more true than that of Celsus? Galen goes even so far as to find some relation between the symptoms of the genital organs and those of the throat. William of Sallicet knew that the primary ulcerations of the penis had been contracted by connections with filthy women; he established perfectly the relations which exist between ulcerations of the genital organs and buboes, etc.

The more exact knowledge of the filiation of the symptoms, of the connections and origin of the primary and constitutional symptoms, is

[1] Letters on Syphilis.

what has been wanting to observers and historians of the pox from the earliest times. But what was the leprosy of that epoch? Was the leprosy of the Greeks or of the Arabs, which we recognize at the present day, similar to this ancient leprosy? In no respect, for the leprosy of that time was often contagious and it was frequently communicated by sexual intercourse. Evidently *it was not our present leprosy.*

Astruc himself had very well understood it. Besides, the descriptions of the authors are sufficiently clear; and poor Astruc, who lived at a time (1740) when gonorrhœa was still looked upon as one of the symptoms of the only virus,[1] *pox*, found himself quite hindered by these formal utterances. Wishing to prove, despite this, that the clap of the Middle Ages was not the clap, he has left us, in his candor, the finest model of a specious argument that could be dreamed. Listen to this:—

It is beyond the possibility of a doubt that women who had had relations with a *leper* found themselves subsequently affected most often with an *erisipelatous inflammation* of the *vagina* and of the *urethra*, with a *difficulty in urinating* which was considerable and very inconvenient, and which was called Arsure,[2] or Burning, and that the men who had to do with women in that condition, or even who had connection with healthy women, but *not having taken care to wash themselves* after having connection with a *leper*, contracted from them, AS BY CONTAGION, a disease in all respects *similar* to that of which we have spoken.

Is not the "as by contagion" a find? Astruc adds:—

During all the time that leprosy existed there existed a disease which prostitution could inflict upon courtesans and which the courtesans could communicate to the debauched, which must have been

[1] *Cf.* B. Bell, On the Venereal.

[2] We have already seen that the word *arsure* in the Middle Ages was one of the numerous expressions which served to designate the local manifestations of venereal disease,—that is to say, virulent sores of the sexual parts or a urethral discharge.

frequent *formerly*, but which has disappeared with the leprosy itself, *of which it was a symptom*. . . . It is self-evident that leprosy was transmitted from an infected to a healthy person not only by living and residing together, but especially by the venereal act.[1]

So it was the venereal disease; and it sufficed, in the fifteenth century, to give it its true name instead of making a new disease out of it. We shall now see, by the termination of the letter of Ricord, that the great syphilographer—who was not exactly a simpleton—did not think that any thanks were due to Astruc for having broken so many lances against windmills.

But the greater part of the contemporaries of Astruc inclined his way, first, because it is much more comfortable to accept the ideas of others than to find some one's self, and because of the reputation of the writer; so true is it that a "made" man may permit himself to write heresies—some would say asininities—without any one, or hardly any one, making a move. Were it only the hangers-on who live off the crumbs which fall from the master's table, the scholars for whom places are especially created with a semblance of competition, some one can always be found to republish the errors of the file-leader, and from that time they are hallowed. We will take the opportunity of calling attention to a certain number when we study the modern authors.

To return to the letter of Ricord. Here is his concluding sentence:—

I have no pretension to retrospective science; the words of Astruc have frightened me too much. . . . But whoever studies syphilis, however little he may have his mind tormented by the anxiety to know, will ask of himself, what I have done a hundred times, *what was this terrible epidemic of the fifteenth century, and where did it come from?*[2]

[1] J. Astruc, De morbo venereis. Lutetiæ Parisiorum, 1740. On Venereal Diseases. Paris, 1740.

[2] Ricord, Letters on Syphilis. Translated by D. D. Slade. Boston, 1853. The French edition appeared in 1851.

This is what we have endeavored to explain in our rather prolix dissertation of which this chapter is composed. The silence of the master, or, if it be preferred, his simple interrogation, proves that the problem is one of those which may be looked upon as difficult to solve. Have we come near the solution? The reader alone is in a position to judge in an exact and impartial manner.

CHAPTER V.

ORIGIN OF THE VENEREAL DISEASE AND THE DIFFERENT NAMES IT RECEIVED IN THE FIFTEENTH CENTURY.

Why the writers of the time almost without exception believed from the beginning in a new disease.—Different opinions and odd theories on the origin of venereal disease; simplicity of the authors of that epoch.—Popular beliefs; curious explanation on the influence of the stars, of the surrounding air, of sexual relations with lepers, of unnatural debaucheries, of the flesh of cadavers used as food, etc.—Incalculable number of words which served to designate syphilis in the fifteenth century; each people gives it a name.—Therapeutics disarmed at the very beginning; the charlatans emerge from the earth.

WE have just seen, in the preceding chapter, how venereal disease, restricted for centuries in the haunts of debauchery whence it sallied, but in an intermittent manner, suddenly threw itself on the entire population and mingled with the epidemic of the fifteenth century. It is, then, easy to explain why the public and physicians themselves, literally overpowered, believed in an unknown disease, for from the very beginning they took nothing but the symptoms into consideration, and only such as were the most terrible of the scourge, which went on growing. The epidemic over, there remained syphilis, which was studied as a new disease, thenceforth classified. Later on, after the first years of excitement, physicians began to think. Some brainy individuals noticed that the current symptoms presented by their patients had points of great similarity to the descriptions of the physicians of antiquity, and especially of those of the Middle Ages, regarding affections of the genital organs. We shall soon inquire into this change of front of scientific men in our study of the sixteenth century.

However that may be, the first impression was in favor of the novelty of the disease, and, as there was a lack of serious data to explain its origin, it was imagination which took care of this. No one could surmise to what fantastic conclusions people may be led—even those reputed to have common sense—when the imagination is given free play upon any point of the arcana of science. If we add to that the influences of environment, and especially if we transport ourselves back to the time when the fables regarding the epidemic of Naples were conceived, written, and repeated,—that is to say, at the close of the Middle Ages,—we can scarcely expect anything reasonable or even credible. Nevertheless, all these fictions are interesting to reproduce, for, as will be seen shortly, it is especially from popular beliefs the most eccentric in appearance that historical truth can be arrived at.

The astrologers, who were very important personages at that period of simplicity and ignorance, were the first to give their opinions, and, quite naturally, attributed the origin of the disease to certain astral conjunctions. But, you may ask, why did the physicians of the fifteenth century—certainly more learned than the mass of their fellow-citizens—encourage the dissemination of such absurdities? The reason is very simple: they were of their times. The maunderings of astrologers have found credit everywhere, even in palaces, and many crowned heads have had recourse to them before and after the fifteenth century. And, to tell the truth, perhaps the physicians of that time were not sorrv to see the origin of the disease, for which they were not in a condition to give a scientific explanation, attributed to the malign influence of the stars or to the maleficent conjunction of planets.

The first author who spoke of the epidemic is Bartholomew Steber,[1] of Vienna, whose manuscript dates from 1494. "It is a new disease caused by the conjunction of planets," says he, without dilating much upon the question of the origin. Next, in chronological order, we find Grünbeck (or Grünpeck), of Burckausen, who gives us the first printed work on syphilis;[2] according to him, the disease is "the unlucky work of Saturn and of Mars."

Coradin Gilini,[3] who comes next, explains, in his little work on the *French disease*, to what the origin of the scourge is to be attributed. He gives more details than Grünbeck:—

> It is to the conjunction of Saturn and of Mars, which occurred January 16, 1496, at about noon, and which presaged a mortality among men; or else to the conjunction of Jupiter and of Mars, which had occurred November 17, 1494, in a warm and moist sign. There had been liberated vapors from the earth and from the water; and Mars, who is hot and dry, had set them on fire. The air was changed and corrupted; thence heated and putrid humors, which have been the cause of this disease.

The only thing to remember, in these maunderings, is that telluric miasms had spread themselves in Italy, probably after the rains and inundations which are noted as having taken place about the time of the siege of Naples.

Gaspard Torella,[4] in his first treatise, relates similar trash, and which must have inspired Molière:—

[1] A mala Franczos, morbo gallorum, preservatio ac cura. Vienna. The French Disease: its Prevention and Treatment.

[2] Tractatus de pestilentiali scorrâ, sive mal de Frazos, 1496. Treatise on Pestilential Scorra (filth); that is to say, the French disease.

[3] Opusculum de morbo gallico, 1497. Manual on the French Disease.

[4] De pudendagrâ. Romæ, 1497.

This disease had been caused, according to the astrologers, by the constellation of superior bodies, because a universal effect must be referred to universal causes; and this by reason of the meeting of Saturn in the sign of Aries. For there is, in the sign of Aries and in that of Pisces, stars which have the virtue of producing monsters.

And that is the reason why your daughter is dumb.

Wendelin Hock,[1] whilst very seriously recognizing the power of the stars, over which he discourses at length, also calls in the intervention of the bile,—an idea which Grünbeck had timidly expressed:—

This disease had begun, to speak correctly, from the year of Our Lord 1483, because in that year, in the month of October, four planets —to wit, Jupiter, Mars, the Sun, and Mercury—had met in the sign of Libra, in the house of the disease, which denoted a disease caused by the corruption of the blood and of the bile; and because Jupiter was burned in the same sign.

Then follows a description, which is simply marvelous, of a crossing and recrossing of stars and planets which, according to the author, had taken place that year, as also in 1486 and in 1487. They were incessant conjunctions of Jupiter, of Mars, of Venus, of Mercury—with two eclipses of the moon, if you please—in the sign of Scorpio, and always in the *house of the disease*, probably more spacious than that of Socrates. Saturn also joined the festivities and took fire, as also Mercury. From which this obvious conclusion—for the author, at least:—

Thus all this announced the corruption of the blood and of the bile, and the corruption of all the humors, as also the abundance of the melancholic humor, as much in men as in women.

These absurdities were hawked about reprinted for over thirty years. For instance, they are found again

[1] De causâ et origine morbi gallici. Brackenaw, 1502. The second edition, entitled "Mentagra," was published in 1514.

in the works of Jean Benoist[1] (1510), of Peter Maynard[2] (1518), of Ulrich von Hutten[3] (1519), of the celebrated Fracastor[4] (1530), of Nicolas Massa[5] (1532), of Laurence Phrisius[6] (1532), and others.

This last one copies Torella almost word for word, with this difference, that, like Wendelin Hock, he makes the sun take part in his astral conjunctions. Like the latter, he also places the beginning of the disease in the year 1483.

Others mention the astral influence only as a recollection, and look into the organism itself for the origin of the virus. Here is the supposition which Grünbeck advances in his letter to Bernard von Walkirch, canon of the cathedral of Angsburg in 1496; that is to say, at the very time of the epidemic:—

> . . . This disease is engendered by the bile; it mixes its poison with the atrabile, then with the mucus. . . . And, when nature wishes to rid herself of this enemy, she pushes it in the direction of the confluence of the veins which are in the neighborhood of the natural parts.

Leoniceno, a physician in Lombardy, also a contemporary of the epidemic, yields but a feeble belief to the expressions of the astrologers and theologians. His testimony is valuable in this respect, that he shows us that the medical body of that time believed rather in the action of telluric miasmata, all the rivers of Italy having overflowed their banks in that year. Without doubt, malaria, and perhaps *influenza* even, played their part in the deaths occurring in short periods. The fol-

[1] De morbo gallico libellus.

[2] De morbo gallico. Two works. Verona.

[3] *Loc. cit.*

[4] Hieronymi Fracastorii, Syphilis sive morbus gallicus. Veronæ, 1530.

[5] First edition, De morbo gallico, 1532. Second edition, De morbo neapolitano. . . . Lugduni, 1534.

[6] Opusculum de morbo gallico, 1532.

lowing is the passage in which the origin of the plague is discussed :—

It is either by divine wrath, as the theologians believe ; or by the influence of the stars, as the astrologers pretend ; or by a certain unseasonableness of the air, as the physicians think.[1]

This last opinion is really the only one which the author takes the trouble of defending. We may add that it was adopted and reproduced by a certain number of practitioners of the fifteenth century, among others Noel Montesauro,[2] of Verona; Ant. Scanarolo,[3] of Modena ; and by Leonard Schmai, or Schmaus,[4] in 1518.

Pomponius Letus, a poet of the time, quoted by Leoniceno, composed a Latin poem, of which we will translate a few verses, on the inundations of the year 1494 :—

In the time of Alexander VI, in the nones of December, the Tiber widened about twelve fathoms.

Each house became an islet, and in the streets the boats suddenly rose to the level of the windows.

Leoniceno adds a few complimentary explanations, and draws therefrom scientific deductions :—

Similar inundations occurred at all points in Italy and even in all Europe. . . . And it is not surprising that, in the wake of such phenomena, the summer atmosphere acquired those hot and moist qualities which physicians and philosophers regard as the generating (*matrem*) cause of all putrid germs. . . . Inundations rapidly develop a general putrefaction of the air and soil. . . . They may not only determine *pestilential affections* (pestilentia) like those *which afflict us to-day* (ad præsens damna), but also prepare for other diseases in the future.

It is seen that the author positively attributes the

[1] Nic. Leoniceno, *loc. cit.*

[2] De dispositionibus quas vulgares Mal Franzoso appellant. Veronæ, 1498. On the Affection which is Commonly called French Disease.

[3] Dissertatio utilis de morbo gallico. Bononiæ, 1498. Practical Dissertation on the French Disease. Bologna, 1498.

[4] De morbo gallico.

causes of the reigning epidemic to marshy miasms; the former evidently did not consist exclusively of venereal manifestations.

But, despite the power of the astrologers and the superstitious terrors which they inspired, their explanations did not delay in appearing insufficient. As regards the opinion advanced by some physicians, in regard to telluric miasmata, no one paid attention to it. In proportion as the plague diminished in intensity the cases of syphilis emerged more and more, for the diseases which had given the epidemic its murderous character became rarer and tended to disappear. The common sense of the public, as we have already said, immediately recognized, in the signs of the current disease, numerous points of resemblance to the leprosy of the Middle Ages. And it is not surprising to see certain authors causing the lepers—or what concerns them—to step in in the origin of the disease. Let us examine closely these new fables, which we have merely hinted at in the preceding chapter.

Jean Manard,[1] whose testimony we have already called upon, relates, in one of his letters, what the most accredited opinion is in regard to the prevailing disease:—

> Some hold that this disease began at Valencia, in Spain, by a famous courtesan, who, for the price of fifty gold ducats, gave her favors to a knight who was *leprous*. This woman, having been contaminated, in her turn contaminated the young men who saw her intimately. From these more than four hundred were infected in a short time.

The author adds that a few young men out of the four hundred followed Charles VIII to Italy, and carried there the pox.

[1] De morbo gallico. Ferrare, 1525. Epistola secunda.

P. Andrew Matthiole,[1] ten years later, relates an analogous occurrence:—

A few have written that the French had first acquired the disease by having sexual relations with *leprous* women at the time they were crossing Mount Salvium.

The writer alludes to the army of Charles VIII on its march to the conquest of the kingdom of Naples.

Paracelsus,[2] the Swiss alchemist, considers syphilis as being the result of a sort of crossing of leprosy with the venereal bubo:—

Pox owes its origin to the impure intercourse[3] of a French *leper* with a courtesan who had venereal buboes; the latter then infected all those who had to do with her. It is thus that the POX, proceeding from the leprosy and the venereal bubo,—about in the way that the mule results from the coupling of a horse and an ass,—spread by contagion throughout the universe.

Andrew Cæsalpin,[4] of Arezzo, physician of Pope Clement VII, relates a still more odd story, which he claims to have received from eye-witnesses, and notably from a soldier of his country who served in the Spanish army. As may be seen once more, authors rarely lost sight of the idea of leprosy as soon as an explanation of the new disease was concerned, no matter how improbable the explanation might appear:—

This soldier related that, the French having besieged, near Mount Vesuvius, a city named Somma, where a great deal of excellent wine which is called "Greek wine" grows, the Spaniards abandoned the place during the night. But previous to this they infected the wine which was there with blood which they had drawn from patients of the hospital of St. Lazarus.[5] The French, having entered the city and gorged themselves with this wine, commenced to sicken and had very bad symptoms *which resembled those of leprosy.*

[1] Opusculum de morbo gallico, 1535.

[2] Theophrastes Paracelsus Bombastes, Chirurgia, 1536.

[3] In 1478.

[4] Artis medicæ, lib. iv, cap. 3.

[5] Where lepers were treated.

Ant. Musa Brassavole[1] states that the pox was sowed for the first time at the siege of Naples by a loose girl, but he does not explain to us how the disease came to this camp-follower. He leaves it to be understood that syphilis arose spontaneously in her, but he makes no positive statement on the subject.

This thesis of the spontaneousness of syphilis has been held by a large number of authors of the sixteenth and seventeenth centuries, who have started from that point to conclude the antiquity of venereal disease. We will recur to this at the proper time. Here is the text of Brassavole:—

> There was in the camp of the French, in 1495, a courtesan who was quite famous and very handsome, but who was affected with a foul ulcer of the vulva. The men who had commerce with her contracted a malignant affection, which ulcerated the virile organ. . . . Several men were infected; as a result, a large number of women who had relations with these men thus acquired the disease, of which they, in turn, made presents to other men.

Up to the present, with the exception of astral conjunctions, the explanations given by authors in regard to the influence, either of telluric miasmata or of the leprosy of the Middle Ages, still have a scientific appearance; but all those which are to follow are from the domain of phantasy; we enter into the field of incoherence. Here, for example, is what Gabriel Fallopius[2] relates, in speaking of the siege of Naples:—

> The Spaniards, being in very small numbers, and wishing to use cunning against the French, whose army was immense, abandoned their intrenchments at night and poisoned the wells. Not satisfied with this spitefulness, they corrupted the Italian bakers, who were in the enemy's troops, and engaged them to put plaster in the bread they made.

[1] De morbo gallico. Ferrare, 1551.

[2] Tract. de morbo gallico. Mutinæ, 1555, cap. 1. Treatise on the French Disease. Modena, 1555.

Thus, according to Fallopius, the appearance of syphilis in humanity would recognize no other cause than the plaster or poison! All this is nothing but puerile; but here comes the grewsome style introduced by Leonardi Fioraventi.[1] The author claims to have received the story from a person named Paschal Gibilotto, of Naples, aged 98 years. This man's father had been sutler, in 1456, in the army of Alphonso V, King of Aragon, who at that time waged war against John, son of Réné, Duke of Anjou, for the kingdom of Naples:—

> Stores having failed in that long war, as well with the Spaniards as with the French, the sutlers of the two armies prepared different dishes with human flesh and sold them very dear to the famished soldiers. These latter soon had all the symptoms of the pox (pustules, falling out of the hair, etc.). The French, forced to return to their country, called this affection the *disease of Naples*, because they had acquired it in that kingdom. The Spanish and the Italians, convinced that the French had brought it, called it *French disease*.

If Fioraventi, much better known by the "baume" to which he has left his name, had limited himself to relating this gossip of a man of the people, he would simply have been credited with foolishness for having believed it. But, unfortunately, he comes and pretends that he has verified the fact by conclusive experiments (!) upon animals. Then this becomes disconcerting. Outside of jackals, hyenas (coyotes), vultures, and ravens we do not know of many animals which will easily take a nourishment derived from carrion, human or otherwise. And, even admitting that the author succeeded in thus feeding a few of our domestic animals, by previously starving them, it must have required, we are sure, a rare willingness on his part to see upon them the classic symptoms of pox.

[1] Capricci medicinali, 1564. Medical Whims.

The same fable is reproduced, with some variations, by a certain Francis Bacon, Baron Verulam[1]:—

The French, from whom the Disease of Naples has received its name, relate that there were at the siege of Naples some knavish merchants who, instead of tunnies, sold the flesh of men recently killed in Mauritania, and that the origin of the disease was attributed to such a horrible food. The thing appears quite probable, for the cannibals of the Occidental Indies, who live on human flesh, are much subject to the pox.

We will be readily believed when we state that it has not been at all proven that cannibalism has produced syphilis in the savages of the New World; on the other hand, it is undeniable that the sailors of different European nations have especially contributed to the dissemination of the pox on the shores they have visited. It is known as a matter of fact that, among primitive peoples, woman has always been looked upon as a beast of burden; so that, for a nail, a piece of glass, or a bead, or even through simple politeness, the natives of non-civilized countries do not hesitate to turn over their wives to strangers who appear anxious to experience the charms of their conversation.

J. B. Van Helmont[2] was of the opinion that pox recognized for its cause bestiality, when the unnatural intercourse was accomplished with a mare affected with glanders. This idea of the glanders of the horse causing syphilis in man had attracted the attention of Ricord. He called attention to the point,[3] without otherwise insisting upon it, that the epidemic of Naples had presented, in its symptoms, certain points of resemblance with the farcy with which we are acquainted to-day. This is what Van Helmont narrates:—

[1] Sylvæ Sylvarum, sive Historiæ Naturalis, centur. i, art. 26.
[2] Tumulus pestis, 1640.
[3] Letters on Syphilis.

A lay saint, endeavoring to guess why the pox had appeared in the past century and not before, was ravished in spirit and had a vision of a young mare eaten by the farcy, from which he suspected that at the siege of Naples, where that disease appeared for the first time, some man had had an abominable commerce with an animal of that species affected with the same disease, and that subsequently, by an effect of Divine justice, he had, unfortunately, infected the human race.

Such are the curious explanations given by the principal syphilographers of the fifteenth and sixteenth centuries. The reader, educated to the false idea that syphilis has come to us from America, will be astonished, with reason, in confirming the fact that the greater number of authors—physicians as well as historians—have called up the most peculiar and odd reasons to explain the appearance of this disease, new to them. As we have said in our first volume, no one, for a period of twenty-five years, ever supposed for a minute that it could have arisen anywhere but in Europe. The theory which consists in making it come from Hayti, rather peculiar at first sight, is not more fantastic, on the whole, than the majority of the fables we have just related; nevertheless, if this idea had not originated in some brains about the year 1518, everything leads to the belief that the New World would never have been incriminated. This question, too important to be disposed of in a few lines, will form the subject of a special chapter, on account of the incredible favor which the hypothesis of the American origin enjoyed at the time, and still commands with the public ignorant of medical affairs. It will be demonstrated, in the next chapter, that this legend, gathered up by Schmaus, advanced by Oviédo, defended by Fallopius, resuscitated by Astruc, and accepted in our times by a few physicians who are still satisfied with it for want of something better, does not possess the power of withstanding the most superficial examination of facts and dates.

Let us further state, without detaining ourselves at this moment, that certain authors have also attributed the origin of syphilis either to venereal excesses or to the successive coitus of several men with the same woman, and they maintain this theory: that the mingling of different seminal emissions in the same vagina is sufficient to produce the virus.[1] These circumstances having occurred at all epochs, the authors in question are most naturally partisans of the antiquity of syphilis. Others have attributed it to the Maranes,—that is to say, to the Jews driven from Spain by Ferdinand the Catholic at the instigation of Torquemada. We will examine these different questions at the proper time.

Now, let us review the long list of different names which the pox received before finding in the person of Fracastor its final god-father, or, rather, before the term "syphilis" was finally adopted. It would be too easy to find, in the incredible number of all those names, the obvious proof that the disease did not come from San Domingo. Is it admissible that, at any time, physicians and historians should put their brains on the rack—and that for a period of twenty-five years—to discover the origin of a virus, when it is publicly notorious that the said virus came from an island recently discovered? We leave it to the reader, who represents common sense, to assume the care of answering this question.

One has been able to see, by the different quotations already given, that authors attribute, for the greater part, the beginning of the venereal disease to the siege of Naples, whatever may have been the reasons invoked.

[1] In the popular mind the semen plays quite an important part in the production of diseased conditions about the genitalia. I have been told on several occasions by patients that the premature ejaculation of semen in the hair of a female's pudenda engendered pediculi pubis, which the male subsequently acquired in a later intercourse with the female. *Si non é vero, é ben trovato.*—O-D.

An epidemic begins, increases day by day, terrorizes peoples, attains its apogee at the exact time of an expedition which has become celebrated on account of that coincidence, rages especially in Italy by the very reason of the movement of troops which this expedition occasions, and all these events occur in the Middle Ages. It does not require more, in order that the poorly-enlightened imaginations of that epoch should see the relations of cause and effect; and the disease, which seems unknown up to that time, receives a first name which recalls the circumstances under which it was noticed for the first time. These are the French troops which invade Italy and besiege Naples; the Italians immediately call it *French disease* (male Francese).

It may be objected that the aforesaid epidemic had already reigned throughout the entire peninsula for several years, under the name of *inguinal plague.* It is true; but that disease, slightly destructive at the beginning, did not then have the characteristics which it assumed later on, or, rather, had not yet undergone the changes which completely altered its nature, about 1494 or 1495, by reason of the addition of new and terrible elements. However this may be, the word prospered for nearly one hundred years, since all, or nearly all, the authors of the fifteenth and sixteenth centuries who have written in Latin entitle their works "*De morbo gallico.*" Was it from a spirit of revenge that the vanquished gave the name of the conqueror to this disease? It is possible. The French, in retaliation, called it the *Neapolitan disease* (mal Napolitain). Nevertheless, the title *De morbo neapolitano* (N. Massa, 1534) is quite rare for the works of that time; but it is fitting to state that the majority of authors who have written on this subject were Germans or Italians.

From that time it was a sort of fashion for the nations of the Old Continent to give the name of the enemy of the time to venereal disease; but, in writings, it is always the expression of *French disease* which dominates. The *male Francese* of the Neapolitans becomes, with the Germans, *Frantzosen* or *Frantzösischen pocken*, *Frantzösische Krankheit*, or *Lustseuche; mala Franczos* (Steber, 1494); *malum Francicum* (ordinance of Emperor Maximilian, 1495); *mala de Franzos* (Grünpeck, 1496); *malum de Francia* (Schellig, 1500); *malum Francum* (S. Pistor, 1500); *virulentia Gallica* (Capivacceus, 1590). For the English it was *French pox*, *Bordeaux disease*, *foul* or *venereal disease*, *bad disorder*. The Swedes say *Franska Koppor*. The Turks and the peoples of the shores of the Mediterranean employ indifferently the names *disease of Christians* or *disease of the French*. The Persians say *disease of the Turks;* the Poles, *disease of the Germans;* the Muscovites, *disease of the Poles*. The Africans and Moors, but poor friends of Spain, very naturally call it *Spanish disease*, as also the Dutch (*Spaanse pocken*, *Venus ziekte*) and the Portuguese (*mal Castillan*). Auger Ferrier (1564) entitles his work "*De lue Hispanicâ.*" Later on the Japanese have called it *Portuguese disease* (nambokassam), and the Danes *Lystsyge*, *Klephodlt*. The Abyssinians still say *disease of the Francs*.

As can be seen, all the peoples exchanged compliments. And, in the midst of this avalanche of names, not once the expression of *American disease* before the year 1518. It is true that, at that time, the virtues of guaiac, a plant which grows in America, were unknown!

At all events, different authors did not adopt the generally admitted term *morbus gallicus*. It is thus that we see Ulsenius (1496) designating venereal disease under the name of *scabies epidemica* (epidemic eruption); Grünbeck sometimes calls it *pestilentia scorra* (foul plague); an ordinance of Charles VIII (1493), a memoir of the Hôpital du Midi (1495), and a decree of the Parliament of Paris, in 1496, have the expression *grosse vérole* (big pox); certain authors write *vairole* (pox), *vairola magna* (Joubert, 1570). In an ordinance of James IV of Scotland we find the word *grand'gor.* Again we read, in certain works, *disease of Naples, Italian disease* (Rondelet), *gorrhe* or *grosse gorrhe*, *galle de mauvais lieu* (eruption of bad places), *goutte honteuse* (shameful gout), *carie vénérienne* (venereal caries), *pustule impudique* (indecent pustule); then *disease of St. Mevins, of St. Sementius, of St. Roch, of St. Reine, of St. Evagrius, of St. Job* (missal of Passan, 1514), etc.; almost the entire calendar could be mentioned.

This custom of taking saints as patrons of the pox comes from the fact that they, invoked by their respective clients, had reaped all the honors of the cure in fortunate cases. Of course, skeptical people insinuated that such were benign cases and that diet alone would have had a beneficial action; this is quite possible, but we will not insist upon it.

For the Genoese it was *lo male de le Tavelle;* for the Tuscans, *il malo delle Bolle;* for the Lombards, *lo male de la Brosule,*—all words which mean *pustules.* The Spaniards also said, ordinarily, *las bubos, buvas, buas,* or *boas* (pustules); and Almenar (1512), with Fallopius and Roverel, employed the odd expression *patursa,* which certain authors consider as formed of the first syllable of the three words *pa*ssio *tur*pis *sa*turnina (shameful disease of Saturn). Torella (1497) has employed the word *pudendagra* (disease of the shameful parts), Gründpeck (1496) sometimes says *mentulagra* (disease of the penis), and Wendelin Hock (1502) resuscitates the expression of the Romans, given by Pliny the Elder, *mentagra.*

From the very beginning of the seventeenth century the expression *French disease* almost completely disappears, and authors then currently employ the word *pox*, or the capital P. . ., or, again, the expression *lues venerea* (or simply *lues*), venereal disease, *plague of Venus*, *vitiated air of the sky* (azote du ciel), *torpeza* (filth), *virulentia venerea* (Minado, 1596), *venereal disease* (invented by Fernel, 1579), *cristalline* (Guillaumet, 1611), *mal joyeux* (disease of joy, de la Martinière, 1664). Cren is about the only one who entitles his book "*De americana lue*"; and he only wrote in 1762! We shall soon see that it is necessary to come to the eighteenth century to find once more the word *syphilis*, about forgotten since the poem of Fracastor (1530).

It would be in poor taste to linger over this nomenclature; the already long list of different appellations which we have already given shows that the physicians, as well as the patients, were completely ignorant of the origin of the disease. Certainly, popular common sense, as we have already said, immediately recognized the relations which connected the new disease with the leprosy of the Middle Ages. Only the epidemic nature of the scourge puzzled and still puzzles scientific men: if the different diseases which gave it this characteristic had not existed, attention would not have been called to venereal diseases, and the leper asylums, scattered today, would have covered Europe for a few centuries longer.

A few judicious minds, such as Fracastor, without going any farther, left it to be understood that the disease must have existed among the ancients. Others, equally contemporaneous with the epidemic,—Leoniceno (1497), Aquilanus (1498),—similarized it to ancient leprosy; and, in proportion as the plague abates, we see authors abandon more and more the fables in fashion—without in any way explaining farther—and certain ones pronounced themselves frankly in favor of the antiquity of the virus. Torella, whilst stating that nobody, in his time (that is to say, before 1497,—the time at which he wrote), was attacked with a similar disease, admits very well that it may have been observed in ancient times, and he cites the case of the Emperor Heraclius, who, according to him, had had the pox.

However this may be, the general impression, after the taking of Naples, at the time the epidemic was in full sway, was a feeling of stupor. It was a veritable panic; the sick were avoided as pestiferous and physicians refused to treat this disease, which completely threw them off the track. This circumstance is explained by the multiplicity of infectious manifestations which was designated by one single name instead of separating, studying, and classifying the different diseases with grave symptoms whose totality constituted the epidemic.

The lepers themselves avoided all contact with the dying, which is easily understood, for the true venereal patients, attacked with relatively benign lesions, could easily have been carried off by the gangrenous ulcers, the typhus, the phagedena, and other infectious principles which rendered the public scourge extremely murderous. Nevertheless, the physicians of the fifteenth century were wrong in deserting their post, for they thus left the field clear to the charlatans. That is why, although very nearly four hundred years separate us from that epoch, the pirates of medicine swarm more than ever, under the paternal eye of those who are supposed to protect public health. Only a syndical association, officially recognized and performing its functions properly, could prosecute these fellows, for the most part vagabonds; but haste was immediately made first to defeat the statute[1] which would authorize physicians to form a syndicate like ordinary mustard-sellers, druggists, hair-dressers, lemonade venders, notaries, or other taxpayers. And still the famous article has passed, after much exertion. However, Professors Smoothem, Goodwind, Daniel the Polyglot, St. Mark of the Firkin, and companions do not appear to have been unduly excited; they have even made recruits since a few months. And we are of the opinion that those in high places could well employ themselves in increasing the internal superficies of the useful kiosks,[2] in order to afford more space to the remarkable prospectuses which decorate these places of meditation. Poor Medical Syndicate! Thou hast now the right to live. Ah! the good card which castration has!

But, of what use to protest? The authors of the sixteenth century also complained. What did they obtain, and what shall we? Nothing, unless it be the apotheosis of the empirics and other good-for-nothings of science who have become the kings of tact. Well, let us be calm; let us pity the fools who get themselves maimed, and let us return to our documents.

[1] The same or a very similar state of affairs prevails in this country. All the efforts aiming at the suppression of quackery have proven nugatory, by reason of the action of legislatures, and the public is as much at the mercy of charlatans as these gentry could desire.—O-D.

[2] Public urinals which in Paris are filled with the advertisements of so-called "specialists" in venereal diseases. The same state of affairs exists in this country, although the cards are necessarily limited to the water-closets of saloons.—O-D.

This is what Torella[1] says in the year 1500:—

No one could succeed in curing this awful disease regularly and properly, no matter how skillful, experienced and old he happened to be. This gave an opportunity to the ignorant and stubborn vulgarian to decry medicine and to insist that it was a vain or imperfect science, since no physician succeeded in curing the disease. . . .

And it was not without cause that this noise was bruited about, since the learned avoided treating this disease, being convinced that they themselves understood nothing about it. It is on this account that the sellers of drugs, the herbalists and people of the lowest trades, vagabonds and charlatans pass themselves off to-day yet as being those who really and completely cure it. And as they know nothing, they hesitate at nothing (*non dubitant*).

Were it not for the style, one would believe that these two last sentences were written in the nineteenth century!

Wendelin Hock,[2] in 1502, repeats about the same thing and almost in the same words:—

The learned (physicians often give us an example of it in these times) avoid treating such a pitiless disease, persuaded that they know nothing of it. This is why the sellers of drugs, the herbalists, and other working-people, as also vagabonds and impostors, pass themselves off for the ones who truly and perfectly cure this disease.

Some more testimony, dating from 1519 and emanating from Ulrich von Hutten[3]:—

The physicians, frightened at this disease, not only took good care not to approach those who were affected with it; they even fled out of their sight, as if it had been the most hopeless disease.

At all events, they concluded to treat the sick, for the same author adds, in the succeeding chapter:—

It is known by experience how much trouble this disease, in particular, causes physicians in our times.

Laurent Phrisius,[4] a German physician, says, a little later, that the quacks have fallen from the sky:—

[1] Dialogus de dolore in pudendagrâ, 1500.

[2] *Loc. cit.*

[3] *Loc. cit.*

[4] Laur. Phrisius, De morbo gallico. Basel, 1532, chap. i.

The poor people who found themselves attacked by this disease were driven from society as being stinking corpses; these miserable beings—abandoned by physicians, who did not wish to undertake the treatment of this disease, who refused to see the sick and even to give advice—were compelled to live in the fields and in the woods. . . . Touched by compassion, He (Jesus Christ) sent them from France and from Naples certain empirics or physicians, who, led by an audacious temerity rather than by effective skill, began to treat persons affected with this disease.

According to Guicciardini,[1] of Florence, who wrote the history of his times from 1494 to 1532, a few physicians did attempt to treat the sick, at the beginning, but they did not seem to have accomplished any great cures:—

The physicians understood nothing of the treatment of this disease; and, instead of the appropriate medicines, they frequently gave remedies which were the opposite, and capable rather of irritating the disease. And this one caused a large number to die, regardless of age or sex; others remained crippled and disfigured.

It could be seen, from the quotations here given, that the first feeling, at the sight of the colossal proportions which the epidemic had assumed in a relatively short space of time, was that of terror. The public, physicians, the lepers themselves,—we have stated why,—everybody fled from the diseased. It was a general excitement; then, the first moment of stupor having passed off, attention was turned to those unfortunates who were rotting or dying, often from lack of care. The charlatans, whom nothing disconcerts, took hold of the patients, and the physicians followed in the lead set by the empirics.

Now there occurred what may be observed in every epidemic. At the beginning all, or nearly all, the patients die; toward the middle the deaths and recoveries balance each other; at the end all remedies are

[1] Francesco Guicciardini, La historia d'Italia. In Vinegia, 1583.

heroic. This means that, the virus becoming attenuated, nearly all the patients get cured, often in spite of the remedies; nevertheless, a few dozen specifics are loudly vaunted, and each one promises himself to make use of them the next time. But, then, as they are given at the beginning of the epidemic, they no longer act; the fashion is past.

The empirics accordingly tried a multitude of products, all extremely complicated and especially odd. Among these were found ointments with a mercurial base, which the courtesans and procuresses employed for venereal affections since feudal times. Those who were affected with syphilis and who had recovered at the time of the height of the plague, or who, contaminated later on, were looked upon as presenting an attenuated form of the epidemic disease, found benefit in the remedy, and the mercurial treatment flourished like a green-bay tree. But we shall see later on that it was used with so little discrimination that it became rather harmful, and, for this reason, it almost fell into discredit. At the present time it still feels the effect of the maledictions heaped upon it in the fifteenth century. At all events, it is sufficiently spicy to notice one fact: the workers who proscribe it to-day are the exact successors of those who started it in the Middle Ages. Other times, other manners. The modern quacks extol the vegetable treatment, whilst the mountebanks of the fifteenth century gave quicksilver. But we know the object of Messrs. Duck, Quack and Co. is the therapeutic always being the slightest consideration.

CHAPTER VI.

The Pretended American Origin of the Syphilitic Virus.

How the legend of the American origin was born.—Absurd fables to which this erroneous belief gave rise.—A simple examination of facts and dates reduces the hypothesis to nothing; negative proof derived from the letters of Christopher Columbus.—Incredible favor which this story has enjoyed and still enjoys with the public.—Its lack of success with the medical profession, among whom it daily loses ground.—The precursors of Pasteur: the syphylococcus suspected at the beginning of the sixteenth century.—The "system of worms," or theory of microbes.

As we have already said, one must arrive up to the year 1518 (twenty-five years after the discovery of America) to find the first written accusation attributing the origin of syphilitic disease to the New World. Up to that time, in fact, all the authors who were partisans of the modern origin, believed in an epidemic disease born in Europe. The cause only brought about a difference in opinions. And no one, before Leonard Schmaus,[1] had positively stated that venereal disease had originated in America. To tell the truth, another German, named Nicolas Poll,[2] physician of Charles V, was the innocent cause of this change of opinion, for he had written, in the preceding year (1517), that guaiac, obtained from the Spanish island, cured venereal disease. Immediately, the majority of physicians, thinking that the disease must inevitably have come from the

[1] De morbo gallico.

[2] De cura Morbi Gallici per lignum Guyacum. On the Treatment of the French Disease by means of Guaiac-Wood.

same country as the remedy, boldly affirmed that the New World was the cradle of the pox, Providence always placing the remedy next to the disease. Schmaus made himself the echo of this grotesque opinion, and almost all the writers of the time followed him like the sheep of Panurge.

It is none the less true that, up to that time, there was no agreement as to the true origin of the disease. The multiplicity of curious theories which were admitted and repeated for nearly twenty-five years proves this in a superabundant manner; and, although the subject is still being discussed, one is forced to admit that *not one* among the learned had given out the shadow of a supposition respecting the American origin of syphilis until 1518, or 1517, if you wish. This is an undeniable fact and, I believe, has never been challenged.

The following year a syphilitic knight, Ulrich von Hutten,[1] who had endured for eight years all the barbarous treatments then in use,—and notably mercurial frictions,—wrote a work on the pox. Having had the fortune of being benefited by guaiac,—or, rather, by the suppression of harmful medication,—he praised the properties of the *sacred wood*, as it was then called, proclaimed with Schmaus that guaiac was the specific for venereal disease, and naturally defended the opinion of the American origin. The hypothesis was decisively admitted, and we know that it prospered, but there was a lack of documentary evidence to prop it up; the supposition of Ulrich von Hutten was therefore entirely gratuitous. Nevertheless, all the peoples of the Old Continent took it up with enthusiasm,—this new idea which, in a way, made them innocent,—for it seemed that it would end the great scientific quarrel regarding

[1] *Loc. cit.*

venereal disease, with which they could no longer mutually reproach each other.

The idea being adopted, there remained nothing more than to relate how the virus had been introduced upon European soil. No one, previous to Christopher Columbus, having set foot upon the American continent,—so called because Amerigo Vespucci did not discover it,—it was quite natural to say that the disease had been brought back by the crews of the Genoese navigator. This even appeared so simple that no trouble whatever was taken to sketch even the semblance of a proof until 1525, the time at which Oviédo began to write his history of the West Indies. This work is the only document upon which the partisans of the American origin of syphilis have been able to support themselves. We will soon see what we should think of it.

Then an attempt was made to explain how the pox arose in America. Astral conjunctions, which had been worn out in Europe, being completely out of style, another thing had to be found. The natives of the Antilles were, in 1493, completely bare of literature; and imagination undertook to publish a series of fables, each one more amusing than the other.

The most curious one emanates from Americus Vespucius, the very one who had the honor of leaving his name to the new world[1] discovered by Christopher Columbus. When the women of that country, says the author, do not find the men sufficiently passionate to satisfy their desires, they resort to artificial methods of exciting them :—

[1] This slight, whose cause is, in general, but little known, is due to a learned man of St. Dié, who corresponded with Americus Vespucius, one of the companions of Columbus. This learned man was the first geographer who made a map of the New Continent; and, as he had made use of the documents of his friend, he gave the new country the name of America; custom did the rest.

They cause the genital organs of their husbands to swell to such proportions that they appear deformed and hideous; this result is obtained by the bite of a venomous animal. As a result of this, a large number of the men subjected to this procedure are condemned to impotency, for no care is taken of them, and the diseases are such that they render all erections, in the future, impossible; accordingly, the greater part of these remain eunuchs.[1]

The author does not state that these practices ever produced the least virus. Nevertheless, such is the anecdote from which Girtanner[2] started out—being a great admirer of Astruc—to establish a system on the American origin of syphilis; it is true that the German physician—just like his fellow-countryman, Grüner—made the *amende honorable* later on, and took back his first opinion.

This story of erection by means of insect-stings smacks too much of the marvelous to be swallowed without any proof. Vespucius appears to us, in fact, to have been the victim of an optical illusion. That circumstances of this sort could have occurred in isolated cases might, possibly, be admitted; but being given the results mentioned by the author (*restant eunuchi*), everything would lead to the belief that the Indian women of the sixteenth century did not long persist in experiments which led to such disastrous results. It would have been a destruction of the very object sought. The most narrow-minded among them would not have hesitated to prefer the mediocrity of their husbands in matters of gallantry—or even the "menuserie de leurs

[1] Faciunt intumescere maritorum inguina in tantam crassitudinem ut deformia videantur et turpia, et hoc quodam earum artificio et mordicatione quorumdam animalium venenorum, et hujus rei causâ multi emittunt inguina quæ illis ob defectum curæ flaccescunt, et multi eorum restant eunuchi. (Amerigo Vespucci, Novis Orbis Region. ac Insular. incognit. Basileæ, 1532.)

[2] Girtanner, Abhandlung ueber die venerische Krankheiten. Göttingen, 1788. Dissertation on Venereal Diseases.

serviteurs,"[1] as Brantôme would have said—to those fantastic dimensions due to morbid œdema, and to that illusory and ephemeral valor (*inguina flaccescunt*), if it really be true that any could be retained under such conditions. On the whole, an eccentric idea. She who first had it must not have found many imitators. Vespucci, no doubt, took for a custom one of those monstrous practices such as witches still advise in certain unenlightened countries, but which few people try, and fortunately so.

Nevertheless, this fable has been received with favor by a few authors partisans of the American origin, among others Pauw, an English author, who saw, in the stings of poisonous insects, the true source of pox.

Another English author, Martin Lister,[2] who wrote toward the end of the fifteenth century, also locates the origin of pox in America, but rejects the preceding story to replace it by another which is not worth much more :-

> It is more reasonable to believe that the venereal disease recognizes for its origin the circumstance that human beings ate the flesh of the *ivana*, or *iguana ;* this animal is a serpend of the family of quadrupeds, and of which the Indians are very fond.

This curious idea has scarcely been quoted since except by three authors,—Vercelloni,[3] who rejects it; Astruc and Ballay, who adopt it. Ballay goes even farther than Lister, for he gives the means of finding the germ of the syphilis inclosed, according to him, in the iguana. In support of his opinion, he formulates an hypothesis[4] which is none other than the theory of *microbes*,

[1] Little things of their lovers.

[2] Dissertation sur la vérole, 1694.

[3] Treatise on Venereal Diseases of Both Sexes. Published in Latin at Leyden, in 1722.

[4] Ballay, Traité sommaire des maladies vénér. Paris, 1762. Short Treatise on Venereal Diseases.

except that he does not use that word, unknown in his time. "If the lizard *ivana*, or *iguana*, of Fernandes and of Lister were to be placed in an infusion, and a drop of this infusion were examined with a solar microscope, there might, perhaps, be seen that species of *small animal* which we call *venereal virus*."

Si l'on mettoit à l'infusion le lézard *ivana*, ou *iguana*, de Fernandés et de Lister, et qu'on observât au microscope solaire une goutte de cette infusion, ou y verroit peut-être cette espèce de petit animal que nous nommous le virus vénérien.

It is by means of the microscope, as a matter of fact, that this microbe was found in syphilitic products, about ten years ago; and it was even christened with the name of *syphilococcus.* But it does not appear that its discovery, foreshadowed in 1762, has done much for the advance of venereal therapeutics. Ballay adds a reflection, plainly debatable, but which still possesses some logic: "We could also add, in favor of the *system of worms*, that mercury would not have the virtue of curing the pox were it not kept up by small animals; for mercury is, in truth, the poison of all small animals; I mean, of all insects."

Nous pourrious dire encore, à la faveur du système des vers, que le mercure n'auroit point la vertu de guérir la vérole, si elle n'étoit entretenue par de petits animaux; car le mercure est en effet le poison de tous les petits animaux, je veux dire de tous les insectes.

It follows from this passage that the microbian theory was already in the air—if I may so express myself—more than a century ago. To tell the truth, the microscope was invented.

Thirty years before Ballay, two French physicians, Deidier and especially Desault, had defended the same theory. "We judge that the venereal leaven consists of *imperceptible worms.* . . . This idea of *poxy worms,* although they do not come under the cognizance of the senses, will not appear so outlandish if one but reflect that modern philosophers believe that lice, fleas, and crab-lice have other insects on the surface of their body,[1] which are as annoying to them as they are to us, and which are so small, in regard to their size, as they are thin and slender in regard to ours."

Nous estimons que le levain vénérien consiste dans des *vers imperceptibles*. . . . Cette idée des *vers véroliques*, quoiqu'ils ne tombent pas sous les sens, ne paraîtra pas si sauvage, si l'on fait réflexion que les philosophes modernes croyent que les poulx, puces et morpions ont encore d'autres insectes sur la surface de leur corps qui les incommodent autant à eux, qu'eux à nous, et qui sont aussi petits, par rapport à leur grandeur, qu'ils sont minces et déliez par rapport à la notre.[2]

This "system of worms," in which the venereal microbe had been perfectly guessed at, was treated as chimerical by the big-wigs of the time. It was Boerhaave who especially took it upon himself to batter it down. De la Metterie, his translator, eagerly lets us know this in his preface, in which microbes, too much ahead of the times, are not spared. "The animalcules of Deidier, the imperceptible worms which Desault has just hatched,—in fine, all the chimerical ideas upon the nature of the venereal poison which have appeared,—disappear before the demonstrations of this illustrious author."

Les animalcules de Deidier, les vers imperceptibles que Desault vient de faire éclore, toutes les chimères enfin qui ont paru sur la

[1] So, naturalists observe, a flea
Has smaller fleas that on him prey,
And these have smaller still to bite 'em ;
And so proceed *ad infinitum*.—HUDIBRAS.

[2] P. Desault, Dissertation sur les malad. vénér. Bordeaux, 1733. Dissertation on Venereal Diseases.

nature du venin vénérien, disparoissent aux démonstrations de cet illustre auteur.[1]

Evidently France was not yet ripe for the theories of Pasteur.

And yet Deidier and Desault did not even deserve the merit of invention, for we must go back to the seventeenth century to find the first author who had this idea; at least, in so far as syphilis is concerned. It was a Dutchman, Etienne Blankard, who wrote in 1684. Besides, he declares himself never having seen this idea expressed anywhere, in which respect he seems to us perfectly right. For Blankard the syphilitic virus is an acid, an alkali, a *salted acid.* This definition may, perhaps, set chemists dreaming, but it must not be forgotten that it dates back two hundred years. "But, outside of our speaking of an acid, we could advance another cause, of which no one, so far as I know, has thought: to wit, that in the seed of men and that moist matter which women carry in their wombs and in their sheaths are found *small animals*, which, being venomous, corrupt not only our genital parts, but even, growing in time to large quantities, thrust themselves everywhere *in our blood*, which they corrupt."

Mais outre que nous parlous d'un acide, nous pourrious encore avancer une cause, à laquelle personne que je sçache a songé : à sçavoir que dans la semence des hommes et cette matière humide, que les femmes portent dans leur matrice, et leur gaine, se trouvent de petites bétes les quelles veneneuses, corrompent non seulement nos parties génitales, mais même accroissent avec le tems en grande quantité, se fourrent par tout *dans nôtre sang*, qu'elles corrompent.[2]

No genuine documents making positive assertions

[1] This "illustrious author" is Herman Boerhaave. (Dissertat sur les malad. vénér., translated by la Mettrie, Paris, 1735.) The original, written in Latin, was published in 1728.

[2] E. Blankard (translated by William Willi), Traité de la vérole. Amsterdam, 1688. Treatise on the Pox.

can be found anterior to this date. Nevertheless, an observation of Ulrich von Hutten,[1] upon which the author does not dilate, leads one to think that, already at the beginning of the sixteenth century, some physicians had suspected certain animalcules of being concerned in some way in the production of the virus. "I remember," says the German knight, in 1519, "that I was forbidden, in certain places, from eating peas, because, they[2] assured me, these grains may inclose small winged insects,[3] whose presence is a cause of infection."

Memini tunc a pisorum esu interdictum quibus dam locis quod in his vermiculi nascebantur alati : unde infici crederetur.

M. Pasteur, whom we consider a savant, without believing us compelled on that account to always share his views, will permit us to repeat with the Bible: "*Nihil sub sole novum!*"[4]

In short, another author of the name of Linder, almost unknown, and whose theories do not seem to have made much noise in the learned world, has derived his origin "of sodomy, formerly practiced between men and large apes, which are the Satyrs of the ancients."[5] We are unable to state whether, in the Golden Age, anthropoid apes had such affections; but, with what present explorers have informed us respecting the quadrumana of certain sizes, we cannot well see a gorilla—or even a simple orang-outang—annoyed by a sodomitic Redskin, and lending himself meekly to the affair.

At all events, this assertion did not meet with much success. It is, on the whole, but a variant of the fables

[1] *Loc. cit.*

[2] The physicians who treated him during the course of his syphilis.

[3] This is the *Bruchus pisi*, a sort of larva found in peas.

[4] "There is nothing new under the sun." Ecclesiastes, chap. i, v. 10.

[5] J. Linder, Dissertation sur les venins, 1706. Dissertation on Venoms.

which were current at the end of the fifteenth century for the purpose of explaining the origin of the epidemic of Naples. We have seen that certain authors invoked bestiality, either of men coupling themselves with pigs, bitches, goats, geese, or of courtesans submitting to the assaults of goats, of dogs, etc. All these idle stories prove, by their improbability in view of the result, that no one could furnish a rational explanation of the unforeseen appearance of a disease inherent to our species, but which it was resolved for the first time to investigate officially.

Such are the absurdities related by a certain number of authors who have endeavored to support the new opinion by all possible means. And no one thought of the fact that the idea should have come earlier. It will be admitted with difficulty that the learned world of the epoch preserved silence for twenty-five years on such an important event solely through indifference. If the return of Columbus—in 1493—had been heralded by several cases of an unknown disease, there would have been found a physician to treat it and some historian to make mention of it. Even admitting, if you wish, that the navigator, but little satisfied with his find, had desired to hush it up, there would certainly have been some gossips among the contaminated sailors: then the mystery would have leaked out. And when the disease became classic, what reason would the Genoese admiral and his officers have had to make a mystery of its origin? A secret may be kept by one man, even by two in case of necessity; it will rarely be preserved by an entire fleet, especially when there exists no especial reason for such action.

Can it be admitted with any show of reason that a man of the standing of Christopher Columbus could have, for years, looked upon a quarrel impassively, a quarrel of nations throwing upon each other the responsibility of the new virus, when he could by a single word—if he had known what to do—have destroyed all these uncertainties? But, no; he died without saying anything,—no more verbally than in his letters; and, when on his third voyage (1498) he speaks of the ravages of syphilis in the Spanish isle, it is in the most simple manner. He speaks of it as of any other disease which might have afflicted the colony. To tell the truth, the disease was known for five years. Moreover, it seems to us that Ferdinand Columbus, who was familiar with all that his father had done, since he had traveled with him, would not have feared to tarnish his memory by relating the circumstance, if that had existed.[1]

Another contemporary of whom we have spoken, Peter Martyrus, of Algeria, had accompanied Columbus to America; now, in none of his writings is it stated that there was found, in the Spanish isle, an epidemic disease of venereal origin. And yet P. Martyrus published, in 1500, his "History of the New World." He was well acquainted with syphilis, since, as we have seen, he pities much, in one of his letters dated 1488, his friend Aryas for having contracted the disease which was already

[1] Ferdinand Columbus (natural son of the navigator), who has written the complete biography of his father, gives a very detailed account of his voyages to America and of the persecutions of which he was the victim. Such is the power of calumny that they dared load with chains the one who had presented a colony to Spain. Columbus always kept his chains and requested that after his death they be placed with him in his coffin, which was done. Let us compare the two men. The one, Ferdinand surnamed the Catholic, who, never aught but that of being the lackey of a Torquemada, reposes, embalmed, in the palace of the Escurial; the other foresaw the existence of a new country, and knew how to discover it: he dies ignored and miserable; with his bones are mingled ignominious chains! Which is the greater?

called by different names (*las bubas*, *morbus gallicus*, *elephantiasis*); and in the last, written in 1507, he deplores the state of another friend afflicted with the same disease, which he there designates, without hesitation, *elephantiasis*. Would he not have named it *American disease* had he observed the existence of this disease in the Antilles, and for the first time? It would have been an easy matter for him to compare and to make a conclusion if he had found on his return, in the disease then prevailing in Europe, the symptoms of a disease current in San Domingo. But no; nowhere, in his works, can the slightest allusion to America, relative to the pox, be found. We will say the same thing in regard to another chronicler of this epoch, Diego Alvares de Chonca, who also was one of the companions of Columbus.

To sum up, the most absolute silence reigns in all the writings up to 1518; and we even see that Schmaus—who takes good care not to prove his assertion, and for a good reason—limits himself to the statement that this opinion was prevalent in his time. Then he intimates that the atmospheric condition in 1494 might have contributed to the development of the disease. Either he does not attach much importance to the noise running about or else he contradicts himself, for he adds that the disease may have easily started in Europe by an epidemic, as his predecessors think, and he attributes this epidemic to the telluric miasmata developed in consequence of inundations.

The system of the American origin, as we have seen, found a few warm defenders, among whom Ulrich von Hutten; then, being no longer sustained and daily losing its only merit, that of novelty, it almost disappeared forever. But it was destined to be rescued from shipwreck, and that thanks to a man who was yet a mere child at the date of the first voyage of Christopher Columbus. As this man became later on, in 1513, inspector of the American mines and governor of San Domingo, and had in a sort of a way the need of justifying himself to Charles V for his lies and tyranny to the natives of the island, the American origin of syphilis was for him an excuse, and, in fact, a Godsend. This man was Oviédo y Valdez.

Las Cases, an eye-witness who was in America at the same time as Oviédo and knew him well, does not hesitate to say so. He treats his work as an "execrable and false history, this man having been one of the tyrants, of the thieves, and of the destroyers of India, and, consequently, the chief enemy of the Indians."

> . . . falsissima y execrable historia, habiendo este sido uno de tiranos, ladrones, y destructores de la India, y por consiguiente capital enemigo de los Indios.

Besides, this is what Oviédo himself acknowledges:[1] he excuses himself by saying that the Indian race is the impersonation of perversity and deserving of all punishments.

This is why were seen to come forth, at intervals of ten years, two voluminous works on the Antilles, in which the American legend was fished up again. As Dervergie[2] says, the system of Schmaus and of Ulrich von Hutten "would probably have fallen in the deepest oblivion had Oviédo not reproduced it in 1525[3] and in 1555."

[1] He represents them as anthropophagi, and he adds that this is why "God permits them to be destroyed." We may conclude from this that he was not favorably disposed toward them. (Fernandez Gonzalez d'Oviédo y Valdez, Historia general y natural de las Indias Occidentales. Sevilla, 1535.)

[2] Clinique de la maladie syphilitique. Paris, 1826.

[3] The first volume of Oviédo was entitled "Sumario d'historia general y natural de las Indias Occidentales."

Up to that time, in fact, the system rested only upon a simple supposition; and Oviédo, a page of scarcely fifteen years of age (he was born in 1478),—that is to say, a boy at the time of the discovery of America,—is the only one positive on a matter of which he was himself ignorant up to 1525. It may even be boldly advanced that, without Schmaus and Ulrich von Hutten, he would have been ignorant of it all his life. But this legend was useful to him, as we have stated, and, as he returned from his visit to San Domingo, in his turn, it was believed that he had been able to verify the fact. The learned men of the time did not ask for more: "*A beau mentir qui vient de loin!*" [who has traveled far can tell good lies] says the proverb.

Besides, it is sufficient to examine a few dates in order to be immediately sure. In Chapter XIII of Book II of his work, Oviédo states that, on the return from the *second* voyage of Christopher Columbus—which took place, as is well known, June 8, 1496—the crew returned contaminated. He begins thus: "It appears to me that I might be accused of carelessness were I to omit speaking of the two new plagues of which Christians had to suffer in this *second* voyage which the admiral made. . . . One of these plagues was carried to Spain on the return from *this* voyage of Columbus, and thence in all the other provinces of the entire world."

Me paresce que de me podria notar à descuydo dexar de decir dos plagas nuevas que los chripstianos, en este segundo viage des almirante, padescieron. . . . Una dellas fue transferida con esla vuelta de Colom a España, y de alli a todas las otras provincias del mundo toto.

Then, a little farther on, in the course of the same chapter, he adds: "Christians suffered from great sores caused by the disease called *las bubas* (which is native in the Indias)."

Padescieron mas estos chripstianos . . . muy crudeles dolores e passion del mal de las bubas (porque el origen dellas sou las Indias).

It was then syphilis. The first plague, of which the author also speaks, was caused by the presence of the *nigua*, a sort of flea. Besides, there can be no question in regard to the date. Oviédo meant undoubtedly to speak of the second voyage, for we again read, in Chapter XIV: "I have said, in the foregoing chapter, that Columbus returned to Spain in the year 1496."

En el precedente capitulo dixe qùe volvio Colom a España el ano de mill e quatrocientos e seis.

Now, in 1496, as we shall see, syphilis already possessed several official names (morbus gallicus, Neapolitan disease, las bubas, big pox), and that for several years.

Christopher Columbus left Palos, as we have already said, August 3, 1492, discovered the land of America October 12 of the same year, and left it January 6, 1493.[1] Overtaken by a storm, he remained eight days in sight of the mouth of the Tagus without being able to enter it. Finally he landed at Palos *March 13, 1493*, if we are to believe Astruc. It will be admitted that, before this date, the crew of Columbus—even if it had brought back syphilis—would have found it absolutely impossible to communicate anything. But we have seen that syphilis was noticed in Europe long before that time. The letter of P. Martyrus to Aryus is dated 1488; in it he speaks of the *French disease;* Fioraventi ascribes its origin to the year 1456; Widmann, who had lived before and after the discovery of America, determines

[1] Columbus died at Seville, May 20, 1506, poor and abandoned; he was ignorant, up to the end, that he had discovered a continent unknown up to that time, for he believed that he had touched the west coast of India.

upon the year 1457, which agrees with the testimony of Fioraventi. Ulrich von Hutten says that "it was not spoken of for two years in all, counting from the time it began," and as, in common with many others, he fixes as the date of the notoriety of the French disease the year 1493, he must have considered it as having really begun in 1491. Fulgose asserts that the disease existed in Italy at least two years previous to the expedition of Charles VIII (which began in 1494),—that is to say, from the year 1492; this fact is confirmed by the letter of Pope Alexander VI persuading the King of France to abandon that expedition on account of the epidemic of *inguinal plague* which was devastating Italy.

It is seen that, if these dates are not all traced one on the other, the testimonies at least agree in essentials, —that is to say, all the authors mentioned above place the beginning of the *Morbus Gallicus* at a time long anterior to the return of Columbus, and do not even allude to the discovery of the New World. The letter of Alexander VI regarding the venereal disease prevailing in Italy is dated April, 1494. Charles VIII could not permit himself to be stopped by a consideration of such slight importance, for the very good reason that syphilis was already known in France and had even received an official name. Witness the following, one month previous—and not one year[1]—to the confidential communication of Alexander VI. It concerns a royal statute whose whole tenor proves that other decrees, issued for the same purpose some time before,

[1] As good faith should be the rule of action of every man of science or of letters who permits himself to write, we make it a duty to once more put the reader on his guard in regard to a cause of error which is but seldom suspected; the document certainly bears the date of 1493, but 1494 should be read, the French year then beginning at Easter. But this remark applies only to French works and for the three months embraced between January 1st and Easter-day.

had been ineffectual. We reproduce textually the passage, which is extracted from the collection entitled "ORDONNANCES DES ROIS DE FRANCE DE LA TROISIÈME RACE."[1]

At Paris, March 25, 1493. Injunctions Regarding Contagious Diseases and Filth.—Inasmuch as by these presents there has been published, cried, and ordered by sound of trumpet and public crier in all the lanes of Paris, so that no one can pretend cause of ignorance, that all those sick with the *Big Pox* shall immediately go without the city, and strangers shall return to their native places, and others reside outside of said city, *under penalty of the halter;* nevertheless, the said sick people, in disregarding said cries, have returned from all parts and converse in the city with healthy persons, which is a dangerous thing for the people and for the seignary which is at present in Paris.

1. It is ordered herewith, by order of the King and of the Lord Provost of Paris, that all suffering from the said disease, men as well as women, do, after the present notice, without delay, evacuate and leave the said city and outskirts of Paris and betake themselves, to wit: the said foreigners to take up their residence in the country and place of which they are natives, and the others outside of the said city and outskirts, under penalty of *being thrown in the river* if they are caught after the day has passed; and all the overseers of the quarters and sergeants are enjoined to seize or cause to

[1] Decrees of the kings of France of the third race, vol. xx, page 436. So far as the letter of P. Martyrus is concerned, some authors have claimed that there was an error in the date; it is a convenient way of setting aside documents which are troublesome to a theory. So far as the decree of Charles VIII is concerned, our impartiality makes it a duty for us to say that there are as many good reasons in support of as in opposition to the exactness of the date, and we will not delay ourselves in a discussion of no profit to anybody.

be seized those who may be found, so as to carry out its execution.

2. *Item.* It is commanded and enjoined that each one having authority cause the cleansing and removal of all dirt and filth, etc.

A Paris, 25 mars, 1493. Injonctions touchant les maladies contagienses et les immondices.—Combient que par cy-devant ayt été publié, crié, et ordonné à son de trompe et cry public par les carrefours de Paris, à ce que aucun n'en peust prétendre cause d'ignorance, que tous malades de la Grosse Vérole vuidassent incontinent hors la ville, et s'en allassent les estrangiers ès lieux dont il sont natifs, et les autres résidassent hors ladite ville, sur peine de la hart; néantmoins lesdits malades en contempnant lesdits cris, sont retournez de toutes parts et conversent, parmy la ville, avec les personnes saines, qui est chose dangereuse pour le peuple et la seigneurie qui à présent est à Paris.

1° L'on enjoinct derechief, de par le Roy et mondit sieur prévost de Paris, à tous les malades de ladicte maladie, tant hommes que femmes, que incontinent après ce présent cry ils vuident et se départent de ladite ville et faubourgs de Paris et s'envoisent, sçavoir: lesdits forain faire leur résidence ès pays et lieux dont ils sont natifs, et les autres hors ladite ville et faubourgs, sur peine d'estre *jectez en la rivière*, s'ils y sont prins le jourd'huy passé; et enjoinct-on à tous commissaires quartenier et sergens prendre ou faire prendre ceux qui y seront trouvez pour en faire l'exécution.

2° *Item.* L'on commande et enjoinct que chacun en droit soy fasse diligemment nettoyer et vuider les bones et immondices, etc.

The first part of this document has been given by our distinguished colleague, Dr. Pignot, in his inaugural thesis.[1] This piece, written almost in the same words as the decree of Charles VIII, has the special title, "Cry touchant les Verollez" ("Cry Regarding Those

[1] Pignot, "L'hôpital du Midi et ses origines," Thèse de Paris, 1885. The Hôpital du Midi and its Beginnings. [He wrote the history of syphilis in Paris from the sixteenth century up to the time of Ricord. His intention was to continue the history up to the death of Ricord, the latter having furnished him with invaluable information. Unfortunately for syphilography, typhoid fever ended the life of Albert Pinot, September 19, 1893, at the early age of 36.—O-D.]

Having the Pox"), and emanates directly from the Provost of Paris; it is found in the Blue-book of the Châtelet, dated June 25, 1498. It is, apparently, a simple revision of the royal order of 1493, for no mention is made of Section 2, in regard to filth, and which occurs in the original. A commentator has remarked, and with reason, that the provost had no right to threaten capital punishment of his own authority. And it is reasonable to suppose that the Provost of Paris, in the presence of proportions assumed by venereal diseases, had the decree of the King, promulgated five years previously, simply copied, having no reason to change its tenor, since the situation was exactly the same. Besides, Dr. Pignot himself admits that the provost did nothing but reproduce the former text; but, according to him, the original document was a decree of the Parliament, dated March 6, 1496, which we give farther on.

As if in confirmation of the date and authenticity of the measure taken by Charles VIII, it may not be useless, perhaps, to give here a note emanating from the Marquis du Pastoret, author of the twentieth volume of "Ordinances of the Kings of France" of the third race:—

"We believe that we can, and even should, insert in this place the ordinances of this year touching contagious diseases and filth. . . . One cannot help remarking, as a peculiar thing, that this injunction, dated in 1493, whether it emanates from the Provost of Paris or from any other, speaks in explicit terms of a disease whose origin we continually refer to the expedition of Naples, which occurred but the year after. If the words were not so plain, *one would be led to believe that reference is made to leprosy.*"

Nous croyous pouvoir et devoir même insérer ici l'ordonnance de cette même année touchant les maladies contagienses et les immondices. . . . On ne pent s'empêcher de remarquer, comme singularité, que cette injonction, datée de 1493, soit qu'elle vienne du prévôt de Paris on de tout autre, parle en termes exprés d'une maladie dont nous rapportous habituellement l'origine à l'expédition de Naples qui n'ent lieu que l'année d'après. Si les mots n'étaient pas si positifs, on serait porté à croire qu'il s'agit de la lépre.

Well, it is fortunate that this time the word "vérole" (pox) is written at full length! Or otherwise carping at the nature of this contagious disease would be indulged in again to an insufferable degree. A few like the Marquis de Pastoret would have seen in it the leprosy of the Middle Ages, which, with the meaning given to the word "leprosy" during the feudal period, would have been correct nine times out of ten. Others would have admitted all the various sorts of disease known and unknown except syphilis. But now the reader is in a position to know how he is to hold himself in regard to this logomachy.

Moreover, another document found in the archives of the Hôpital du Midi (now Hôpital Ricord) proves that the venereal disease was classified among the prevailing diseases since the year 1495; this date is even anterior to that of the decree of Parliament. It concerns an account of furnishings for the bedding of the *very precious poxy*—for Rabelais—and presented by the superioress, Sister Jehanne Lasseline. Dr. Pignot has had a fac-simile printed in his remarkable monograph.[1] The following is a copy of this curious bill:—

"Item for having furnished, besides the sheets and ordinary bed-clothes, which she mentions in her accounts, for those sick with the *big pox of Naples*, and for making over the greater part of said sheets and bed-clothes

[1] *Loc. cit.*

which have been spoiled and will be of no further use, the said prioress has been damaged and put to cost at several and different times, even to the sum of eighty Paris pounds."

Item pour avoir fourny oultre les draps et convertures ordres (*ordinaires*) dont elle fait mention en ces comptes pour les malades de la grosse vérole de Naples et pour refaire la peupart des dicts draps et convertures qui out été gastez et qui jamais ne serviront, icelle prieuse a endommaigé et mis en fraye à plusieurs et diverses fois jusques à la somme de IIIIxx (80) livres Parisis. *Sœur Jehanne Lasseline, religieuse et prieuse de l'Ostel-Dieu de Paris. Registre commencé au 1er jour d'octobre mil-quatre-cent quatre vingts et quinze et finissant au dernier jour de septembre suivant.*[1]

Let us now examine the famous decree of the Parliament of Paris, dated March 6, 1496, of which we have spoken on page 175. The first sentence clearly shows that it does not concern a novelty, for it immediately mentions the "contagious disease, called the Great Pox, which *for fully two years gone by*, has prevailed greatly in this kingdom, as much in this city of Paris as in other places."[2] In this decree is found the ordinance of 1493, interpolated, with some additions; but there is no mention made of the filth, which, most probably, was more easy to remove than the pox. We reproduce the principal passages of this instrument to permit the reader to make comparisons and form a personal opinion:—

". . . Which ordinance, enacted in the Châtelet and delivered to the Provost of Paris, has been executed and up to the present well kept.

"To provide for the inconveniences which occur

[1] Sister Jehanne Lasseline, nun and prioress of the Hôtel-Dieu of Paris. Record begun October 1, 1495, and ending on the last day of the succeeding September.

[2] Archiv. Nation, X, 1*a*. Registres du Conseil du Parlement de Paris, tome xl, fol. 74 *et seq.*

daily from the visits and intercourse of patients, who are at present in great numbers in this city of Paris, ill of a certain contagious disease called the Big Pox, it has been advised, concluded, etc., . . . the Points and Articles which follow :—

"In the first place it shall be publicly cried, from the part of the King, that all those affected with this disease of the Big Pox,—*strangers*, as well men as women,—who are not living in and residents of this city of Paris when the said disease has attacked them, four and twenty hours after such cry has been made, shall depart from and leave the said city of Paris for the country and places of which they are natives, or in that place in which they resided when the disease came upon them, or elsewhere wherever they may please, under pain of the halter. And that they may leave the more easily they leave by the gates of St. Denis and St. Jaques, where they will find people stationed who will give each one four cents Parisis in taking the name in writing and forbidding them, under the penalty given above, to return to this City until they are completely cured of that disease."

. . . . Laquelle ordonnance portée en Chastelet, et délivrée au Prévost de Paris a esté mise à exécution et jusques cy bien gardée.

Pour pourveoir aux inconvénients qui adviennent chacun jour de la fréquentation et communication des malades, qui sont de présent en grant nombre en ceste ville de Paris, de certaine maladie contagiense nommé la Grosse Vérole, ont été advisez, concluds, etc., ... les Points et Articles qui s'ensuivent.

Premièrement sera faict cry public de par le Roy, que tous les malades de ceste maladie de Grosse Vérole, estrangiers, tant hommes que femmes, qui n'estoient demourants et résidents en ceste ville de Paris, alors que ladite maladie les a prins, vingt et quatre heures aprés ledit cry fait, s'envoisent et partent hors de ceste dite ville de Paris és pays et lieux dont ils sont natifs, ou là où ils faisoient leur residence quand ceste maladie les a prins, ou ailleurs où bon leur semblera, sur peine de la hart. Et à ce que plus facilement ils pussent partir, se retirent ès porte Saint-Denis et Saint-Jaques, où ils trouveront gens députez, lesquels leur delivreront chacum 4 sols Parisis en prenant leur nom par escript et leur faisant défenses sur la peine que desus, de non rentrer en ceste Ville jusques à ce qu'ils soient entièrement garis de ceste maladie.

The document ends with an express recommendation to the inhabitants of the city, if they be contaminated, to retire to their respective homes; and, above all, not to go to collect, at the designated gates, the famous *4 cents Parisis*, by passing themselves off as strangers.

As may be seen, the new compilation is more detailed than the first and somewhat modified; whereas, the ordinance consigned to the records of the Châtelet by the provost in 1498 is simply an exact copy of the first paragraph of that which Charles VIII caused to be published in 1493. Besides, it will be noticed that the decree of the Parliament enacted in 1476—that is to say, in an intervening epoch—refers to *strangers only;* whereas, in the original text all patients, without distinction, were to leave the city: travelers did not even have the opportunity of getting four cents for their traveling expenses. And, as the ordinance of 1493–94 equally forms a part of a collection of authentic documents, we are forced in the same manner to notice the original text as having served for a groundwork as much for the decree of 1496 as for that of 1498, for these last are, after all, but an old measure again put in force.

The pox, then, was clearly designated not only before the taking of Naples, but even before Columbus had returned from his second voyage. As Oviédo himself positively asserts that the infection of the crew of the admiral took place only after the second expedition,—that is to say, in 1496,—it is sufficient to know how to read in order to obtain the material proof that European syphilis did not originate in America.

It should not be supposed that it is our object to show, in opposition to everything, that syphilis existed only in Europe before the end of the fifteenth century, and was unknown in America. Far from us is the thought. We said, if it will be remembered, that, in our opinion, syphilis must have existed since the most remote antiquity, everywhere where a group of human beings sufficient to constitute a people could be found. So that we are convinced—and we have furnished the proofs—that if venereal disease reigned in Europe, in Asia, and in Africa before the voyages of Columbus, it did not flourish any the less in America. We will go even farther. Oviédo attributes to the second voyage—that is to say, to the year 1496—the infection of the crew of Columbus. Well, we will grant that the contamination of which he speaks may have taken place from the very first incursion upon American soil, or in 1494. Amongst the Spanish sailors, a certain number, he says, returned infected. We admit it the more readily, as the contrary would have been more surprising. But what does this prove? Nothing, unless it be that they had not yet contracted syphilis at the time of their departure. As to those who had it—the so-called lepers—it is probable that they communicated it to the Indian women who had not yet acquired it, for the others ran no risks.

It is known that there are, to-day, terrible cases of syphilis in the colonies; those of our [French] soldiers and sailors who come back with it recover with difficulty.[1] Was it even imagined to see in this a new in-

[1] The same thing was observed during the Mexican war. Cases of syphilis acquired in Mexico by American soldiers were more virulent and

fection? Of course not. So that we repeat what we said on page 32 of Chapter III of our first volume: "The truth is, that syphilis is and was everywhere, but not as intense in all countries and at all times, and, above all, but little known, not to say unrecognized."

Thus we have seen that, up to 1518, the authors who wrote on pox were divided into two camps:—

1. Those who believed, like the public, in the epidemic nature of venereal disease, and attributed to it, as the date of its origin, that of the expedition of Naples; they constituted by far the greater number.

2. The partisans of the antiquity of syphilis,—that is to say, those who do not admit that a trouble of such a nature could have arisen from all parts, and who wished to seek if really it was unknown before the fifteenth century.

Then, in 1518, as we have said, Schmaus created a third opinion,—that of the American origin,—which Oviédo knew how to exploit so well. In spite of that, this ingenious explanation, favorably received by the public, was not defended, until the eighteenth century, but by a very limited number of syphilographers. The most celebrated, beyond all doubt, is Fallopius, who wrote at the same time as Schmaus (1518). In reality, it needed the authority, the fame, and—let us admit—the erudition of Astruc to succeed in imposing this legend. Accordingly, after 1740, the majority of authors are satisfied to accept, without question, the ideas of their celebrated precursor, imagining that the last word has been said on the origin of venereal diseases. We shall see, later on, that a complete change of opinion did

chancres as well as chancroids were inclined to become phagedenic. It is a common saying with the laity that the worst varieties known are the Mexican and the Chinese pox. Possibly, the reason is that an additional infection of virulent micro-organisms takes place.—O-D.

not delay in manifesting itself in the medical profession, and that, in the nineteenth century, when there is more annoyance produced by the desire of wishing to know, a few revolutionary spirits have not feared to except against the voluminous brief containing the proofs bolstered up with so much difficulty by Astruc.

But the mob, which, in general, takes no interest in all things pertaining to archæology, is not familiar with this scientific quarrel. It infinitely prefers those things which are marvelous to those which are exact; and he who has demolished a secular legend has been rarely well received. This is why the fable which places the origin of the pox in America still enjoys high honors in the mind of the public, whilst, a century hence, perhaps, a search will be made for the physician who has remained faithful to this belief.

APPENDIX A.

THE MARANIC PLAGUE.

BEFORE concluding this volume, devoted to the Middle Ages, we will say a few words concerning a theory which was abandoned almost as soon as enunciated, but which is interesting on account of the historical event with which it is connected. We wish to speak of the *maranic plague*—that is to say, epidemic—which raged in several localities, and notably in Ethiopia, among the Jewish refugees. Some authors have endeavored to see the origin of syphilis in this.

In 1492, Ferdinand, King of Spain, influenced by a base cupidity disguised under the appearance of zeal for religion, or taken with an acute attack of Catholicism, as you may wish, exiled all the Jews,[1] which, perhaps, was prudent, and seized their riches, which was not noble. The latter, to the number of 800,000 (17,000 families), were conducted, under the name of *Maranes*, —otherwise called *hogs*,—into France, Italy, Greece, and especially Africa. Stripped of everything, plunged in a state of misery to which they were unaccustomed, they were in excellent conditions for an epidemic trouble to develop among them. It is but right to add that, according to the testimony of historians, some of the exiles had *leprosy*. Thirty thousand among them (J. Nauclerus, G. Fabricius) died of a cutaneous disease, which developed rapidly, and was called *pustular itch*,

[1] Since the year 1483 two thousand Jews had been given to the flames; and, in the district of Seville alone, one hundred thousand were immolated.

contagious pustules, *malæ pustulæ*. The Ethiopians most naturally called it the *Spanish disease*.[1]

According to Jackson, the Jews of Spain, in establishing themselves in Morocco, permitted the inhabitants to sleep with their daughters and wives.[2] Since that time the entire country has been infected with this disease, which they call *the big disease*, or *the disease of women*. The inguinal plague, which prevailed in Rome before the expedition of Charles VIII, was due to the presence of the Maranes, according to Infessura.

[1] Léon l'Africain, Descriptio Africæ, vol. i.

[2] For money, of course. Several of our patients, who have traveled on business in Morocco, in Algeria, in Tunis, and in Egypt, have related to us that it was very hard to have any relations with Moslem women, for whom the *roumi*—that is, the Christian in general—is an hereditary enemy to be fled from,—when he cannot be murdered. On the other hand, it is very easy to obtain, by paying the price, young Jewish girls, even of good family. The chambermaid or the governess, according to the surroundings, manages the meetings, which take place in the virginal chamber, at the home of the parents. The latter are not to be feared, for they are never seen; the price being agreed upon, they take good care to disappear for a sufficient length of time not to be in the way. Business is business!

APPENDIX B.

UKHAT.

SYPHILIS IN NINEVEH AND BABYLON AMONG THE ANCIENT ASSYRIO-CHALDEANS, 700 B.C.

The Tablets of the British Museum at London; Assyrian bricks, cylinders, and seals.—Cuneiform inscriptions on tablets derived from the royal library of Sardanapalus recently interpreted.—The legend of Istar, the goddess of voluptuousness.—Pustules, scales, alopecia, and ulcers of venereal origin of Izdubar, the hero of Babylonian fable.—The disease *uχhat*.

IN our first volume[1] we stated that Chaldea, whose capital was Babylon, was for centuries in connection with Syria and Egypt, the centre of all debauchery. We judged at the time that it was impossible that these nations should have been spared from syphilis, and we were of the opinion that India and Chaldea were its cradle. Latin citations from Lucilius demonstrate that Syria was infected with it in the time of Antiochus the Great; that is to say, nearly two centuries B.C. We have also been enabled to see that Pliny the Elder positively designates Egypt, the near neighbor of India, as being the source of venereal affections. Martial, who relates in such a clear fashion the method and manner in which the *obscene disease* (indecens morbus)—that is to say, venereal disease—is acquired, reproaches the debauchees for their *Syrian tumors;* and Moses, in Deuteronomy, menaces libertines with anal papules and the *Egyptian ulcer.* It was from this that we had the

[1] Syphilis in Ancient and Prehistoric Times. F. A. Davis, 1891.

idea of examining Egyptian hieroglyphics. We cited several texts—of necessity vague and obscure—on the pathology of the ancient Egypt of the Pharaohs; but up to February, 1890, we had been unable to find anything, in works dealing with cuneiform characters,[1] which related to medicine. At all events, the proof whose existence we suspected was published too late for it to be possible for us to utilize it in our first volume. This is the manner in which it came into our hands :—

In December, 1890, our American *confrère*, Dr. Ohmann-Dumesnil, Professor of Syphilography in the Marion-Sims College of Medicine, requested from us the authority of translating into English our history of syphilis, the first volume of which had just appeared. The translation of this volume was made and we received a copy of it at the end of December, 1891. What was our surprise and at the same time satisfaction to find, appended to the chapter concerning the Egyptians, a paragraph of fifty lines on syphilis among the Babylonians.[2] As this was an addition of too much

[1] Among other publications which are curious, but in no way medical, we quote the following :—

Saulcy, Recherches sur la chronologie des empires de Ninive, de Babylone et d'ecbatane. Paris, 1850. Researches on the chronolgy of the empires of Nineveh, Babylon, and Ecbatana.

J. Ménant, Annales des rois d'Assyrie. Paris, 1874. Annals of the Kings of Assyria.——Babylone et la Chaldée. Paris, 1875. Babylon and Chaldea.——La bibliothèque du palais de Ninive. Paris, 1880. The Library of the Palace of Nineveh.——"Rapport sur les cylindres Assyro-Chaldéens," publié dans les Archiv. des missions scientif. et littér., 3e sér., tome vi, 1880. "Report on the Assyrio-Chaldean Cylinders," published in the Archiv. des missions scientif. et littér., 3d series, vol. vi, 1880.——Empreintes de cachets Assyro-Chaldéens relevées au Musée Brittanique. Paris, 1882. Imprints of Assyrio-Chaldean Seals Obtained at the British Museum, Paris, 1882.

J. Halévy, Documents religieux de l'Assyrie et de la Babylonie. Paris, 1882. Religious Documents of Assyria and Babylonia. Paris, 1882.

[2] Syphilis in Ancient and Prehistoric Times. Philadelphia. F. A. Davis, 1891, page 81.

importance to pass by in silence, we have—after certain personal researches—placed an analysis of it at the end of the present volume. We hope that our readers, in view of the originality of the subject, will pardon this addition, which can only be presented as a side issue. The following are the points furnished by Dr. Ohmann-Dumesnil:—

"This subchapter is added as a supplement to the preceding chapter, as not only bearing upon the subject, but on account of the similarity the story bears to the myths of other nations, explanatory of the origin of venereal diseases. I am indebted for this to an article published in the *Monatshefte fuer Praktische Dermatologie*, May 1, 1891, by J. K. Proksch, who has laid under contribution the translations of Zahnpfund and Jeremias, the interpreters of the cuneiform inscriptions found on Babylonian bricks."

Before examining this translation we will say a few words on the discoveries of our philologists concerning Assyria.

It is known that the British Museum has possessed for a long time tablets originating from the ancient land of Assur and covered with inscriptions. M. Joachim Ménant, a learned Assyriologist, was commissioned by the French government to examine these tablets and give their interpretation. Our countryman made several stays in England and his studies were embraced in two reports to the minister in 1863 and in 1880. These researches, which were very interesting from an historical point of view as relating to ancient peoples, did not give any new facts regarding the thesis which we are defending; it is for this reason that we had passed them over in silence. This is not the case with the Assyrian tablets recently translated. Have these which are in the British Museum escaped the investigations of savants up to the present time, or are they of more recent importation to Europe? We are unable to answer this. At all events, M. Ménant in none of his works speaks of the interesting legend reported in the German medical journal. It is, nevertheless, worthy of notice from several stand-points, for, according to Dr. Proksch, the author of the article, the tablets which contain it formed a part of the royal library[1] of Assur-bani-pal (Sardanapalus).

Here arises a question of intense interest. Like the German translators, we have placed "Sardanapalus" in parenthesis. But is this king, whose annals have been found on Assyrian bricks, really the Σαρδανάπαλος of the Greeks? Despite the similarity in consonance which exists between the two names, M. Ménant is inclined to believe that it is not the same individual. The learned philologist bases his opinion on the fact that the Sardanapalus who is concerned here, and who is designated by the following

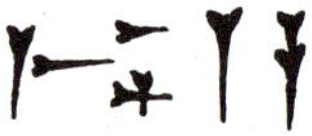

giving the phonetic sound *Assur-bani-pal*, is represented in cuneiform inscriptions as a valiant warrior; whereas that of the Greeks is famous only for his life of debauchery and, especially, his mode of death. The annals of the time acquaint us with the fact that Assur-bani-pal, having ascended the throne during the life-time

[1] The tablets constituted the books of that period (seventh century B.C.). The Assyrians wrote upon brick-clay by means of an iron wedge, and subsequently placed this in an oven; after being baked the cuneiform characters, impressed in the clay, became ineffaceable. At times very important events were engraved on marble or granite. [A fine example of cuneiform engraving in marble may be seen in the rooms of the St. Louis Mercantile Library.—O-D.]

of his father Assurhaddon (*Assur-akh-idin*), in the year 667 B.C., established his royal residence at Nineveh (Ninua) and conferred the vice-royalty of Babylon (*Bab-iln*, gate of God) upon his youngest brother Sallummu-Kin. This prince revolted against his elder brother and was vanquished. His defeat is related on the monuments of the time in which the history of this campaign was written by order of the King of Nineveh. The last paragraph is contained in these lines: "I, Assur-bani-pal, King of the Legions, King of the Land of Assur . . . I have punished the rebels and spared the other children of Bab-iln . . . I have permitted them to remain in Bab-iln . . . I."

This Assur-bani-pal was not the last king of Assyria, for he had a successor, about 625 B.C., Assur-edil-ili,[1] his son, who ends the list of known monarchs. Besides, Nineveh was destroyed 605 B.C.; so that it is permissible to inquire if the Sardanapalus of the Greeks was not a myth,[2] for we cannot find, in the royal chronology of the

[1] Although the exact date of the assumption of the throne by Assur-edil-ili is not known, Assyriologists are agreed in fixing the length of the reign of Assur-bani-pal at forty-two years. This latter had, consequently, ceased to be king twenty years before the destruction of Nineveh.

[2] The following is what M. Ménant states in his introduction in "Annales des rois d'Assyrie," ("Annals of the Kings of Assyria"): "Let us not forget that the Greeks had no relations with Assyria until long after the fall of Nineveh. It is certain that they could not read the writing whose interpretation we are making to-day; it is even evident that they had before their eyes inscriptions whose terms they mutilated, and of which we can reconstruct the elements despite the mutilations which have been handed down to us." According to another tradition reported by M. Langlois ("Archiv. des missions scientifiq.," tome iv), the monarch, after the ruin of Nineveh, should have retired to Cilicia and there founded the city of Tarsus (*Tarsous*). This diversity of opinions confirms us in the idea that the Greek imagination once more supplied the supposed facts of history. It is but right to add that certain historians reckon two or even three Sardanapaluses, which has caused Fréret to say ("Mém. de l'Academie des Inscrip. et Belles-Lettres," tome v) that this name was nothing but an honorary title. This in no manner detracts from the merit of the painting of M. Louis Chalon, "The Death of Sardanapalus," which attracted so much attention in the Paris Salon of 1891, for we know that the domain of the artist is most often that of fiction.

Assyrians, outside of Assur-bani-pal, any personage bearing an analogous name. Besides, among the inscriptions discovered up to the present, none mentions, in connection with any king of Assyria, the well-known circumstances of that horrible death, unique in its kind, but sublime and beautiful in its horror. However this may be, if we must accept the Greek version, it is fortunate for contemporaneous retrospective science that the precious tablets escaped the holocaust to which the cerebrated neurotic, in a last delirious conception, offered himself as the principal victim!

The legend consigned to the archives of the palace of Assur-bani-pal presents certain analogies, in its details, to the Greek fable. There are to be found about the same beliefs, and often the same personages, whose names alone differ. For instance, we shall see the goddess Istar, incarnate Venus, and accessorily Juno, Ceres, Pallas, etc.; the Sacred Bull, who almost immediately steps in on the stage, seems to us to be a cousin-german of the Bull Apis of the Egyptians; Sit-Napiôtim plays the rôle of Pluto; Arad-Ea, with his boat, is none other than the Charon of the Greeks, and it would not be difficult to find analogies in the other characters.

Now, it is related in the Assyrian tablets that Istar (star—note the analogy with the English word), goddess of criminal love, of fertility, of war, etc., and mother of the gods and of men, asked Izdubar[1] (Nimrod) to take her for his wife; the hero, no doubt very brave, but

[1]According to M. Ménant, in "Babylone et la Chaldée" ("Babylon and Chaldea"), Izdubar is the hero of the Chaldean epoch, and some of his exploits recall the labors of Hercules. He was born a short time after the deluge, of which a fabulous personage—in another legend—narrates the recent changes, and notably the details concerning the building of the ark, the entrance of the animals, etc. This recital, of which nothing but fragments remain, has been found on bricks also preserved in the British Museum of London.

little gallant, repulsed this tender proposition in a manner more than impertinent. Rage of Istar, who asked her father Anu to wreak vengeance for the outrage. This request had the effect of the immediate dispatch of the Sacred Bull against Izdubar and his friend Eabani.

We cannot easily understand why this Eabani, of whom nothing has been said so far, and who plays no part in the matter, should be included in the vengeance of Istar and should be equally made a target for the horns of the celestial ruminant. The sequel will show us that he takes the joke from the wrong side and outrages the goddess in the most cruel fashion. At all events, we cannot but admire such a proof of physical strength, for certain impressions of cylinders serving as seals, and found in the ruins of Nineveh and Babylon, represent Eabani holding one of the horns of the animal with one hand and the tail at its root with the other. On the side can be seen Izdubar piercing the heart of the Bull with a weapon which is badly defined.

Istar, too much vexed to pay any attention to the powerful muscles of Eabani, hurls a terrible imprecation; Eabani replies by tearing out the penis (*ibattu*)[1] of the Bull and hurling it in the face of the goddess. The injury is doubly marked, as well on account of the act itself as on account of the nature of the projectile. It is easy to surmise the degree of exasperation to which Istar arrives, and the new imprecation which she launches causes the entire planetary system to tremble. This time Istar is the mistress of the battle-field, for Eabani, struck to the death, succumbs at the end of twelve days and Izdubar is attacked by a long and painful disease which a certain translator regards as having been leprosy.

[1] The female genitalia were designated in Assyrian by the word *lalû*.

It is at this point that the story will become interesting in regard to the subject we are considering. Eabani is dead. Izdubar wanders aimlessly until he has reached the infernal regions. There he is given a magic remedy for his disease; but it does not succeed,—either from a lack of susceptibility or some other cause,—for Izdubar had to deplore the loss of his sexual organs, which were attacked by gangrene. Seeing this, Sit-Napiôtim, god of the Infernal Regions, places him in the hands of the boatman Arad-Ea with orders to conduct him to the *Fountain of Life*,[1] and he adds:—

> The man whom thou hast just taken has his body covered with *pustules; scales* have altered the fairness of his body. Take him, Arad-Ea, to the *cleansing-place*, where he can wash his pustules clean as snow, and take off his *skins;* the sea will carry them off; his body will appear well. The *coverings of his head will be renewed*, as also the *covering of his shameful parts;* by the time he returns to his country there will be no folds; all will be new.

The text then relates that Arad-Ea conducted his passenger to the place of purification, and that all occurred as had been predicted; the patient became as white as snow.

This account recalls to us King David begging the Almighty to cure him, and almost in the same words: "Sprinkle me with hyssop, and I shall be *purified;* and I will become *whiter than the snow* (super nivem dealbabor)." The last two phrases, as Dr. Ohmann-Dumesnil

[1] M. Ménant, who has written a work on the library of Nineveh according to the Assyrian tablets of the British Museum, gives another legend of Istar, and reproduces the translation of M. Oppert, a distinguished Orientalist. According to this story, Istar herself descended to the Infernal Regions, under forced circumstances, in search of her son; there she was attacked by *the thirty-six diseases*, of which she could not get well, says the fable, except by drinking of the waters of the *Fountain of Life.* At this time the recent interpretation of the tablets of the British Museum was unknown; this is why, in our first volume, published in 1890, we did not speak of these legends, which seemed to bear no relationship to our subject.

very justly observes, can only be interpreted in the following manner: "The covering which invested his pudenda, and 'shall show no folds,' 'must be new,' cannot be understood as meaning anything else than that the covering over or about his genitals must not become unclean through pathological secretions and become corroded or fold-like (cicatricial); it must be made new,—*i.e.*, clean."

The symptoms which are described, their cure without leaving a trace, the genital seat of the greater part of them, the marked alopecia,—everything conspires to cause the disappearánce of the least hesitation in making a diagnosis. In the whole series of diseases, be they venereal or cutaneous, syphilis alone answers to the Assyrio-Chaldean description. The diagnosis of *simple psoriasis*, which the stubborn will claim, would certainly prove insufficient, in view of the classical phenomena which accompany this dermatic affection and the intervention of Istar,—that is to say, the *Venus Salacia* of the Babylonians.

Dr. Ohmann-Dumesnil is of the opinion that Eabani also had syphilis, and bases himself on the text, according to which Eabani had spent six days and seven nights in the arms of his well-beloved Uχhat.[1] As our American *confrère* remarks, with reason, venereal diseases, for the Orientals of antiquity, were always the result either of an erotic furore caused by Divine wrath or of sexual excesses. "The name of the hierodulus—*Uχhat*—points very plainly to the *Uχhet* disease,—the *uχedu*, or *uχetu;* that is, syphilis of the ancient Egyptians."

We know that, in antiquity, allegory was the basis

[1] The text, impressed with the simplicity and *naïveté* of the ancients, who ignored the art of glossing and called things by their names, without malice, is in these words: "And Eabani had spent six days and seven nights dallying with the lalû of his well beloved."

of all literature, and that, amongst all peoples, the monuments which have served to reconstruct history were especially written in a symbolic form. That long poem, the Bible, is nothing but a series of allegories intermingled with precepts; Greek mythology has personified all human affairs in the same manner as the Hindoo fable from which it is derived; there would, then, be nothing surprising that the inhabitants of ancient Babylon—where no one seemed to weary—should have adopted the custom of designating a venereal individual by the expression, "He has *caressed Uχhat.*" We have seen, on page 48, that the English of the Middle Ages said, in the same sense, "He has *been bitten by a Winchester goose*," because the Bishop of Winchester had the brothels under his jurisdiction at that time. When we say, to-day, that a gentleman has had "a scrimmage with Venus," no one makes a mistake. Now, Istar was the Assyrian Venus, and we have just seen that Izdubar and especially Eabani had had serious encounters with her. Izdubar treated himself, because, as he says himself, he did not wish to die like his friend, which tends to prove that they were affected by the same disease.

The allegorical meaning given to the term *uχhat* confirms that which we attributed to an absolutely analogous Egyptian word. Those who have read our first volume will remember that, in the chapter devoted to the medicine of the land of the Pharaohs, we extracted from an Egyptian-Coptic-Latin glossary a few words which appeared to us to have a certain relation to venereal manifestations. The first one of these words was an hieroglyph, giving the sound Aχat, and answering to the Latin expression, *morbus vulvæ*,—that is to say, *disease of the vulva*. At that time we asked ourselves, in default of more ample information, of what nature that disease could be. To-day there can be no doubt, for the term *Aχat* seems to have ties of relationship, which are very close, with the symbolic name of the companion of Eabani, the dangerous *Uχat*.

VOLUME III.

SYPHILIS IN MODERN TIMES.

SYPHILIS
IN MODERN TIMES.

CHAPTER I.

AFTER THE EPIDEMIC OF NAPLES; SYPHILIS RECOGNIZED AND CLASSIFIED.

Syphilis is an established fact: the name *Morbus Gallicus*, or *French Disease*, prevails.—Manners of the time: patients of note.—Scandalous life of the popes and of the clergy in general.—Heredity of long date and the action of the air invoked to explain the presence of syphilis in the convents of the sixteenth century.—The first trials in therapeutics: the greasers of pox.—The mass of the poxy.—Passing the pan (*la casserole*).—The raising of shields against mercury.—Fernel, the last rampart of antimercurialism.—The opinions of physicians of the time on the nature of the venereal virus.—More or less rational medications employed during the course of the sixteenth century; their effects.—The pills of Barbarossa.—Rôle attributed to mercurial salivation.—Sudorific plants proclaimed, each in turn, to be universal panaceas.—Grandeur and fall of *guaiac*, of *Smilax China*, of *sarsaparilla*, and of *sassafras*.—A return to mercury is made in 1560.—Different theories regarding venereal pathology in the sixteenth century.

WE have now arrived at the end of the fifteenth century. Syphilis is recognized as a morbid entity and described, together with its different symptoms, under the name of *Morbus Gallicus*. At all events, from this time on there is no more any possible discussion regarding the nature of the disease: so that we can be permitted to follow its history from the works which have come down to us, without being obliged—as in our two first volumes[1]—to commence by proving its existence.

Without desiring to take up the question of the numberless names which served to designate the pitiless disease, we may say that the authors of the time employed indifferently the expressions of *French disease* and *Neapolitan disease.* However, that of *French disease* prevailed, as we have already stated: so that, in order to conform to the usage of that epoch, we will retain that designation every time that we meet with it.

It might have been believed, after what has been read on that curious period of the Middle Ages, that the customs would take on a change in a manner more favorable to hygiene and become edifying, if not by reason of an elevation of the intellectual plane, at least from necessity. In truth, the different epidemics of sexual origin which we have narrated were anything but alluring; and that of 1493, which had but just raged (it is known how!) could seem to be supplied with all the qualifications requisite to deter the most rash. Unfortunately it availed nothing, and the end of the fifteenth century had nothing to envy—from the point of view of manners—of the most frightful times of the Roman fall and of the feudal epoch of the year 1000, of which we have spoken. As it would be tiresome to be continually repeating the same thing, —for the debauched of all ages have done nothing but imitate each other, with some variations,—we will limit ourselves this time to calling attention to diseased persons of prominence. The most famous examples are furnished to us by monarchs and princes of the Church;

[1] Syphilis in Ancient and Prehistoric Times, and Syphilis in the Middle Ages.

so that we will begin with the popes: the greater the lord, the higher the honor!

To the honest and illustrious Pius II succeeded, in 1464, the Venetian, Paul II, aged 60 years. The latter liked small boys; he did not disregard women either, with which he had simply filled the Vatican. According to Attilio Arezzo,[1] "the pontifical palace had been transformed into a sewer."

. . . Paulus II ex concubina domum replevit, et quasi sterquilinium facta est sedes Barionis.

"So far as manners are concerned," says the same author, "Sixtus IV, successor of Paul II, in 1471, was an abominable pontiff; worse than was Alexander VI himself, perhaps." He required an enormous amount of money to pander to his vices. And he undertook the purchase of sins and even of crimes. He caused to appear two books on this subject,—the "Taxes de la Chancellerie Apostolique" ("Taxes of the Apostolic Chancery") and the "Taxes de la Pénitencerie" ("Taxes of the Penitential Court"). Under his pontificate everything could be done with money. "Now," says Guillaume Ranchin, lawyer of Montpellier, "there remains naught but to be rich in order to have freedom and impunity to do evil and a passport to Paradise for one's self and one's evil deeds." His nephew, Peter, whom he created Cardinal of St. Sixtus, cost him heavily: it is true that the young debauchee repaid in favors which were much pleasing to the pontiff.

Sixtus IV was the first pope who dared to patent prostitution and levy a tax on courtesans. He was soon restrained in this by the higher clergy. Quite frequently prelates exploited houses of debauchery on their own

[1] Letters (in Baluze); Miscellanea, vol. iv, p. 519.

account and made no secret of it. It is thus that Agrippa, of Nettesheim,[1] one day heard the Bishop of Rome relate, in a cynical manner, that his profits consisted in "two benefices, a cure of twenty gold florins, and *three girls in a stew* bringing twenty jules a week!"

. . . duo beneficia, unum curatum auroreorum viginti et tres putanas in burdello, quæ reddunt singulis hebdomadibus julios viginti.

All this without prejudice to the concubines which the clergy permitted themselves, and the bastards which popes, cardinals, prelates, and ordinary frock-wearers publicly raised. At least, among them the paternal fibre vibrated; it is an attenuating circumstance.

Debauchery was general; and, as we have shown on a former occasion,[2] it had penetrated in the cloisters of nuns. "The women in convents," said Savanarola, "become worse than the courtesans."[3] But they were the exclusive object of monks. They were imprisoned and persecuted if they had any relations with laymen; whereas, if they were willing to join themselves openly with monks, masses were sung and joyous and solid banquets were held. At least, so we are informed by J. Burchard,[4] who has obtained his information from a good source. Masuccio, an eye-witness quoted by this author, claims to have "been present at the thing,—not once, but several times. The nuns thus coupled," adds he, "give birth to gentle and pretty little monks, or else they cause abortions to be performed. And if any one were tempted to uphold that this is not true, he

[1] De Vanitate et incertitudine suintiarum, cap. 64. On the Vanity and Uncertainty of the Sciences.

[2] Syphilis in the Middle Ages, chap. iii.

[3] Sop. Amos (48th predic., April 13, 1496). Venice, 1519. Folio 219, *r.*

[4] La civilization en Italie au temps de la Renaissance, tome ii, p. 227. Civilization in Italy at the Time of the Renaissance.

need only search the privy-vaults of the convents of nuns and he will find there quantities of children's bones,—about the same as in Bethlehem in the time of Herod."

. . . assisté à la chose, non pas une, mais plusieurs fois. Les nonnes ainsi accouplées mettent au monde de gentils petits moinillons, ou bien elles se font avorter. Et si quelqu'un était tenté de soutenir que ce n'est pas vrai, il n'a qu'à fouiller dans les cloaques des convents de nonnes, il y trouvera quantité d'ossements d'enfants, à peu près comme à Béthlehem, au temps d'Hérode.

A dealer in paints, of the city of Soissons, made a discovery of this sort in 1867. I was then at college and I bought different chemical products, for experiments, at his place. Now, he related that, in having a cellar dug, he had found an incredible quantity of bones derived from children which had arrived at term. I was too young at that time to attach any great importance to the fact; but, later on, I explained to myself the presence of the said bones. The house of the paint-dealer is adjoining to the estates of the cloister of Notre Dame, the largest of the city, and the latter still served as a barracks in 1870; in it there was regularly lodged a regiment of infantry. Now, this cloister had in former times been a celebrated convent of nuns, and the house in question was built on the site reserved for the cemetery.

It is no cause of astonishment that syphilis should have spread to a certain degree at this epoch. Scarcely is it officially recognized when we see successfully attacked, in chronological order, Cardinals Cesar Borgia (the son of the pope), Bartolomeo Marti (1497), Ascanio Sforza Visconti; then Julien de la Rovère (1499), the future Jules II, "prominent debauchee who, become pope in 1503, will not take his shoe off on Good Friday for the adoration of the cross, because his foot was eaten by the French disease,"[1] and Pope Leo X (1513). To mention again the cardinal of St. Denis, Villiers de la Groslaye, who died of the pox August 6, 1499, etc. etc.

Roman sodomy had been resuscitated in the fifteenth century; it was called the *Italian vice.* No pope of this epoch was exempt from it: Paul II (1464), Sixtus IV (1471), Innocent VIII (1484), Alexander VI (1492), and especially Jules II (1503). We will except from this list the Cardinal of Sienna, elected under the name of Pius III (1503); but it must be said that he wore the tiara but twenty-seven days.

Alexander VI, the celebrated Borgia, varied his pleasures; outside of his pederastic exploits and of a few poisonings between times, he diverted himself with several mistresses. The most famous was his own daughter Lucretia, whom he made pregnant. She also had incestuous relations with her brother, Cesar Borgia. As may be seen, all this took place in the family and was a strictly family affair. A little-known author, Pontano, attributes to astral combinations the mad debauchery of this time and cites celebrated examples, among others that of Alexander VI.

> In our times the sovereign pontiff no doubt followed the example of Lot, whom the Hebrew historians state had known his daughter carnally and rendered her pregnant; it is the opinion of the parish and of the entire city of Rome. I will not dilate any further upon this subject on account of the majesty of the pontifical seat, upon which so many holy priests, with such great virtue—I would almost say with divinity—have seated themselves at times, and, I am sure, will again seat themselves.[2]

[1] Hesnaut, Le mal français, à l'époque de l'expédition de Charles VIII en Italie. Paris, 1886. The French Disease at the Time of the Expedition of Charles VIII into Italy.

[2] " . . . Temporibus nostris Pontificem maximum secutum fortasse Lothi exemplum, de quo Hebraïcis in historiis fiat mentio, filiam suam et cognovisse et gravidam fecisse opinio est et aulæ totius et urbis Romæ universæ. De quo tamen parcius, propter sedis pontificiæ majestatem,

As Hesnaut very justly observes, "the very terms of which the writer makes use exclude all idea of satire and of systematic malice." We will add that, at that time, facts of this kind did not appear as enormous as might be supposed, and especially if we take into consideration the unlimited power which the popes enjoyed, temporal as well as spiritual. Besides, the fact is too notorious to take the pain of bolstering it up with proofs. There is only a choice to be made among the documents of the time, and with the nauseating history of the deeds and acts of this Nero, crowned with the tiara, a large volume could be filled.

Every one knows that he caused to be repeated, for his personal benefit, the floral feasts,[1] of which the Romans were so greedy. The famous painting "Borgia S'amuse," which it was judged proper to refuse—I ask myself why—at the Salon of 1887, was certainly anodyne in comparison with the realistic scenes which Canon Burchard, secret chamberlain of the pontiff, was ordered to organize from time to time. The purveyor of the private pleasures has related day by day in his "Diarium"—and without prejudice, so natural did he regard it—the more or less low-necked caprices of his illustrious hierarchic superior. It was feared, no doubt, that in admitting the painting of Garnier attention would be directed upon Borgia and the other popes of whom the Holy See is not proud; the jury did not wish to appear to approve officially that which the interested still desire to pass as fiction.

But we cannot permit ourselves to be deterred by considerations of such slight importance; so that we

in qua tot sanctissimi sacerdotes, tanta cum integritate et pene dixerim, divinitate, et olim sedera, et, ut mihi persuadeo, etiam sedebunt." (P. J. Pontani opera, vol. iii. De rebus cœlestibus, lib. 28, fol. 294.)

[1] See Syphilis in Ancient and Prehistoric Times, chap. xi, p. 172.

will give a few interesting extracts from the journal of Burchard. Certainly, we have no more ill-feeling toward Borgia than to any other unpunishable assassin, and, consequently, unpunished; he was of his time, of his miserable time. If he still lived, our indignation would, no doubt, astonish him. It is exactly like Behanzin, the black who reigned in Dahomey; he must often ask himself in what respect human sacrifices, which amused him so much, could disturb us so much. And is it not a feeling of hatred or of prejudice which moves us to act as we do? If we speak at such great length of the departed Holy Father Alexander VI, it is because his excesses serve us as a type for the description of the manners of his century. As all examples, good or bad, always come from above, one may, on reading the biography of the head of the Church, form some idea of the morality of his flocks and subjects. Let us hear Burchard:—

> The last Sunday of the month of October, in the evening, there supped with the Duke of Valentinois,[1] in his apartment of the apostolic palace, fifty honest prostitutes who are called courtesans. The latter, after the meal, danced with the servants and others of the company, at first dressed, and, later, stark naked. Then there were placed on the floor the candelabra of the table with lighted candles, and all around them were thrown chestnuts, which the courtesans, naked and on all fours, picked up as they passed in the midst of the candelabra, in the presence of the Pope, of the Duke, and of Lucretia, his sister, who looked on. To terminate the feast gifts were offered, consisting of silk cloaks, pairs of hose, caps, and other things, to those who should know carnally the greatest number of these courtesans. The latter were known carnally in public, in the court of the palace, at the will of those attending, the prizes distributed to the winners,[2] etc.

This is enough, it seems to us, to edify the reader.

[1] Cesar Borgia, son of Alexander VI and brother of Lucretia.

[2] Joh. Burchardi, Diarium sive rerum urbanarum commentarii (1483–1506). Diary or Account of City Occurrences. MSS. published under the care of L. Thuasne in 1883.

As for that matter, the gallant fêtes of the Vatican have been renewed at the Petit-Luxembourg by the Regent of France. These latter have remained famous under the name of the *festivals of Adam* (fêtes d'Adam). There is no writer who denies them, and no one doubts either the incestuous relations of Phillip of Orleans with his daughters, and notably with the Duchess de Berry; but he did not poison. As may be seen, he was a Borgia on a small scale; on this point may be found, in Dulaure,[1] most interesting details.

At all events, the regent had a certain amount of remorse,—a thing unknown to Borgia. He confessed as much to Cardinal Dubois, of gloomy memory, his professor of perversity. "What will history say? It will represent the orgies of my regency as it does the fêtes which we all know of the *court of the favorites* of Henri III. Our dark fêtes will be shown in the full light of day; posterity will know the details. . . . At least it will be known that all occurred at the solicitation of a cardinal!"

Que dira l'histoire? Elle représentera les orgies de ma régence comme les fêtes que nous connaisons tous de la *cour des mignons* de Henri III. Nos fêtes ténébreuses seront mises au grand jour, la postérité en connaîtra les détails. . . . On saura du moins que tout se passait à l'instigation d'un cardinal!

In regard to the celebrated patients belonging to the clergy, we will recall the case of Bishop Jean de Spire, who died in 1104 from the results of a venereal ulcer; that of Pope Boniface VIII, which formed the subject of a pamphlet in 1294, without prejudice to the popes and cardinals of the end of the fifteenth century, whose names we gave at the beginning of this chapter. To mention once more the tragic end of Cardinal Wolsey,

[1] Histoire de Paris. Paris, 1834.

the intriguer, who in 1529 paid with his head for the counsels, both matrimonial and political, which were but little relished by Henry VIII of England. The syphilis with which the prelate was affected was the pretext used.

Then come a host of archbishops and of bishops whose names are mentioned by authors only by reason of their qualities as syphilitics. Such is the case of the bishop who ruled in Hungary at the end of the fifteenth century, and for whom Montagnana expressly wrote a small work on the *French disease.* This work is entitled "Medical Advice to Peter Zeno, Venetian, for the Most Illustrious and Reverend Bishop and Viceroy of Hungary. Padua, 1499." The pox had not respected the Most Reverend! We may equally mention Gaspard Torrella (1493), who combined the two professions of bishop and physician. Peter Pinctor (1500) claims to have cured, by means of mercurial inunctions, the Cardinal of Segovia, Canon Centez, and Pope Alexander VI (Borgia). In regard to the last we may say, more than in any other case, that the syphilis was well merited.

Is it not to Cardinal Bembo that Fracastor, in 1530, addressed his famous poem on syphilis? Let us not forget the celebrated Dubois, whom it would have been scandalous to know had been spared by the virus. It is concerning this adventurer that the Jesuit, Lafiteau, who was sent to propose him to the regent as prime minister, elicited this answer: "What the devil, then, does your cardinal want? I leave him all the authority of the prime minister; he is not satisfied if he has not the title also! Well, what will he do with it? For how long a time will he enjoy it? He is *rotten with the pox.* Chirac, who has seen him, assured me that he would not live six months!"

Que diable veut donc ton cardinal? Je lui laisse toute l'autorité du premier ministre; il n'est pas content s'il n'en a pas le titre! Eh! qu'en fera-t-il? Combien de temps en jouira-t-il? Il est pourri de vérole. Chirac, qui l'a visité, m'a assuré qu'il ne vivrait pas six mois!

Miserable epoch! Miserable people!

As to the small fry,—that is to say, abbés, canons, deacons, subdeacons, monks, nuns, and other specimens of the kind,—we are sufficiently edified concerning their manners, and history has not preserved the names of those who had license to go with the goddess of voluptuousness.

Each time that syphilis has flourished in the midst of monasteries, the fact has been noted in an incidental manner and the communities designated as a whole, the legal state of those interested being, for posterity, of nothing but mediocre importance.

But such was the power of the clergy in the Middle Ages—and even long after—that the physicians of those times, who were not solicitous of falling out with the temporal power, attributed the syphilis of the nuns to causes more or less imaginary. They would rather have declared it fallen from heaven than dare breathe a suspicion concerning the manners of these persons, who were deified in a sort of way. It is fortunate that the ecclesiastical writers (Nicholas de Clemenges, Burchard, and others) took it upon themselves to enlighten us on the subject. We may, accordingly, content ourselves with a smile at the following passage from Victorius (1551):—

The French disease may arise outside of all relations of man with woman, and *vice versâ*. There have been brought to me honest and saintly nuns, confined in monasteries protected like fortresses, under incessant surveillance, and whom nothing could deceive, who, in consequence of the *temperature* of that time and of their *putrid humors*, joined to a state of *weakness* of their limbs, and by a terrible fatality, contracted the French disease.[1]

Victorius was ignorant of or pretended to ignore the subterranean passages which connected the convents of the male and of the female religious; certain ones communicated with each other simply by gardens. This author had probably not read the work of Burchard, on the manners of the Renaissance, which we have quoted on page 202.

Almenar (1502) and T. de Bethencourt (1526), who treated, several years before Victorius, a respectable number of clerks and of monks, had found another explanation. As they could not advance, for their clients, the guarantee of monasteries "protected like fortresses," they imagined heredity showing itself after a long period of time. For them syphilis was incurable, was inevitably transmitted to children, and could even, in these latter, not show itself until *adult life*. And, say they, this origin must be admitted, in all charity (*pie credendum est*), when it concerns men and religious women. It was, perhaps, prudent tactics in the sixteenth century, but it is not strong as etiological diagnosis. No matter how skillful a similar method might be in our time, in which the reputation of the *well meaning physician* is a source of profit, we would not resign ourselves to put science under an extinguisher in that manner. How much more do we prefer the position of Ricord! He never would consent to seem to be the dupe of the hypocrisy of his sacred-saintly pat-

[1] "Gallicus propignitur morbus, adhuc millo præexistente commercio viri cum muliere et contra. Sane occurrerunt mihi honestæ et sanctæ noniales, fortissimis claustris obturatæ, sub ardua quippe et inviolabili custodia, quæ ex præsentis cœli statu atque ex statu humorum ex eis putrescentium, cum statu imbecillium membrorum, malo fato, in Gallicum cecidere morbum."

ronage. Every one knows the story of that ecclesiast who blamed his gown—made of material which was too coarse—of having caused an abrasion of the glans. At all events, the witty answer of the master, who doubted the good habits of the said gown, is a little too naturalistic for us to be able to reproduce it here.

However, the authors of the sixteenth century were not all satisfied with these agreeable explanations. It is thus that we see Fallopius rejecting the *pie credendum est* of T. de Bethencourt and clearly state, in 1555, that syphilis was acquired neither by air nor by water, but really from a real contact,—that is to say, a contact difficult to ignore:—

"Although certain persons of great renown have desired, in taking up the defense of the chastity of women, to say that they had been infected in taking holy water, this infection assuredly came to them by a very different sprinkling."

Quoi que quelques gens d'un grand nom ayent voulu, prenant la deffense de la chasteté des femmes, dire qu'elles avoient été infectées en prenant de l'eau-bénite, cette infection leur est assurement venüe par une aspersion bien différente.[1]

As to the laymen, who did not see the necessity of showing themselves more virtuous than the ministers, they were not spared either by the common scourge. And the virus which had crossed the portals of the Vatican saw itself in as good a condition under the imperial cloak as under the rags of the beggar; under the purple of the cardinal as under the most simple robe. To mention only monarchs and the members of royal families, we will recall the death of the drunkard, Wenceslaus, King of Bohemia, at the beginning of the fourteenth century; that of Hubert VII, Prince of

[1] Quotation from Vercelloni, translated by Devaux.

Padua, in 1345; of John of Gaunt, Duke of Lancaster, brother of Richard II, King of England, in 1399; of Ladislaus, King of Poland, in 1414; of Henry V of England, in 1422, and others.

Finally, every one knows the adventure of Francis I with *la belle Ferronnière;* and it is also known that the outraged husband, not being able to obtain direct revenge from the King of France, voluntarily contracted syphilis, which he transmitted to his wife and, as a natural result, to his powerful rival. The king finally died[1] in the course of a few years. The celebrated Charles V and Charles IX of France, if we are to believe Trenille,[2] as also Henry III, according to Astruc, would come to join that long list of syphilitic kings of which the venerable David, until we receive better information, remains the eldest. No doubt there have been many

[1] A chronicler of the time composed, on this subject, a sort of epitaph, which must not have caused great effort of the imagination :—

"Ce fut en quinze cent quarante-sept,
Le sept du mois de juillet,
Que le Roi mourut à Rambouillet
De la vérole qu'il avait."

['Twas in the month of June, the seventh,
In fourteen forty-seven,
At Rambouillet, with pox as cause,
The king went up to heaven.—O-D.]

As we are at doggerel verses, we will also risk a quatrain, asking the reader's pardon in advance :—

Quand Vénus te ravit la couronne de France,
Le pouvoir absolue, le trône à fleur de lis,
Ignorais-tu, François, dans ta concupiscence,
Que nous sommes egaux devans la syphilis ?

[When Venus robbed thee of the crown of France,
Of regal power, the throne of flower de lis,
Did'st thou forget, in thy concupiscence,
We're equals, Francis, in front of syphilis ?—O-D.]

[2] Traité pathologique et thérapeutique des maladies vénér. Paris, 1845. Treatise on the Pathology and Treatment of Venereal Diseases.

others, and there will be many more; but it would appear captious to dwell any longer upon a subject of such paltry importance.

Such were the manners at the beginning of the sixteenth century; syphilis was in full sway and spared no one. As a poet of the past century was enabled to say,

> "Et la garde qui veille à la porte du Louvre
> N'en défend pas nos rois."[1]

From this time on we no longer have the care, in pursuing our study, of demonstrating the existence of syphilis, for it is official. And our task will soon be terminated. We will take good care not to give a list of all the authors who have written on the subject; such an enumeration, even without the slightest commentary or semblance of analysis, would assume the dimensions of an encyclopædia. If a work of this character should, perhaps, be of value to the reader or investigator, it would possess no interest for the practitioner, who wants details—especially conclusions—and has no use for eight or ten thousand references to authors whom he has neither the time nor, often, the power to consult. Besides, such a catalogue has appeared under the title "Bibliography of Venereal Diseases,"[2] and comprises no less than five 16mo volumes. We will refer the reader, desirous of looking up the sources, to this work.

It, therefore, remains for us to follow the history of the principal theories advanced, as well upon the nature

[1] And the guard on duty at the Louvre
From it does not protect our kings.—O-D.

[2] Proksch, Die Litteratur ueber die venerischen Krankheiten. Bonn, 1889. [The Index-Catalogue of the Surgeon-General's Library and the Index Medicus also contain a very extensive bibliography on syphilis and venereal diseases.—O-D.]

of the virus as upon its progress in the organism, and that of the trials and gropings in the dark of therapeusis, from the time of the expedition of Charles VIII to the present. At all events, let fear be dissipated; we will not repeat here the history of the epidemic of Naples, with which we have occupied ourselves at sufficient length. We will likewise pass over the authors of the end of the fifteenth century, whose principal passages we have already quoted. Therefore, leaving aside the question of the origin of syphilis, which has been sufficiently studied, we will now search as to what was the opinion, at the beginning of the sixteenth century, of the medical profession on the nature of the new morbid entity which was henceforth clearly defined.

Let us say at once that syphilis in the fifteenth century implied no idea of disgrace, even in the eyes of the clergy. Later on it was judged proper to see in it Divine punishment, without noticing that this imputation was irreverent to the Creator. In fact, what would be thought of a divinity who had *blindly* scattered a plague capable of afflicting both the innocent and guilty, if guilty there be? What sort of a *providence* is one which, even in its wrath, *does not foresee* the consequences of its acts? For, although history does not mention it, we like to believe that the infants tainted with hereditary syphilis, and the unfortunate nurses contaminated at this source, were not included in the upbraidings of the clericals of the sixteenth century. Let us not forget that, quite recently yet, in certain provincial dispensaries managed by Sisters, there were no mercurial preparations, under the pretext that *shameful diseases* should not be treated. For this reason we give up to the meditations of the successors, fortunately disarmed by Torquemada, this quotation from Corlieu[1]: "To be affected with syphilis was looked upon at that time as a misfortune, *and not as a crime.* . . . There even existed, it appears, *a mass for the poxy;* it is the mass of St. Job, *contra morbum gallicum,* and the gospel was most naturally taken from St. Luke."

Être affecté de la syphilis était considéré alors comme un malheur et non comme une faute. . . . Il y avait même, parait-il, une messe pour les vérolés; c'est la messe de Saint-Job, contra morbum gallicum,[2] et l'evangile était pris tout naturellement dans Saint-Luc.

For nearly fifty years, dating from the great epidemic, the different opinions in regard to the origin and nature of venereal disease were practically the same. We have examined the writings of the principal authors and we have seen, if it be remembered, that some saw in the matter the consequences of a celestial witchcraft, of astral conjunctions; that others, more skeptical, blamed telluric miasmata; and that certain ones—the smaller number—took it upon themselves to find the symptoms of leprosy,[3] and concluded, in consequence, in favor of the antiquity of the disease. Among all these opinions there were some differences; it was believed that in this there was seen a degeneration of ancient leprosy, and Ricord himself was not far from attaching himself to this hypothesis. In conclusion, we will limit ourselves to recalling the *Maranic plague*, in which certain authors of the beginning of this century have desired to see primitive syphilis. But there was no echo.

In the beginning, patients, in order to conceal their debauchery, did not confess how they had come by

[1] Traduction des opuscules de Gruenbeck, imprimés en 1496. Paris, 1884. Translation of the books of Gruenbeck, printed in 1496.

[2] Missale Romanum. Venetiis, 1521.

[3] There exist some writers to-day who contend, in a more or less imperfect manner, that syphilis is a modified form of leprosy, despite the fact that both diseases are occasionally seen to exist in the same individual.—O-D.

their disease: this circumstance contributed to render more credible the opinion that the disease was of epidemic nature. A multitude of reasons was sought for to explain its production, and we have seen to what absurdities scientific men permitted themselves to be drawn. At all events, Torella (1500) appears to have been the first one to suspect the true mode of propagation of the virus, for he says that this disease "ordinarily came about by way of transmission." Jacques Catanée (1505), George Vella (1508), and Nicholas Massa (1532) advanced the same opinion, as also Fracastor.[1]

We consequently come to 1530, a time at which the theory of the American origin still enjoyed great popularity: being still scarcely 10 years old, it still derived the benefit of a general favor. That year, 1530, is interesting, inasmuch as it saw the birth of the much celebrated poem of Fracastor,[2] in which the author gave the name as *lues*, at first not much noticed; of SYPHILIS, which it was destined to retain. The scope of the work of the physician of Verona is not known; and we will content ourselves with recalling the principal points.

The shepherd, Syphilus, who watched the flocks of King Alcithous, one day reproached Apollo with drying up the trees, of draining the springs in such a manner that his flock was dying through want of shade and of water. He swore that in future he would sacrifice to his king and no longer to the sun. Apollo, enraged, loosened upon the whole land a shameful disease which attacked first of all Syphilus, and spread everywhere

[1] De morbis contagiosis. Venetiis, 1546. On Contagious Diseases. Venice, 1546.

[2] Hieronymi Fracastorii, Syphilis, sive Morbus Gallicus. Veronæ, 1530. Hieronymus Fracastor, Syphilis, or the French Disease. Verona, 1530.

without sparing the king himself. "Syphilus has his body covered with shameful ulcers; he was the first to know nights without sleep and cramps in his limbs; it was he who gave his name to this disease, which was called *syphilis* from that time, on account of this circumstance."

> Siphilus ostendit turpes per corpus Achores;
> Insomnes primus noctes, convulsaque membra
> Sensit, et a primo traxit cognomina morbi,
> Syphilidemque ab eo labem dixere coloni.

Fracastor terminates his poem in a manner agreeable to the accepted opinion of his times. Indeed, Syphilus finds the nymph Americis, who orders him to sacrifice a white cow to Juno if he desire to be cured of his sores. The shepherd obeys, and from the blood of the victim springs guaiac, the famous sudorific wood. The allusions here are sufficiently clear for us to be able to look upon ourselves as excused from furnishing any explanation. At all events, certain passages lead us to think that Fracastor did not believe very strongly in the American origin, although he did sacrifice to the fashion of the day.[1] The proof of it is in the following verse: "However, if belief is to be placed in well-observed facts, this opinion *must be abandoned.*"

> At vero, si rite fidem observata merentur,
> Non ita consendum.

He adds that he has seen the contagium arise spontaneously in virgins, outside of prostitution, and he concludes in admitting the possibility of contagion by the

[1] This opinion, although extensively spread among the people, was little shared in by scientific men. It is thus that Alphonsus Ferry ("De morbo gallico." Naples, 1537), whilst not admitting the antiquity of syphilis, recognizes the fact that the majority of physicians of his time regarded this disease as being as old as man.

air, ignorant at that time that the kiss, chaste or otherwise, may be sufficient.

Farther on he clearly defines himself a partisan of the antiquity of venereal disease, and, desiring to explain what may have led to the belief in the novelty of syphilis, he gives a reason which is perhaps the best of all: "One is led to think that it is not the first time that it has been seen on earth, but that it has made frequent appearances, although up to the present it has not been known by any special name. The night of ages, which holds everything concealed in its bosom, ends by effacing things and even their names."

> Non semel in terris visam, sed sæpe fuisse
> Ducendum est, quamquam nobis nec nomine nota
> Hactenus illa fuit: quoniam longa vetustas,
> Cuncta sinu involvens, et res et nomina delet.

In another one of his works, published later on,[1] Fracastor also says, regarding the epidemic of Naples, that "it is impossible that a disease of slow progress and development should have been able to disseminate itself in such a short time, and that it should be enough for a fleet disembarking in Spain for all Europe to be invaded at once." Here is a remark which is very just; and one is painfully surprised to see the author, later on, join himself to the errors of the majority of his contemporaries. In fact, he attributes the origin of syphilis to the conjunction of Saturn, Jupiter, and Mars, in the sign of Cancer.

Fracastor recommends a large number of plants used in the form of infusion, such as mint, hops, thyme, and, above all, guaiac. Sweating must be promoted by means of bedclothing, and he insists upon this method

[1] De morbis contagiosis. Lib. iii. On Contagious Diseases. Book iii.

of treatment, for, says he, "when one perspires the rottenness leaves the body with the drops of sweat."

Dum sudes fœdæque fluant per corpora guttæ.

He also speaks of purging and of bleeding, and praises, above everything, mercurial frictions pushed to salivation, which was, according to him and the other physicians of that time, one way of curing. In our day this untoward complication is avoided.[1]

Let us now say a few words concerning this famous method of mercurial inunctions which the physicians of the fifteenth century inherited from the empirics.

Employed in Europe from the feudal epoch, either for *leprosy* or for the *thick scurf* (*gale epaisse*),—or whatever other name it pleased them to give to venereal lesions,—these inunctions were also in use among the Arabs, who employed them against lice and perhaps, also, for syphilides, which they recognized at that time under the different names of *bothor*, *asafati*, etc. The Arab preparation was called *unguentum saracenicum* (Saracene ointment), and contained but one-ninth of mercury. The empirics, during all the Middle Ages, had used it only with prudence, and, when physicians decided to use it in their turn, it was only in very small doses; thus, the ointment of Torella was one in forty. But the quacks, who are always bold, wished to do better and more rapidly; they administered it in a blind fashion. The first results being encouraging, no limits were known; the frightful stomatites and debility which resulted were considered, from the very start, as so many symptoms of syphilis.

[1] It may be in France, but in Hot Springs, Ark., mercurial inunctions are pushed to such an extent that salivation is by no means infrequent. Many of the patients suffer from marked mercurial ptyalism, and suffer in consequence.—O-D.

The following was the *modus operandi:* Instead of recommending to patients, as it is done in our days, very small and accurately-weighed doses of blue ointment, the patient was smeared, *from head to feet*, with a sort of semi-fluid mixture, in which mercury formed a large proportion. A varnishing brush was used, and the ointment was spread without the least regard to quantity, as is shown in a curious vignette of the time, which we have reproduced and placed as a frontispiece to this book. The apothecaries or others entrusted to apply mercurial ointment were called "greasers of the pox" (*graisseurs de la vérole*), as Rabelais informs us. Then, the *smearing* having ended, the patients were made to get in—only the rich—large sweating-vats;[1] but the latter were heated to such a degree that a few were asphyxiated. The poor were simply piled in ovens, in which they were sometimes forgotten for too long a time; and it was not a rare occurrence to find a certain number who had passed into the condition of half-burnt charcoal. At all events, it appears that this method boasted of successes, "with the exception," says Yvaren,[2] "of a few scorched and a small number roasted." This was a direct method of cooking the humors; that of the patient sometimes followed.

The therapeutic object was to eliminate the virus by way of the saliva and sweat; this is what was then called *passer par la casserole* (go through the pan).[3]

[1] This is almost the identical method (*mutatis mutandis*) which is employed at the celebrated Hot Springs of Arkansas, to-day, by so many of the practitioners located at that place; and it is about as empirical as in the fifteenth century.—O-D.

[2] Traduction en vers français du poème de Fracastor. Paris, 1847. Translation in French Verse of the Poem of Fracastor.

[3] At the beginning, as the patients drooled night and day, they were given, for this use, a special basin, which was called *la casserole* (the pan), from which arose the expression. Later, this term was employed to the entire course of treatment; it has even been retained in French military

The course of treatment generally lasted from twenty to twenty-five days;[1] but few patients could continue this treatment until the end, to which horses even could not all have successfully resisted. Three-fourths of the patients, according to the testimony of Ulrich von Hutten, debilitated either by these extreme sweatings, or by the absorption of mercury in such toxic doses, or by the disturbances of stomatitis, died in a few days. The others dragged out a miserable existence, and scarcely one in a hundred got out of the scrape. "It may well be said," remarks Patton,[2] quite justly, "that these patients got well in spite of the medicine!"

Accordingly, some patients refused mercury. The results, as a matter of fact, were not very encouraging. The sight of the unfortunates in whom the mouth was nothing but a large ulcer, of foul odor, continually slobbering, suffering in a horrible manner, almost unable to take food, scarcely able to stand up,—such a hideous sight must have made the most intrepid turn back. Accordingly, we believe in the word of Ulrich von Hutten[3] when he avers that the patients "howled." He himself had had syphilis, and, although he was but 20 years of age at the time, we must be astonished that he could have followed such a treatment for *eight years.* As in spite of this he was not cured, he came to the point of accusing mercury of being not only inefficient, but even harmful. We know that the poor

hospitals, in which it is synonymous with *mercurial treatment;* but the soldiers, who to-day still speak of "*passer par la casserole*," are, of course, ignorant of the origin of this phrase.

[1] Torrella was satisfied, for his patients, with fifteen consecutive days of the oven; they had to enter it fasting.

[2] Translation of Ulrich von Hutten's work, La maladie française. Lyons, 1865. The French Disease.

[3] *Loc. cit.*

metal is not yet cleared of this accusation, apparently true, but really false. Ulrich von Hutten, who lauds guaiac, owed his cure most probably to the suppression of all active remedies. The aversion of the German knight to mercury is but too well justified, so far as he was concerned, at least; but we may feel surprised, with Patton, that physicians of the worth of Ricinius, Scopus, and Stromer—friends of Ulrich von Hutten—should not have understood that it was not the mercury in itself, but the abuse of it in its use and the deplorable manner in which it was administered, which brought about the troubles.

At all events, in the face of the categorical refusal of patients, the physicians were forced, through loss of patients, to abandon little by little the classic "casserole" which syphilitics no longer would have. From that time they limited themselves to sweatings in blankets and with the aid of sudorific drinks. The frictions were made with a greater degree of measure and the troubles due to mercurialism diminished in intensity. As these latter, from the very beginning, had been attributed to syphilis, it is easily understood why all authors note, at the end of twenty-five years, a great modification in the symptoms observed.[1] Ulrich von Hutten, who was in a better position than any one to verify the facts, also states that the scourge had considerably diminished in 1519,—the time at which he wrote. He was not a physician, it is true, but all the more thanks are due to him for having described the lesions of mercurial stomatitis, for having risen against the erroneous opinions of certain physickers who ac-

[1] It is even presumable that syphilis had reduced itself to proportions which were not of an alarming nature, for, if we are to believe Erasmus, a learned Dutchman who died in 1536, "it was quite the thing, among people at court, to be affected with it."

cused mercury of producing gummata, syphilitic tubercles, alopecia, etc., and for having observed—which is not bad for the time—the disastrous effects of alcohol and of venereal excesses in the syphilitic, formerly leprous.

Then it was thought of to administer mercury by the stomach. Peter Andrew Matthiole was the first (1533) who dared give it internally in the form of pills. These pills were composed of *crude mercury.* A celebrated pirate of the island of Lesbos, Kheireden, better known under the name of Barbarossa, brought some to Francis I, so that it was the king who inaugurated this mode of treatment in France.[1] But if the stomatitis were less severe than with the inunctions, they always went to the point of salivation, without which the learned faculty of that time considered medication useless. Let us immediately add that it is necessary to come to 1718 to find an author, Chicoyneau, chancellor of the University of Montpellier, try to demonstrate the uselessness of salivation. Naturally no one listened to him, and this idea only triumphed later, hardly a century ago.

At all events, before the use of mercurial pills, therapeusis was not limited to inunctions of mercury followed with sweating in ovens. From the very beginning of the sixteenth century, as we have stated, the habit of piling patients like ordinary pans in ovens was discontinued little by little: less barbarous, if not more

[1] The following is given, as a matter of curiosity, as the composition of these famous pills:—

℞ Crude mercury,	. . . .	6 parts.
Rhubarb,	. . . .	3 parts.
Ambergris,		
Musk,	. . . . āā	1 part.
Wheat-flour,	. . . .	2 parts.

Mix with lemon-juice and make into pills as large as a pea.
Sig : One pill daily.

rational, methods were adopted. It is thus that certain physicians dieted their patients, bled them, or applied leeches to them: it will be admitted that this was, to say the least, quite an odd method of preparing them to combat the syphilitic anæmia.

Then they were purged, and they were made to swallow a mass of cooling drinks with a basis of wild chicory,[1] of borage, of parsley, etc. Then, when the physician judged that he had well "digested and taken out the temper of the humors," he again gave, from time to time, a stronger purgative. It is to be supposed that men, at that time, were more vigorous than they are now, for the therapeusis of to-day has replaced with tonics all these debilitating treatments.

For the cutaneous troubles baths of lukewarm water were ordered, to be followed by inunctions of a liniment with a sulphur, litharge, cream of tartar, orris-root powder base, etc. For the osteocopic pains there were prescribed rubbing in of decoction of hyoscyamus, of laurel-oil, of chamomile, of saffron, etc. Some few imaginative physicians,—perhaps the homœopaths of the times,—such as Aquilanus (1498), Cataneus (1505), Matthiole (1535), Benedictus or Jean Benoist (1510), prescribed the use of boiled or fried *viper*, or else viper-bouillon, syrup of the decoction of vipers, etc. If the disease resisted these diverse means, which must have sometimes happened, recourse was had to the famous vats and ovens. Or else an issue was made to the head, to an arm or a leg, in such a manner as to afford an emunctory for the vitiated humors. Coradin Gilini (1497), Wendelin Hock (1502), and Benedict Victorius (1551) express themselves as having been well pleased with this method.

[1] Cichorium intybus.—O-D.

Then, in 1519, Ulrich von Hutten made guaiac the fashion: at the very beginning nothing else would be taken, but the fascination was not long-lived. It is the story of all new remedies. In the beginning they cure everything; after a few years they are forgotten. This is what happened to guaiac. As it was believed to be absolutely harmless, it was indiscriminately given to all patients. In other words, an abuse was made of this diaphoretic, and the subjects with a delicate organism did not long resist these profuse sweats, which debilitated them. Witness the following passage from Peter Andrew Matthiole[1]:—

> I have observed that those with the pox of a dry nature have been attacked by hectic fever and consumption through the use of the decoction of guaiac.

The reign of guaiac had not lasted twenty years.

But it is always necessary that popular enthusiasm should be directed to some panacea. Chinese *smilax*, a sort of tuberculous root imported into Europe by Chinese merchants, inherited the worship which had at first been devoted to the *sacred wood.* And that which aided in giving it popularity was its use by Charles V for his gout, according to Vesalius.[2] Then, in its turn, it fell into discredit, dethroned by *sarsaparilla.* Vesalius himself, in the letter we have just mentioned, considered smilax as very inferior to the sacred wood.

> Of a certainty, decoction of smilax is much below that of guaiac for the excrescences or tumors of the bones and for malignant syphilitic ulcers.

This way of looking at the matter is shared in by Jerome Cardan (1548), Antony Musa Brassavolus

[1] Opusculum de morbo gallico, 1535. Hand-book on the French Disease.

[2] Epistola de Radice Chinæ. 1546.

(1551), Antony Fracancianus, Julian Paulmier (1578), and especially by Fallopius,[1] who clearly states:—

This root should not be employed in the pox; for, having tried it three or four times, I obtained no result whatever.

In our days *Smilax China* is forgotten; guaiac is but little used except in the form of powder or of an extract in some pills; and sarsaparilla is, with iodide of potassium, the basis of the *special* depurative syrup of nearly all of the pharmacists of France and of Navarre.

Then there comes from Florida a new specific, *sassafras*, an aromatic substance about forgotten to-day.[2]

After all, the physicians following Ulrich von Hutten were not always satisfied with sudorific roots; when a cure delayed in showing itself, they had recourse to mercurial inunctions. However, they made use of them with greater care and in quantity less than the quacks, those *executioners of humanity*—according to the expression of Gilini—whom nothing deters, not even the death of their patients. Alphonse Ferry[3] gave the assurance that it was necessary "to return to inunctions after having tried the sacred wood two or three times in vain." We shall see farther on that Fallopius acted after the same principles.

But the true promoter of this reaction was Theophrastes Paracelsus. This surgeon was the first to proclaim, in 1536, that mercury was the *only* and single specific. It required a certain amount of courage: guaiac had lost its prestige, it is true, but there re-

[1] De morbo gallico. 1560.

[2] This may be true of France, but in the rural districts of the United States it still enjoys great popularity as a blood "purifier." All the members of the farmer's family are made to undergo a course of sassafras "tea" every spring to "clean" the blood, and this custom bids fair to persist for some time to come.—O-D.

[3] De ligno sancto. 1538. On the Sacred Wood.

mained the struggle against the growing favor of smilax and of sarsaparilla. Paracelsus, like a true revolutionary spirit, overthrew the theory of the *four humors* and maintained that libertinage was the only origin of syphilis. Later on Fernel adopted this way of looking upon the matter so far as the origin of venereal disease was concerned, but remained inflexible in respect to mercury.

We have now come to the second half of the sixteenth century: this is marked by a slight progress in medical science. There is no longer, so to speak, any mention of astral conjunctions or planetary influences. Physicians are now occupied in finding how syphilis develops itself, the symptoms are studied, their value is discussed, and, if the explanations which are given make the physicians of the nineteenth century smile, they at least bear testimony to the constant efforts made in the desire to discover scientific truth. Then a few authors begin to write in French;[1] and, one sees frequently recurring the expressions *apostème* [abscess], *matière mélancolique* [melancholic matter], *phlegme* [phlegm], *pituite* [aqueous humor], etc.: it must not be forgotten that the humors reigned at that time. This may be judged of by the different extracts we will give from principal authors whose treatises are exclusively devoted to venereal diseases.

Let us first listen to Benoit Textor,[2] who wrote in 1550: if he do not announce the duality of the chancre from the stand-point of the nature of the virus, he at least knew that chancres were to be divided into two

[1] To tell the truth, the first French author who wrote upon syphilis is Jaques de Béthencourt, in 1527; his predecessors, from the time of the epidemic of Naples, are all Germans or Italians.

[2] Textor, De la nature et cure du chancre. Lyon, 1550. On the Nature and Cure of the Chancre.

classes which were quite distinct from a symptomatic point of view.

"At the beginning the matter is quite obscure and difficult to know. . . . When it is touched, at times it provokes pain, at others it does not.

"There are two principal varieties of chancres. One is without ulceration, commonly called aposthumous. . . . The other is ulcerated and excoriated."

Au commencement la matière est fort obscure et difficile à cognoistre. . . . Quand on lattouche, aucunefois elle meine doleur, aucunefois cela n'advient pas.

Il y ha deux principales différences de chancres. Lun est sans ulcère vulgairement appellé apostemeux. . . . Lautre est exulcéré ou escorché.

He had certainly observed *extra-genital* chancres, for he recognizes the fact that chancres may be situated upon different parts of the body, especially upon soft, glandular parts.

"The which are quick to receive this coarse melancholic humor, as are the nostrils, the lips, and the breasts."

Les quelles sont promptes à recevoir ceste grosse matière de melancholie, comme sont les narines, les lèvres, et les mammelles.

He looked upon the chancre as incurable, or, at least, as very difficult to cure, and he boldly advises extirpation,—a method already proposed by Celsus, in the century of Augustus, and again taken up in our days. The future will inform us as to what must be thought of this method.

The author describes, in addition, a *non-ulcerated chancre* (*!*) of the mamma, which he seems to have confounded with some carcinoma or other tumor of the breast at its initial period.

"It is quite a large tumor which is resisting to the

touch. . . . It is of an ashen color tending to a purplish, violaceous, or dark color. When looked at it seems to be soft, but to the touch it is found very hard."

C'est une tumeur fort grande qui résiste au touchement. . . . Elle est de couleur cendrée tendant à couleur purpuree, ou violette, ou de couleur obscure. Selon le regard, elle semble estre molle, mais au toucher elle se treuve très dur.

For the venereal chancre Textor advises emollients and a host of resolving ointments. The internal treatment is, to say the least, curious :—

" The blood of duck or gosling to be drunk warm from the freshly-killed animal, . . . or crawfish-gruel with asses' milk taken for the space of five days, eating crawfish for as many days, which is marvelously useful."

Sang de canard ou doison à boire tout chaud de la beste frai tuee, . . . ou brouet descrevisses avec laict d'Asnesse prins par lespace de cinq iours, en mengeant autant de iours des escrevisses, ce qui est merveilleusement utile.

Agreed ; it was at least as good as the famous *casserole* of his predecessors. He lays great store by his crawfish treatment, for he recurs to it upon several occasions: perhaps it is on account of the Latin name, *cancer*, which means *chancre* and *crawfish* equally.[1]

Five years later, in 1555, Gabriel Fallopius[2] clearly described the primary lesion, and gave the chancrous induration as a pathognomonic symptom of the pox. He also had recourse to mercurial inunctions, but only in grave cases.

I make use of mercury in rebellious poxes and desperate ones, especially when I have previously employed all other means.

[1] This strongly suggests a foreshadowing of the homœopathic doctrine of *similia similibus curantur*, which even to-day has such a large circle of believers. Truly, it may be said, *nil novum sub sole !*—O-D.

[2] G. Fallopius, De morbo gallico liber absolutissimus. Patavii, 1564.

Besides, it is toward this period of 1560 that physicians, recognizing the inefficiency of exotic plants, all returned little by little to the use of mercury. Fracancianus [1] acknowledges it very frankly.

Another way of treating the disease is to employ mercurial inunctions. Although they seem to cure it sometimes, they had, nevertheless, been abandoned as too violent and dangerous a remedy. But the disease having become difficult and stubborn, many very skillful physicians have been obliged to return to it within two years.

At all events, Jean Fernel remained firm. Frightened by the miserable results obtained by the empirics, he declared himself a deadly foe to mercury, and composed two opiates, the *small* and the *great*,[2] having a basis of purgative plants, without mercury or guaiac, and which he looked upon as heroic. It is useless to state that the remedy was absolutely inefficient.

As we have seen, mercury was at first used in the form of liniment and of ointment for inunctions or frictions. Then, in 1506, Bolognini proposed a mercurial cerate: several were tried, prepared in different ways. The most celebrated of all is that which was described by Jean de Vigo in 1514, and which is still much used in our days under the name of *emplastrum de Vigo.* Mercury was also given in fumigations: there was, at that time, mixed with different perfumes either cinnabar or mercury rubbed up with the essence of turpentine or saliva. To-day the cinnabar fumigations are especially employed, in hospitals, for the destruction of lice. Then came the method of *washing*, consisting of lotions of sublimate (20 grammes to the litre of distilled water [2-per-cent. solution]), and of which Auger Ferrier appears to have been the first to speak, in 1553. These

[1] De morbo gallico. 1564.

[2] De curatione Luis Venereæ, 1556. On the Cure of Venereal Lues.

lotions were applied to the limbs for ten days, from one to three times daily. Then sweating was produced, in bed, by means of hot stones. As soon as the symptoms of stomatitis were quite plain, the treatment was stopped: it was, after all, the object of the medication.

"By this the gums rotted and ulcerated, as in the cases in which the liniments and the perfumes were employed: it was this which indicated the end of the treatment."

Par là les gencives se pourrissaient et s'ulcéraient, comme dans les cas où l'on employait les liniments et les parfums: c'est ce qui indiquait la fui du traitement.[1]

Let us add, however, to be exact, that a certain number of physicians—sufficiently small in number to have been easily counted—rose against mercurial salivation from the very beginning of the sixteenth century, and gave the means of arresting or even of preventing it. For that purpose they advised purgatives as soon as the first signs of salivation showed themselves, and to prevent it they recommended using the inunctions only every three or four days. These physicians, as we have stated, were the exceptions; it is hardly one every five years that can be found, and the sixteenth century cannot boast of twenty for its share. And, like Astruc, we will hand down their names to posterity. First of all we find Wendelin Hock (1502), then Jean Almenar (1512), Peter Maynard (1518), Jaques de Béthencourt (1527), Nicholas Massa (1532), Jean Paschal (1534), Louis Lobera (1544), Anthony Musa Brassavola (1551), Thierry de Héry (1552), Amatus Lusitanus (1556), Guillaume Rondelet (1560), Leonard Botal (1563), George Dordon (1568), Ambrose Paré (1575), Julian

[1] Auger Ferrier, De lue hispanica. Parisiis, 1564. On the Spanish Lues. Paris, 1564.

Paulmier (1578), John Wier (1580), John Zecchius (1586), Jerome Mercurial (1587), Luke Ghini (1589), and Peter Torrez (1600). There are to be mentioned, in addition, John Hartmann (1611) and Louis Septal (1614), who belong to the seventeenth century.

Certainly, the authors of which we have just given a list preached in the desert; but, as the inunctions were abandoned little by little and replaced by internal medication, the lesions due to mercurial stomatitis were no longer as formidable nor as frequent.

In the second half of the sixteenth century the physicians were not yet enlightened in regard to the progress of the venereal virus in the economy; and, as they were ignorant of the existence of and accordingly of the rôle of the lymphatics, they referred the ganglionic engorgements to purely external causes. It is thus that Guillaume Rondelet (1560) explains the origin of inguinal adenitis by a lack of hygienic attention and care: "If the froth or thin matter touch the groins, then the venereal bubo forms."

> Si l'escume ou la sanie touche les aines, lors le bubon venerien s'engendre.[1]

He was acquainted with blennorrhagia, which he called, indifferently, *gonorrhœa*, *pisse-chaude*, *chaude-pisse*, and he describes it separately; but in all the cases in which it is coincident with syphilis he makes of it the initial symptom of that disease.

Like Thierry de Héry (1552), he had clearly noticed that the bubo which is indolent and which does not suppurate was a sign, so to speak, pathognomonic of syphilis:—

"If one have venereal buboes which have not run,

[1] Rondelet, Traité de vérole. Treatise on the Pox. Translated by Maniald. Bordeaux, 1576.

but have gone in or have indurated themselves, we may assure such a one with certainty of having the pox, even if he deny it."

Si quelqu'un a bubons qui n'aient point jetté, mais soient rentrez en dedans, ou se soient endurcis, nous pouvons certainement asseurer celuy la avoir la vérole, encore qu'il le nie.

Rondelet appears to be the first author who observed sternalgia;[1] he lays great stress upon this symptom:—

"The front of the chest brings pain in this disease, which is one of the surest marks."

Le devant de la poitrine ameine douleur en ceste maladie, qu'est une des plus asseurees marques.

This phenomenon was doubtless more frequent in the sixteenth century than it is to-day, for, in spite of our unceasing investigations during the entire period of our residence at the Hôpital de Lourcine, we have never been able to note it but once in a manner beyond a doubt. We have been less fortunate in this respect than one of our contemporaries, who imagines, among other things, that he has invented sternalgia. Let us leave it to him: Rondelet will not claim it; no more will Baglivi.

From a therapeutic point of view, Rondelet is to be counted with the physicians of the sixteenth century who re-instated mercury.

"From the things stated above it appears that quicksilver is an antidote and a remedy highly proper for the pox, inasmuch as it has cured it, in whatever manner it be applied, for it produces sweats and dries up by reason of the subtlety of its parts."

[1] Baglivi later on (1704) made of this a pathognomonic sign of venereal diseases; but it is erroneously that Jourdan considers him the first to mention the symptoms, since Rondelet had already spoken of it in 1560.

Des choses dessusdictes appert asses l'argentvif estre antidote et remede fort propre pour la vérole, pour ce qu'il la guerit, en quelque sorte que soit applicqué, car il esment les sueurs, et deseche acause de la subtilité des ses parties.

On this point he was seconded by Anthony Chaumète,[1] who wrote in the same year:—

"Those who so strongly condemn the use of mercury have never used it in the proper manner. . . . I have always been satisfied with it, and I have cured by this remedy a large number of persons affected with inveterate cases of pox."

Ceux qui condamnent si fort l'usage du mercure ne l'ont jamais employé comme il faut. . . . Je m'en suis toujours bien trouvé et j'ai guéri par ce remède un grand nombre de gens atteints de véroles invétérées.

Ambrose Paré (1575)[2] also shared in this opinion, which he expresses in about the same words as Rondelet:—

"The method of inunctions is the most useful and the surest of all. . . .

"Mercury is the true antidote of pox; when it is properly given it has an admirable virtue, and in whatever manner it be applied it cures that disease by drying, by reason of the smallness of its parts, and by inducing sweats."

Le mercure est le véritable antidote de la vérole; lorsqu'il est donné à propos, il a une vertu admirable, et de quelque façon qu'on l'applique il guérit cette maladie, en dessèchant, par la petitesse de ces parties, et en provoquant des sueurs.

The illustrious surgeon had, like Fallopius, noticed the specific nature of the indurated chancre:—

"If there be an ulcer on the penis, and if hardness

[1] Method. morbi venerei curandi, 1560, chap. v. On the Method of Curing Venereal Disease.

[2] Lib. xix, chap. ix and x.

remain at the site, such a thing infallibly shows the patient has pox."

S'il y a ulcere à la verge et s'il demeure dureté au lieu, telle chose infalliblement montre le malade avoir la vérole.

We will limit our quotations to the foregoing, for, in multiplying them, we could not give the reader any more information: the latter must have his faith settled in regard to this curious period of the sixteenth century. Up to the year 1600, and even beyond it, it is always the never-ending quarrel between the mercurialists and the non-mercurialists; mercury taken up and abandoned time and again; salivation considered as a method of treatment by the greater number of mercurialists, and this latter stifling the timid voice of a few minds, too much ahead of their times, who dared denounce the misdeeds of stomatitis. In medicine, as in everything else, and at whatever epoch it may be, Dame Routine was, is, and always will be powerful; the revolutionary spirits will always be confounded with the rebels and treated as such: every new idea is destined to be repulsed at the very beginning, no matter what its value may be. If it be really good, it will never have worse adversaries than those in the highest places,—that is to say, those who most appreciate merit. Why? Because, not having found it themselves, they consider themselves as outraged, and such things are never forgiven.

CHAPTER II.

VENEREAL PATHOLOGY IN THE SEVENTEENTH CENTURY.

What was understood, in the seventeenth century, by the expression "*crystalline.*"—The astral conjunctions again.—The types of physicians who inspired Molière.—The "*joyful disease.*"—The theory of the *fermentation of seeds* and that of venereal excesses.—Return in favor of the ancient origin of syphilis.—First idea of mediate contagion.—*Universal syphilis* and *particular syphilis.*—Syphilis reduced to its true proportions.

As we have already said incidentally in the preceding chapter, the first half of the seventeenth century does not differ materially from the end of the sixteenth in regard to the progress made in venereal pathology then prevailing. It is even necessary to come to 1664 to find, in medical treatises, a new idea or an important remark which has not been previously made. Up to that time it is the same theories more or less antagonistic, accompanied by the same errors. However, we will quote, as belonging to the first half of the seventeenth century, T. Guillaumet, one of the first who made use of the expression *crystalline* as regards venereal lesions. As the word is still pronounced in our days by the public—without a knowledge on the part of those who use it as to what it really refers—we will give a few explanations.

The author seems to have been desirous of so designating the œdema which sometimes attends the initial symptom of syphilis. He explains to us that the irritation of the mucous membrane brings on swelling of the parts, and these latter are then tense and shining like crystal, whence the name *crystalline.*

"The which inflation [swelling] is so great and strongly stretched that it glistens through, and especially if light be brought to bear upon it."

Laquelle inflation est si grande et fort tandue qu'elle reluit à travers, et sur tout si l'on y opose la lumière.[1]

Later on, certain authors, such as Cockburn (1713), Vercelloni (1722), and others, have designated, under the name of *crystallines*, small, transparent bullæ which seem to have been simple vesicles of vulvar or preputial herpes. Guillaumet concludes by saying that this affection is nothing else than the pox, representing the same symptoms, but with this difference, that those of the crystalline are more violent. His little work is a treatise on syphilis; the author makes a horrible jumble and creates terrible confusion between the latter disease and certain affections which have no relations to it. It is thus that in his descriptions may be recognized, among other inflammatory diseases, urethritis and cystitis. He is a partisan of the antiquity of syphilis, for, for him, it was the leprosy of the time of Moses. He recommends the treatment by mercurial ointments.

The work of de la Martinière (1664)[2] presents us with a curious mass of incoherent and of judicious remarks. An uncompromising enemy of mercury, he advises purgatives and sudorifics; guaiac and sarsaparilla are his favorite remedies. He distinguishes, like at the present day, three periods in the progress of syphilis: the *preceding*, *following*, *unexpected* signs [signes *precedans*, *suivans*, *survenans*] which he describes correspond to our three periods,—*primary*, *secondary*, *tertiary*. The multiplicity of the manifestations of the

[1] T. Guillaumet, Traité de la Cristalline. Lyon, 1611. Treatise on the Crystalline.

[2] Traité des malad. vénér. Paris, 1664. Treatise on Venereal Disease.

secondary period disconcerting him slightly, he concludes by recognizing *four species* of syphilis, each one distinct. To explain the genesis of pustulo-crustaceous syphilides, which he calls his third species, he gives himself up to a dissertation so original in character that it would be a pity not to quote it:—

"The cause of those round pustules which appear upon the body of him who is attacked by the third species of pox is due to the circumstance that the poison of this disease communicates itself successively to the liver by the veins, to the heart by the arteries, and to the brain by the nerves; and that which causes these pustules to appear preferably on the head than on other parts is due to the circumstance that the poison, being very subtle, searches for spirits rather than for the mass of the flesh; and as there are more spirits in the brain than in the other parts of the body, and as it is of a more moist and less heated substance, it receives much more readily the impressions of the malignity of the poison."

La cause de ces pustules rondes qui paroissent au corps de celuy qui est attaqué de la troisiéme espece de Vérole, procede de ce que le venin de cette maladie ce communique successivement au Foye par les Veines, au Cœur par les Arteres, et au Cerveau par les Nerfs; et ce qui fait que ces pustules paroissent plûtost à la Teste qu'és autre parties, provient de ce que le venin estant fort subtil, recherche plûtost les esprits que la masse de la chair; et comme dans le cerveau il y a plus d'esprits que dans les autres parties du corps, et qu'il est d'une substance plus humide et moins chaude, il reçoit bien plûtost les impressions de la malignité du venin.

Decidedly Molière exaggerated in nothing.

The author then describes the indurated chancre under the name of *schyrre* [scirrhus], and shares in the error of his contemporaries in the sense that he makes *clap* one of the initial symptoms of syphilis.

But some thanks are due to him for having noticed that gonorrhœa was not always followed by secondary symptoms. And he takes care to state that one must be guarded against *treating as Poxy* (*traiter en Verolez*) those who only have a simple clap. However, by the side of this observation, which he was one of the first to make, we see the astral conjunctions re-appear. It is in connection with nocturnal headache that he gives us this disillusion. He might have been thought in advance of his times: well! not at all. In a chapter entitled "The Reason Why the Syphilitic Humor Emits Itself at Night and Ceases in the Day,"[1] he assumes that the night engenders bad influences by means of the *stars* and of the *shadow of the earth*: it follows that the *malignant exhalations of the earth* are attracted by the body of man, which puts the *humor* in motion, etc. Farther on he declares that those who acquire syphilis on the *day of Venus* are more affected than the others, and that one must not be treated on the *day of Saturn*. There is no use talking. Science was still in the midst of the Dark Ages.

De la Martinière concludes in these words:—

"The seed has taken birth everywhere, to such an extent that at present it is called the *joyful disease*, the which was formerly named the *disease of Naples*."

> Cette graine a prîs naissance partout, tellement qu'à-present on l'appelle le *mal joyeux*, lequel autrefois se nommait le *mal de Naples*.

Was it not rather the circumstances in which the disease was taken which were joyful? If not the expression might be considered as ironical, for it seems credible that if the patients laughed it was on the other side of the mouth.

[1] La raison pourquoy l'humeur vérolique s'esmeut le soir et cesse le jour.

In 1673, an English author, Maynwaringe,[1] wrote the history of the question of origin. He is of the opinion that this disease is the result of venereal excesses—an opinion which had been already advanced before him, and notably by Arelius Minadoüs[2]—and he adds: "That Venery thereof being antique, the product Lues we may well judge antique also."

The Dutchman, Stephen Blankard, equally treated of, a little later (1684), the question of the origin of syphilis.[3] According to him, the disease has been known from the most ancient times and treated under other names. But Blankard still admitted the usefulness of mercurial salivation,—a thing of which we cannot approve.

Le Monnier (1689),[4] like his predecessors, advises salivation as a therapeutic measure, and classes gonorrhœa among the primary symptoms of syphilis. He recognizes the fact that the disease is very contagious and that a simple contact (infected glass) outside of coitus is sufficient. He adds that it may also be taken " . . . without congress, in sleeping with a luetic subject, . . . which may occur even by the vapor which arises from the bed and sheets in which he has rested."

> . . . san le congrez, en couchant avec un sujet vérolé, . . . ce qui peut se faire même par la vapeur qui s'élève du lit et des draps dans lesquels il a reposé.

This last explanation is more than debatable, but it is an improvement on the theory of contagion by the

[1] The History and Mystery of the Venereal Lues. London, 1673.

[2] De virulentia venerea. Venetiis, 1596. On the Venereal Poison. Venice, 1596.

[3] Traité de la vérole (Treatise on Syphilis). Translated from the Dutch by William Willis. Amsterdam, 1688.

[4] Nouveau traité de la maladie vénéreenne. Paris, 1689. New Treatise on the Venereal Disease.

air. Then, attacking the question of origin, he defends an opinion, which is odd enough, which he states having found in several authors, but whose names he does not mention. According to these authors, a perfectly healthy woman might observe syphilis arise in her from the fact of having submitted herself to several men in a short space of time, even supposing her partners perfectly healthy. It is the theory of the *fermentation of the seeds.* The explanations furnished by le Monnier have all the more relish, as it is felt that he is convinced:—

"It may happen that a healthy woman be surprised with it, when, at the same time, she has had commerce with several men, although healthy ones, because the different qualities which compose the different seeds she has received, joined to the acrid and salty parts of which her own is composed and to the moist and very warm disposition of the place which receives them, much increased by the continuation of the rubbing or confrication, excite, in their mingling, so rapid a movement, so violent an irritation, and a *fermentation* so prompt, that they subsequently change themselves to corruption, which is the more pernicious as these kinds of matters are subtile and charged with a great number of spirits: *corruptio optimi solet esse pessima.*"[1]

Il peut se faire qu'une femme saine en soit surprise, quand en même temps elle a eu commerce avec plusieurs hommes, quoy que sains, parce que les différentes qualitez qui composent les différentes semences qu'elle a reçûës, jointes aux parties acres et salines dont la sienne est composée, et à la disposition humide et fort chaude du lieu qui les reçoit, augmentée de beaucoup par la continuation du frotement ou confrication, excitent à leur rencontre un mouvement si rapide, une irritation si violente et une fermentation si prompte qu'elles se

[1] The corruption of that which is the best generally produces that which is the worst.

déterminent ensuite à la corruption, qui est d'autant plus pernicieuse que ces sortes de matières sont subtiles et chargées d'un grand nombre d'esprits : *corruptio optimi solet esse pessima.*

This thesis has been maintained since by Ucay, Nicholas de Blégny, de Saint-Romain, Vercelloni, Dibon, Jourdan de Pellerin, and some others.

Le Monnier then advances a correct idea, which we have not found in any other author before him. He admits that a healthy woman, having had recent relations with an infected individual, may transmit the virus to one or more others without being herself contaminated. It is mediate contagion. Besides, he finds the manner of seeing of his predecessors defective, in that they recognized four species of syphilis. He brings back the virus to one single type; he suspected, without clearly saying so, that the soil alone caused the differences in the intensity of the manifestations.

"It must be admitted that this cause is everywhere the same; that there is nothing more than the more or less of venereal virus which has made a larger or smaller progress in the mass of the humors and in the parts, which makes its effects and its different characters."

On doit convenir que cette cause est partout la même, qu'il n'y a que le plus ou moins de virus venerien qui a fait un plus grand ou moindre progrez dans la masse des humeurs et dans les parties, qui fait ces effets et ces differens caracteres.

For him gonorrhœa and buboes are the signs of syphilis; but he calls attention to the fact that genital ulcers are not all alike, and he distinguishes three kinds. The first, which corresponds to our herpes, he calls "a small, whitish blister, which ulcerates and enlarges, but which also heals easily in a short time."

. . . une petite vescie blanchâtre, qui s'ulcere et qui s'élargit, mais aussi qui se guerit facilement en peu de temps.

The second he calls *œil-de-perdrix* (soft-corn), according to the expression prevalent, because "of its roundness and of a slight redness and whiteness which occurs in its middle." This appears to be the primary lesion of syphilis. As to the description of the third kind, it can only be referred to the soft chancre and to the phagedenic chancre, which are non-infecting. "It eats, spreads, and causes an eschar; the color of the ulcer becomes livid, its shape irregular, the edges callous and everted; the inflammation which surrounds it is great; the matter which it suppurates melts and rots the flesh and the neighboring parts."

Il ronge, ambule et fait exare; la couleur de l'ulcere devient livide, sa figure inégale, les lèvres calleuses et renversées, l'inflammation qui l'environne est grande, la matière qu'il suppure dissout et pourrit les chairs et les parties voisines.

He advises salivation by means of inunctions or mercurial pills, concurrently with purging, bleeding, and baths. However, he does not approve the cauterizations, which were in common use at that time, by the aid of acids (sulphuric or nitric), for they produced eschars and, as a result, losses of substance, which were not always easy to cure.

Lopez Pinna[1] (1696), who declares himself a partisan of the antiquity of syphilis, recognizes as its source venereal excesses.

Gervais Ucay (1699)[2] says that syphilis is almost as old as the world, for it has as its origin the corruption of several seeds in the same vagina. For him the fact is beyond doubt, and all other hypotheses are ridiculous.

[1] Tratado de morbo galico. Sevilla, 1696. Treatise on the French Disease. Seville, 1696.

[2] Traité de la maladie vénér. Amsterdam, 1699. Treatise on the Venereal Disease.

"The cause of syphilis may be plainly explained by means of corrupted seeds in the wombs of public women. . . .

"It is well known that, if a perfectly-healthy girl—and a virgin, if you will, in order that there may be no suspicion of any venereal disease—mingled with a dozen lads as healthy as she, and debauched herself with each one in turn, either some or others would soon have the pox, and all together would finally acquire it by the repetition of the venereal acts."

On peut expliquer clairement la cause de la vérole par le moyen des semences corrompues dans les matrices des femmes publiques. . . .

On sçait que si une fille parfaitement saine et pucelle, si on veut, afin qu'il n'y ait aucun soupçon de mal venerien, se mêloit parmi une douzaine de garçons aussi sains qu'elle, et se débauchoit tour à tour avec eux, ou les uns ou les autres auroient bientôt la vérole, et tous ensemble la contracteroient enfin par la repetition des actes veneriens.

In the same manner as Thierry de Héry, Fernel, le Monnier, and others, he admits for syphilis an incubation of ten years and more; and thus, like his predecessors, he considers as syphilitic all sexual diseases. Let us not forget that, at that time, there still existed physicians who did not hesitate to state that syphilis was the "totality of all diseases." And we hasten to testify to the fact that G. Ucay made a real progress when he declared that certain chancres and buboes and some gonorrhœas were purely local diseases. To tell the truth, he leaves them their name of *pox*, since he believed in the identity of the virus, but he establishes quite distinct forms:—

"There is, nevertheless, an accidental difference, which consists in that the great Pox generally invades the entire body, because the mass of the blood is infected; that is why it may be called *universal;* and that clap, chancre, and the bubo occupy but a single part, either because the syphilitic ferment has not been carried farther since it was communicated, or it has been expelled by the force of nature, by means of imperfect crisis, as is seen in buboes, or, in fine, by some other accident; and it is for this reason that it may be called a *particular* Pox."

Il y a pourtant une difference accidentelle qui consiste en ce que la grosse Vérole occupe généralement tout le corps, à cause que la masse du sang est infectée; c'est pourquoi on la peut appeler *universelle;* et que la Chaude-pisse, le Chancre, et le Bubon n'occupent qu'une seule partie, soit parce que le ferment vérolique n'a pas été porté plus loin, depuis qu'il a été communiqué, soit qu'il ait été expulsé par la force de la nature, par manière de crise imparfaite, comme on voit dans les Bubons, ou enfin par quelque autre accident, et c'est pour cela qu'on peut appeler cette Vérole *particulière.*

The author looks upon mercury as the only specific. At all events, he spared children and the aged from salivation; in a general way, he treated patients according to indications, and not by the rules of a blind theory. He advises, for instance, to bleed only plethoric persons. He also looked upon syphilis as a very ancient disease. As to the different ways of contracting the disease, he enumerated three,—heredity, coitus, and contact,—which make two altogether, the second variety being included in the third. He had noticed, besides, that the patients who succumbed were carried off by late complications, by consecutive changes of essential organs, and not by the syphilitic virus itself:—

"Pox is not ordinarily a mortal disease; people are seen who have carried it thirty years and more; and, when one dies of it, it is not so much by this disease as it is by others which are attracted by the disturbance caused by the syphilitic ferment."

La Vérole n'est pas ordinairement une maladie mortelle, on voit des gens qui la portent trente ans, et davantage; et lors qu'on en meurt, ce n'est pas tant par cette maladie que par d'autres qui sont attirées par le désordre que fait le ferment Vérolique.

But these correct ideas do not go without some fantastic theories. It is thus that, surprised at seeing, among several men having had relations with the same woman, here a chancre, there a gonorrhœa, and nothing in the others, he enters into explanations, which are quite original, in which the *prostates* and the *parstates* play a very important part. Then he asks himself why some of his predecessors have looked for the cause of syphilis in the conjunctions of Jupiter, Mars, Saturn, Venus, Mercury, etc., and he shoots several shafts of humor at them:—

"No doubt the origin of these opinions comes from the old fable, in which we see, among those pretended divinities, a large number of adulteries, rapes, and amorous passions; and, as the stars bear the names of these gods, they believed that there occurred among these stars some prostitution. I do not know why it has not been said that they themselves take the pox, and that they subsequently communicate it to men by their influences, since one is the consequence of the other."

Sans doute que la source de ces opinions vient de l'ancienne fable, ou lon voit, parmi ces prétenduës Divinitez un grand nombre d'adulteres, de viols, et de passions amoureuses: et comme les Astres portent les noms de ces Dieux, ils auront crû qu'il se passoit parmi ces Astres quelques maquerellages. Je ne sçai pourquoi l'on n'a pas dit qu'ils prenoient eux-mêmes la Vérole, et qu'ensuite ils la communiquoint aux hommes par leur influences, puisque l'un est la suite de l'autre.

With a few judicious observations on venereal pathology, which we have noticed above, Ucay completes, with honor, the list of writers of note of the seventeenth century.

CHAPTER III.

IN THE EIGHTEENTH CENTURY.

Sydenham and Boerhaave exhume the fable of the American origin; Astruc consecrates that legend.—*Larvated syphilis* and the *mercurial disease*.—Baron Van Swieten; his liquor.—Swediaur launches the word *blennorrhagia*.—Hunter describes the *hard chancre*.—Bell defends the doctrine of the non-identity of the two viruses, gonorrhœal and syphilitic.—The therapeutic value of salivation is denied by the majority of authors; pretended immunity of pipe-smokers in regard to mercurial stomatitis.

THE first writer of the eighteenth century worthy of mention is Jacques Vercelloni,[1] of Ast, in Piedmont. He maintains, in 1722, about the same theses as G. Ucay, and shares the opinions of the latter on many points. He adopts the theory of *fermentation of the seeds*, advises guaiac, sarsaparilla, and sassafras, and is a partisan of mercurial therapeutics; but he finds that salivation is a means which is of "small reliability." Finally, in this work, there is made mention of the *speculum matricis*, of which preceding authors say but little. At all events, Ambrose Paré (1575) has described a *speculum magnum*, which is nothing else than the *dioptrus* of Paulus Ægineta (sixth century),—that is to say, a dilator of the vagina which permits an examination of the deep parts. Let us not forget, also, that an identical instrument was found in the ruins of Pompeii, about 1819.

In 1728 appeared the work of the Dutchman, Boer-

[1] Traité des maladies qui arrivent aux parties génitales des deux sexes. Paris, 1730. Treatise on the Diseases Affecting the Genitals of Both Sexes. Translated in French by Devaux, from the Latin edition of Leyden.

haave[1], a distinguished physician of that time of whom we have already spoken: in it we see shadowing forth some differences of opinion from contemporaries and predecessors. The author, for instance, states that gonorrhœa, which up to that time had almost always been a symptom of syphilis, rarely occurs in connection with it at the time in which he writes. From this he concludes that the symptomatology of syphilis has been modified in a marked manner. To believe him, clap would even be a sort of vaccination against the great pox:—

"On the contrary (which ought to console those who have none but similar gallantries) it is almost always the preservative."

Au contraire (ce qui doit consoler ceux qui n'ont que de pareilles galanteries) elle en est presque toujours le préservatif.

Happy times! In the nineteenth century one does not prevent the other.

He laughs at Vercelloni—and with reason—who explains syphilitic ulcerations of the throat, in woman, by a sort of sympathy existing between the womb and the gullet. But he does not do much better than the Italian author when he assumes that the patients acquired more "*poison*" as they displayed more passion in coitus, and that because of the heat developed during the act:—

"The fire of love is a true inflammation of the entire body, and principally of the genital parts, in which it seems to concentrate itself."

Le feu de l'amour est une vraye inflammation de tout le corps, et principalement des parties génitales, ou il semble se concentrer.

Perhaps he was wrong in ridiculing so much the system of the *worms* and *animalcules* of the venereal

[1] Hermann Boerhaave. Sur les maladies vénéréennes. Paris, 1735. On Venereal Diseases. Translated from the Latin by de la Mettrie.

virus which Deidier and Desault had just advanced, for they seem to have had a presentiment of the microbe.

However, coming to the question of origin, Boerhaave adopts the opinion of Sydenham,—to wit, that if syphilis were brought to Europe by the companions of Columbus (as a matter of fact it comes from Africa), it had been introduced on the New Continent by slaves from the coast of Guinea. Sydenham and Boerhaave did not consider the fact that African negroes were not sent into slavery in the New World until long after the epidemic of Naples and the voyages of Columbus. The syphilitic virus had not much need, it will be admitted, of passing by the Antilles to return to Europe, the only part of the world pretended to be spared up to that time. It was much easier for it to follow the coast of Africa and to pass in by Gibraltar or Brindisi.

But Boerhaave has his own idea; for him syphilis is endemic among negroes; and, to sustain his dictum, he calls in the authority of one Bosman. At best, he does not notice that the facts reported by that author are nothing else than arguments in favor of the theory of the *fermentation of seeds*,—an opinion which he, himself, vigorously rejected at the very beginning of his work. He says, as a matter of fact, that he does not admit, like his predecessors, that syphilis could arise "from the congress of several healthy men with a healthy woman." And it is precisely on a case of this sort that Bosman[1] bases himself. This latter author relates that he has seen vagabonds—of which the number is occasionally considerable—buy a girl, whom they ravished one after the other. Most often she died in the course of the operation, in view of the number

[1] William Bosman, Lettres, 8 and 12. Description of the Coast of Guinea.

of her assailants, and those who had not had their share *continued with the dead body.* This, for Bosman, is the origin of syphilis, and Boerhaave does not express the shadow of a doubt in regard to the matter.

Dibon,[1] two years later, determines that gonorrhœa is never or very rarely cured by the use of mercury. To-day we understand the reason, but the author himself was astonished at it. He advised "aperitive and cooling teas" (*les Ptisanes apéritives et refraîchissantes*), emulsions, tinctures, turpentine; and, as a local treatment of the chancres, cauterizations with nitric acid, with nitrate of silver, and dressings with red precipitate. Internally, he gave mercury in the form of pills; it was necessary, he said, that the mercury be well prepared and properly administered.

That famous preparation, of which he speaks so much, is chemically-pure mercury,—that is to say, freed of lead, arsenic, and other substances it might contain. He had obtained his secret from a certain chemist, somewhat of a physician at opportunities, who treated syphilitics and cured them. This empiric rose up against the practice of salivation, which he looked upon as disastrous,—one good point for the chemist. The following are the circumstances under which the author was brought to ask his help:—

Having heard of the successes which the healer obtained with his drug, he came to him offering to bring him a rich merchant, from among his patients, who was not improved by the ordinary means. The learned man preferred to disclose the remedy and refused all payment, adding, however, that if the merchant, since he had property, desired to show himself grateful, he would

[1] Dissertation sur les maladies vénériennes. Paris, 1724. Dissertation on Venereal Diseases.

not oppose him. Dibon assured him that his patient would not fail to do so, for he looked upon him as a very honest man. The chemist, who had learned to know the human heart, expressed his doubts. "He answered me that they were all honest people when they were ill, but, once cured, they were no longer the same."

Il me répondit qu'ils etoient tous d'honnestes gens lorsqu'ils étoient malades, mais que guéris, ce n'etoit plus de même.

This is a remark which promises to hold good for a long time to come.

In the second part of his work, published in the succeeding year,[1] the author repeats about the same things which have been said before him. Like Ucay, he distinguishes two kinds of syphilis. By *particular pox* he understands all the sexual local lesions, including the bubo. He says that the name may change according to the seat of the genital affection, but it is always the pox. "It will bear the name of clap in the discharge which occurs from the penis or vagina."

Elle portera le nom de chaude-pisse dans l'écoulement qui arrive à la verge ou au vagin.

General pox (la vérole générale)—which G. Ucay called *universal*—is that which extends to all portions of the body. He also admits incubation of several years. It is probable that this error arose from the fact that some patients really contracted syphilis a long time after a gonorrhœa. The secondary lesions appearing, for example, eight or ten years after the gonorrhœa—then looked upon as syphilitic—must inevitably have given rise to fatal interpretations. Dibon is of the opinion that syphilis is as ancient as the world; he adds

[1] Descript. de la nature et des causes des malad. vénér. Paris, 1725. Description of the Nature and Causes of Venereal Diseases.

that it may arise from venereal excesses, "*especially when there is a mingling of several seeds.*"[1] For him it was ancient leprosy.

P. Desault (1733) rejects mercurial salivation, for he does not admit that it is the "*flux from the mouth*" alone which cures. Although he agrees in this with Fernel, he does not share in the horror of that physician for mercury.

"Fernel and his disciple, Palmarius, celebrated physicians of the Faculty of Paris, deterred by the cruelty of the treatment of syphilis by the flux of the mouth, endeavored to cure it without producing it; they adopted the plan of renouncing mercury, and of saying as much evil of it as we shall praise it."

Fernel et son disciple, Palmarius, celebres Medecins de la Faculté de Paris, rebutez de la cruauté du traitement de la Vérole par le flux de bouche, tenterent de la guerir sans le procurer; ils prirent le parti de renoncer au mercure, et d'en dire autant de mal que nous en ferons d'éloges.

As we have seen (vol. ii, chapter vi), he was one of the promoters of the *system of worms.* This proves only one thing,—that these two diseases have, at all times, given rise to errors in diagnosis.

Janson,[2] who writes in 1740, draws a terrifying picture of syphilis and describes as current symptoms of the disease the grave and happily exceptional manifestations. He looks upon syphilis as very ancient and as the result of venereal excesses; then he gives curious explanations on the nature and progress of the virus:—

"Syphilis is composed of molecules whose nature is

[1] ". . . *surtout lorsqu'il se fait conjonction de plusieurs semences.*" Dissertation sur les malad. vénér. Paris, 1733. Dissertation on Venereal Diseases.

[2] Tableau des malad. vénér. Amsterdam, 1740. Picture of Venereal Diseases.

tartareous, inclining to the acrid, and so penetrating that it inserts itself in the pores of the skin, and, passing thence into the substances composing us, manifests itself more often on the genital parts of both sexes than elsewhere."

La Vérole est composée de Molecules dont la nature est tartareuse, tirant sur l'aigre, et si pénétrante qu'elle s'insère dans les pores de la peau, et de la passant dans les substances qui nous composent, se manifeste plus souvent aux Parties génitales des deux Sexes qu'ailleurs.

Farther on he again states that the syphilitic virus consists "in a tartareous acid, participating of the acrid, and tending to the coagulation of the blood and of the humors."

. . . dans un acide tartareux, participant de l'aigre, et tendant à la coagulation du sang et des humeurs.

The author, no doubt, thinks highly of this explanation, for he recurs to it to satiety. It may not be superfluous to recall the fact that, at the time Janson wrote, Molière[1] had been buried more than sixty years!

That same year, 1740, is memorable in the annals of science, for it witnessed the appearance of the work of the celebrated Astruc,[2] of whom we have spoken time and time again. This work had such fame throughout all Europe that we cannot refrain from dwelling upon it for a short period of time. In order that the reader may be able to obtain a clear idea of the effect produced by this work, we will condense in a few lines the different scientific opinions which have been given out in regard to the origin of syphilis since the epidemic of Naples.

As was shown and could be proven, the opinions, at

[1] Molière died in 1673, at the age of 51 years.

[2] De morbis venereis. Lutetiæ Parisiorum, 1740. On Venereal Diseases.

the end of the fifteenth century, were at first quite different. The astrologers saw in this epidemic a new disease attributable to the maleficent conjunctions of the planets; a few physicians made of it the resultant of telluric miasmata, and each nation accused its enemy of having brought the scourge. The public and certain physicians, when the epidemic had diminished,—that is to say, when it had been freed of heterogeneous elements,—simply saw in it the contamination of the eternal *leprosy.*[1] Others believed in a transformation of the latter disease. In 1518 the noise traveled that the disease came from America. Oviédo took up the fable, which was useful to him, and gave it an aftermath of fact. But, at the end of twenty-five or thirty years, like guaiac, which had given birth to it, it fell in the most complete forgetfulness. In the second half of the fifteenth century we come to mercury, and the *French disease* is called the *venereal disease:* the question of its origin is discussed but very little, and there is hardly one or two authors who mention, as a memorandum, the New Continent.

During the entire course of the seventeenth century there is, so to speak, no more mention of the *French disease* or of the *disease of Naples;* the *venereal disease* even begins to be called *pox* (vérole) toward the year 1660, authors once more bringing forward the question of origin, and almost all making of it an ancient disease continuing leprosy or derived from it. Toward the end of the seventeenth century a new theory makes its appearance: syphilis created with all its parts, without contagion, by the fermentation of several seeds in the

[1] There are some to-day even who pretend that leprosy is simply a modification of syphilis or *vice versâ*, despite the fact that both diseases are observed affecting the same individual, syphilis being engrafted upon a leper.—O-D.

same vagina. Authors admit that libertinage and venereal excesses may produce it, and they proclaim the antiquity of syphilis. These theories are taken up and repeated by all the authors during the entire first half of the eighteenth century, and it is the opinion favorable to the antiquity of syphilis which dominates at the time in which the celebrated Astruc writes.

This physician undertook to resuscitate the legend of the American origin, and displayed, in that task, a patience and an activity incredible in quantity for an epoch in which researches must have been much more laborious than in our days. Whilst incomplete and presenting arguments most often defective and wanting from the very foundation, this work is, none the less, the most remarkable which the eighteenth century presents to us on this matter. The author was certainly acting in good faith; but, carried away undoubtedly by his belief, he has permitted several *naïvetés*—not to say more—to escape him each time that he has found himself confronted by documents too unfavorable to his cause.

Taking one by one the texts upon which his predecessors had supported themselves, he has compelled himself to demonstrate that passages aimed at had reference to I know not what fantastic disease, having all the symptoms of syphilis, plainly contagious, but which has disappeared at the siege of Naples. We will certainly not seek here to retort to the arguments advanced by Astruc, for it would be necessary to write a work longer than his, which would be undoubtedly in bad taste and without any practical utility. Nevertheless, we would advise the reader, who is desirous of obtaining more light upon this burning question, to read, before arriving at any conclusions, the "De morbis venereis." He can compare his argumentation with ours, and may perhaps thus arrive at a positive opinion.

However this may be, Astruc acquired a fame which was almost universal. Practicing physicians not having the time to verify the dicta of those who write big books, almost all the disciples of Æsculapius believed Astruc on his word and followed him in their writings like so many sheep of Panurge. As Jourdan says, in 1826, "his historical romance on syphilis succeeds and soon counted as many partisans as it had readers." From the faculty the American legend came back to the public, where it still remains. And, as nothing is harder to destroy than a legend, there will be many sunny days to come for this fairy-tale.

It was especially about this time (middle of the eighteenth century) that the doctrine of *disguised venereal diseases* flourished. All the unusual morbid phenomena which could not be explained at that time were attributed to a concealed venereal disease,—that is to say, without venereal symptoms. It is thus that Furstenan[1] went so far as to place hysterical phenomena to the credit of a venereal virus *driven back in the body* by a badly-directed treatment! But it was especially Rosen (1764) who made himself the apostle of this doctrine. For instance, he accepted as hereditary some symptoms of recent syphilis in two patients aged 30 years. Van Swieten, in refusing to admit the heredity of syphilis, momentarily checked this theory, but Stoll restored it to its place of honor and Fabre was one of his warmest partisans.

It was then that war was again waged on mercury, and they went so far as to assert, Ritter among others

[1] Dissertatio de contagio et morbis contagiosis. Rintelæ, 1742. Dissertation on Contagion and Contagious Diseases.

(1747), that the dangerous symptoms of syphilis were more the effect of the treatment than those of the disease itself. In fact, a *mercurial disease* was accepted, distinct from the venereal disease, and to whose account was charged almost all the classic signs of syphilis.

However, it was toward 1743 that the Dutch baron, Van Swieten, made himself a name in syphilography by means of the liquor of his composition, which is yet in current use in practice. He thus popularized the employment of corrosive sublimate. The present formula differs slightly from that of the author, but the principle is exactly the same, as may be seen by comparing the two, which are given below:—

LIQUOR EMPLOYED BY VAN SWIETEN.	LIQUOR OF VAN SWIETEN OF THE "CODEX."
℞ Hydrarg. bichlor., 0.80 gr.	℞ Hydrarg. bichlor., 1 gr.
Spts. frumenti, 1.00 kilogr.	Spts. vini rectificat., 100 grs.
M. Sig.: Two spoonfuls a day.	Aquæ destillat., 900 grs.
	M. Sig.: A tablespoonful a day.

At this time we begin to find a certain number of authors opposed to salivation. It is with sole reference to this that we will mention Guisard,[1] who was, notwithstanding, an antimercurialist who felt convinced. He was wrong in this respect, that he fettered elimination as much as possible; but one must not be too exacting in regard to the physicians of the nineteenth century.

"The true way of reaping the benefit of the cure of venereal diseases consists in making mercury roll about a long time in the body, and to keep away everything which might drive it away too fast. And it is with this object in view that an effort is made to prevent the mouth-flux, almost as much as is studied the prevention

[1] Dissertation pratique sur les maux vénér, 1743. Practical Dissertation on Venereal Diseases.

of diarrhœa, in the conviction which prevails that evacuations of such a nature will scarcely ever fail to bring the enterprise to naught."

Le vrai moyen de tirer parti de la cure des maladies vénériennes consiste à faire rouler long-tems le mercure dans le corps, et à eloigner tout ce qui pourroit le chasser trop vite. Aussi est-ce dans cette vûe qu'on tâche de prévenir le flux de bouche, presque qu'autant qu'on s'étudie à détourner la diarrhée, dans la persuasion on l'on est que des évacuations de cette nature ne manqueroient jamais de faire échouer l'entreprise.

Jourdan de Pellerin[1] is one hundred and fifty years behind the times, for he again brings forward the question of astral conjunctions, of which no more was said since the end of the sixteenth century. De la Martinière is, as a matter of fact, about the only one, in a space of two hundred years, who exhumed that theory, already dead of old age. At all events, Jourdan de Pellerin does not say that syphilis had been directly engendered by the meeting of planets ; he merely considers these latter as capable of favoring the extension of the disease. But it is even too much for a contemporary of Voltaire and of J. J. Rousseau. "I will merely say that this malign influence could only be looked upon as a partial cause and of occasional occurrence, inasmuch as it facilitates and increases the fermentation."

Je dirai seulement qu'on ne pourroit regarder cette maligne influence que comme une cause partielle et occasionelle, en tant qu'elle facilite et augmente la fermentation.

He also admits that venereal excesses may suffice to produce syphilis. "It may arise in two healthy persons who, in their congress, may not place limits to their voluptuous sensuality and who may outrage nature."

[1] Traité sur les maladies vénériennes. Paris, 1749. Treatise on Venereal Diseases.

Elle peut survenir chez deux personnes saines qui, dans leur congrés, ne donneront point de bornes à leurs voluptés sensuelles et qui outreront la nature.

In addition he adopts the theory of the *fermentation of seeds*, and, always very little of a progressive turn, he advises the *essence of viper*, recommended by Aquilanus, Cataneus, Matthiole, and others, more than two hundred years before. But let us give him credit for not having blindly adopted the conclusions of Astruc, and for having declared himself a partisan of the antiquity of syphilis.

In 1752, an anonymous author,[1] who is no other than Sanchéz, caused to appear an opuscule intended to refute the opinion of the American origin defended by Astruc. The author takes pains to demonstrate that the disease began in Europe by an epidemic, and he bases himself upon the authority of contemporaries such as Fulgose, Cumanus, Bourdigné, Fracastor, and others.

In 1758 Fabre[2] lays before us the doctrine of his master, J. L. Petit. As we have already said, he maintains the thesis of *larvated syphilis*, without prejudice to a large number of other heresies which we shall have occasion to take up. We read, for instance, in regard to a certain particular case, this astonishing sentence: "The discharge of old gonorrhœas renewed itself through the effect of mercury, *as this sometimes happens*."

L'écoulement des anciennes gonorrhées se renouvella par l'effet du mercure, *comme cela arrive quelquefois*.

This is not all. A little farther on, among the hereditary accidents of syphilis, he includes *scurvy*. He makes of *gangrene*, *cancer*, *ovarian tumors*, *hydatids*,

[1] Dissertat. sur l'origine de la malad. vénér. Paris, 1752. Dissertation on the Origin of Venereal Disease.

[2] Essai sur les malad. vénér. Paris, 1758. Essay on Venereal Diseases.

etc., symptoms of syphilis. It goes without saying that gonorrhœa and vegetations are, for him, classical signs.

The author treats by means of mercurial inunctions, which he employs to the point of salivation, without which, according to him, the remedy is robbed of "the principal efficacy which makes a specific against the pox"; it is by the *mouth-flux* that quicksilver expels the "luetic leaven."

Jauberthou,[1] who writes in 1766, does not share in the view of Fabre. Whilst being a mercurialist, he clearly states that salivation is harmful.

We have stated that mercury was again decried about the middle of the eighteenth century. It was on account of certain medical pretenders who, seeing nothing in the treatment of venereal diseases but a pretence to make money, administered it at random. At that time, says Follin, syphilis was exploited by a cloud of charlatans, all physicians to the king, with pensions,—Daran, Armand, Goulard, Keyser, Bellet, and others. With the exception of the king's pension—which has ceased, from the lack of a king—I am not aware that these unscrupulous persons have disappeared to-day, or even that their number has perceptibly diminished.

It was about this time that the first medicated bougies made their appearance. Solid sounds, of wax, otherwise called *bougies*,[2] were already known. There followed emollient, then melting bougies, which were introduced into the bladder, and which were left *in situ*. Thion de la Chaume[3] informs us that a surgeon

[1] Traité des maladies vénériennes. Paris, 1766. Treatise on Venereal Diseases.

[2] In French *bougie* signifies a wax candle or taper. As the urethral sounds were made of wax at the beginning, the name which is now employed was applied to them and has continued to the present day.—O-D.

[3] Tableau des malad. vénér. Paris, 1773. Picture of Venereal Diseases.

of Paris, Haran, introduced melting bougies of his make, which were much in vogue, and enriched the inventor. A princess of the House of France, having heard him spoken of, one day inquired of M. de Bièvre as to what constituted the specialty of this surgeon. It was a difficult thing to explain; but the courtier extricated himself out of the difficulty in a very witty manner. "Madame," said he, "he is a man who wishes to make us believe that bladders are lanterns."[1]

De Cézan,[2] in 1774, still defends the theory of the *fermentation of seeds;* his work contains, in addition, a few bits of information which we give as a matter of curiosity:—

"A physician of the name of M. le Duc, who has traveled in the Levant, states that at Smyrna the women are in the habit of taking two drachms of running mercury every day, to become fat and fresh and to give themselves nice natural colors."

Un médecin, nommé M. le Duc, qui a fait le voyage du Levant, dit qu'à Smirne, les femmes son dans l'usage de prendre deux gros de mercure coulant tous les jours, pour devenir grasses et fraîches, et pour se donner des belles couleur naturelles.

This is an assertion which cannot be accepted except under benefit of inventory. The author then brings up once more the question of the *crystalline*, which he looks upon as an affection peculiar to pederasts. "There are small pimples filled with a whitish matter and hard, whence comes the name of *crystals;* they crown the anus."

[1] *Faire croire que les vessies sont des lanternes* is a French expression equivalent to "pulling the wool over one's eyes." The literal translation as given above shows the wit of the courtier, since the surgeon introduced *bougies* (wax candles) into the bladder just as candles were formerly placed in lanterns. The ingenuity of the answer is certainly admirable.—O-D.

[2] Manuel antisyphilitique. Londres, 1774. Antisyphilitic Hand-book. London, 1774.

Ce sont des petits boutons remplis d'une matière blanche et dure, d'où leur vient le nom de Cristalins ; ils couronnent l'anus.

Among the authors of that time who have drawn a good picture of venereal diseases we will mention Schwediaver, more generally called Swediaur,[1]—a name which he himself adopted to render its pronunciation easier for the French, as he says. He rejected the idea of infection by the air and by bed-sheets, although the latter mode of contagion, no doubt quite rare, may occur as a possibility; it would certainly not be prudent to place an excoriation in direct contact with clothes soiled by syphilitic products. Swediaur does not admit hereditary syphilis; for him syphilis is directly acquired by the child at the time of its passage to the vulva; and he bases himself upon the fact that symptoms are seldom produced before the second month of extra-uterine life. It was Swediaur who created the word *gonorrhœa* (blennorrhagia); clap had, from that time on, a definite scientific name.

In 1786 there appeared in London a work which eclipsed all the preceding ones; it was that of John Hunter,[2] whose works are still justly celebrated. The English surgeon brought up a multitude of new questions and clearly established that the induration of the chancre was the pathognomonic symptom of syphilis; the indurated chancre is still sometimes designated in our day under the name of *Hunterian chancre.* To tell the truth, Fallopius, Ambrose Paré, in the latter half of the sixteenth century, and Nicholas de Blégny, a hundred years later (1673), had observed the hardness and callosity of syphilitic ulcers at the beginning of infection;

[1] Practical Observations on Venereal Complaints. Edinburgh, 1784. [*Conf.* A Practical Treatise on the Symptoms, Effects, Nature, and Treatment of Syphilis. Philadelphia, 1815.—O-D.]

[2] A Treatise on the Venereal Disease. London, 1786.

but Hunter had the credit of describing the indurated chancre and of classifying it in a positive manner. However, he committed grave errors. It is thus that he denied the contagiousness of secondary lesions; but it must be said that all his experimental inoculations were made on syphilitic subjects. The bold inventor cauterized the chancre with the object of preventing general infection.

Hunter still believed in the specific nature of gonorrhœa, although Tode,[1] a Danish physician, had already, twelve years before, denied the possibility of the infection by the clap. But it was especially Benjamin Bell[2] who defended the doctrine of the non-identity of the chancre and gonorrhœa. At all events, Bell did not conceal the fact that his opinion would be opposed; he says so in his book, which he wrote more especially to demonstrate that gonorrhœa and syphilis are derived from two different viruses, which essentially differ in their nature. At that time such a theory could not but be considered, in learned quarters, as nothing short of an enormity.

A contemporary, of the name of Lombard,[3] opposes salivation, and in this regard he brings forward a rather original observation which he had frequently made, but which no one, for a century, seems to have made a note of. "I have observed that pretty generally the use of the pipe was, for those who are addicted to it, a preservative against mercurial salivation; this may be found very extraordinary, but it is none the less true."

[1] Vom Tripper in Ansehung seiner Natur. Copenhagen, 1774. Concerning Gonorrhœa Respecting its Nature.

[2] A Treatise on Gonorrhœa Virulenta and Lues Venerea. Edinburgh, 1793.

[3] Cours de Chirurgie pratique sur les malad. vénér. Strasbourg, 1790. Text-book of Practical Surgery on Venereal Diseases.

J'ai observé qu'assez généralement l'usage de la pipe étoit pour ceux qui en ont l'habitude, un préservatif contre la salivatîon mercurielle; on peut trouver cela fort extraordinaire, mais il n'en est pas moins vrai.

We leave to the author the monopoly of this stillborn discovery, and we will continue, until further orders, to prescribe chlorate of potassium—in preference to tobacco—at such times as we may have reason to fear a mercurial stomatitis.

Thus ends the eighteenth century, whose scientific balance-sheet may be summarized, as regards the subject occupying our attention, into two main events:—

1. The *indurated chancre*, well described by Hunter, is henceforth recognized as an indisputable sign of specificity.

2. Bell establishes the fact that *gonorrhœa* and *syphilis* are each one due to a virus essentially distinct from the other.

Of course, there appeared, during this period of a century, other important works, such as those of Vacca Berlinghieri, of Mahon, etc., which we have not subjected to analysis; but we have been forced to make a choice, for it is, above all, in the domain of history that it is indispensable to limit one's self.

CHAPTER IV.

SYPHILIS IN THE NINETEENTH CENTURY.

The scientific chaos at the beginning of the nineteenth century.—Caron denies extra-genital contagion.—The *fermentation of seeds* once more.—Theory of the non-existence of the venereal virus.—The *identists* and the *unicists*.—Ricord; his work. The revolution of which he was the instigator.—The *chancrous duality*.—The *mixed chancre*.—*Syphilization*.—The *disease of Brünn*, the *disease of St. Euphémie*, the *pian of Nérac*, and the *disease of Chavanne*.—The *radesyge*, *sibbens*, the *disease of St. Paul's Bay*, the *Falcadine* and the *disease of Scherlievo*.—The *Amboyne buttons*, *frambœsia*, *yaws*, and *pian*.

WE now come to the truly scientific epoch of venereal pathology. Before the nineteenth century, in fact, the truth could not assert itself, and we have just seen three long centuries of gropings and errors unfold themselves before us. It is scarcely without a struggle that, at the end of the eighteenth century, the domain of phantasy is left—if not of phantasmagoria—to enter upon the only scientific path, that of experience. "If I had to write the history of syphilography since the sixteenth century up to our days," said M. Mauriac[1] in 1883, "I would divide it into four periods, and I should designate each one of these under the names of: 'The Creative Period,' 'The Dogmatic Period,' 'The Experimental Period,' 'The Scientific Period.'"[2] This classification is per-

[1] Leçons sur les malad. vénér. Paris, 1883. Lectures on Venereal Diseases.

[2] Si j'avais à faire l'histoire de la syphiliographie depuis le seizième siècle jusqu'à nos jours, je la diviserais en quatre, périodes, et je désignerais chacune d'elles sous les noms de: période créatrice, période dogmatique, période expérimentale, période scientifique.

fectly rational in so far as it concerns the four centuries in which the existence of syphilis is not disputed.

M. Mauriac puts the *creative period* from the epidemic of Naples up to 1508. It is known that our distinguished colleague is not as yet a partisan of the ancient origin of syphilis. The *dogmatic period*, which includes almost three centuries, extends up to Hunter and even beyond that time. The author says, with reason, that "it was a period of confusion and of sterile dogmas, a sort of small Middle Age." The *experimental period*, which begins with Hunter, continues well into the nineteenth century, about up to the middle. Finally, the *scientific period* is essentially modern. The last period, in fact, includes scarcely more than forty years, for, as we will show very shortly, Ricord himself, at the beginning of his career, taught some errors, were they only the non-contagiousness of secondary symptoms and the specificity of the soft chancre. It is to Bassereau that the honor is due for having conclusively separated, in 1852, the syphilitic from the chancroidal virus. But let us not anticipate.

We have said that Bell, in 1793, had proclaimed the non-identity of syphilis with gonorrhœa. His theory was combated, as he foresaw it would be, and would perhaps have long remained in the background had not Hernandez,[1] in 1810, considered this question in a brilliant manner when it was made the subject of a competition by the Société de Médecine of Besançon. It was this author who created the theory of *larvated syphilis* in man and in woman.

Nevertheless, by the side of these innovators there is

[1] Essai analytiq. sur la non-identité des virus gonorrhéiq. et syphilitiq. Toulon, 1812. Analytical Essay on the Non-identity of the Gonorrhœal and Syphilitic Virus.

seen from time to time a laggard. A certain Caron comes and pretends, for example, that syphilis can be acquired only in coitus, and that contagion through abrasions in accoucheurs and midwives, in the same manner as by glasses, spoons, and other utensils, is nothing but a "joke." And he adds the following monumental sentence :—

"It is demonstrated, whatever may be said to the contrary, that venereal pus, placed in immediate contact with the lips and the mouth, is never contagious."

Il est démontré, quoi qu'on en dise, que le pus, vénérien, mis en contact avec les lèvres et la bouche, n'est jamais contagieux.[1]

After that we shall hardly be astonished to see come up once more—but this will be the last time—the famous theory of the *fermentation of seeds*. The author is one Lacombe,[2] who declares himself a partisan of the ancient origin and admits, with many of his predecessors, that a healthy woman, having had commerce with several healthy men, may acquire syphilis by the very fact of the multiplicity of males, and of the meeting of their seminal products in the *vas naturale*. The fact upon which he bases himself shows, upon the part of the writer, a simplicity which touches closely upon candor. He relates that four young seminarists, fearing the "pox," had resolved upon having the same mistress at their common expense during the course of their theological studies. It may be seen that these embryo spiritual advisers did not neglect the temporal. By excess of precautions, says the author, they even took a young virgin girl. But they, none the less, contracted syphilis, and about at the same time. Lacombe naturally

[1] Caron, Nouvelle doctrine des malad. vénér. Paris, 1811. New Doctrine in Regard to Venereal Diseases.

[2] La Vénusalgie. 1814. Venusalgia.

concludes in the fermentation of the four semens as the etiological cause. The idea of a fifth rogue,—this one syphilitic, however,—who might have delighted the leisure moments of the charmer, seems to us much more acceptable.

At that time, as it has been possible to see, there was groping still, and the true nature of syphilis was far from being known; nevertheless, during this chaos, which already included three centuries, no one had thought of denying the existence itself of syphilis. But, about 1825, certain authors began to maintain a curious theory, that of the non-existence of the venereal virus: for them the word "pox" was only applied to an artificial group of very different diseases. The apostles of this doctrine were especially Jourdan, Richond des Brus, Desruelles, in France; Abernethy, Fergusson, Guthrie, and Thompson, in England. For them the primary lesions of syphilis were due to *irritation;* the secondary symptoms were explainable by *sympathy.* This thesis had the fate of all eccentricities: it made much noise, but was of short duration.

We come to 1830, a time at which syphilographers are still divided into two great schools.

The first, *school of the identists* (*école des identistes*), always admits the identity of the different venereal viruses: for them syphilis may begin by a chancre, a gonorrhœa, or a bubo, or even appear at the first onset (*d'emblée*), without being preceded by any of those local phenomena. The most noted file-leaders are Lagneau, Baumés, Gibert, Vidal (de Cassis), Cazenave, Devergie, Vepeau, and even Bazin.

The second, *school of the unicists*, recognizes but one syphilitic virus and rejects certain venereal symptoms which it considers as not pertaining to syphilis.

This school is represented by Cullerier, Hardy, and the most distinguished syphilographer of our century. I have named Ricord.

Two very distinct phases are to be studied in the scientific life of Ricord. In the first, which lasted twenty-five years, he propagates certain false ideas, on the one hand; on the other, he confirms some exact theories advanced by his predecessors, and establishes, in 1832, his famous laws on the evolution of syphilis. In the second, which dates from 1857, he acknowledges his errors, profits by the discoveries of others, which he develops and improves upon, and he has the good luck of acquiring universal fame without having, so to say, ever found anything himself. Let us hasten to add that he had the undeniable merit of founding, in a sort of way, venereology, and, if he were not always creative, he at least showed himself an excellent organizer.

It may be said of Ricord that he about ended the conflict which reigned in science for three hundred years, and that, among so many different doctrines, he almost always knew how to choose those that were good, which is much better than to invent bad ones. It is thus that he took from Bell and from Hernandez the absolute distinction between the chancre and gonorrhœa, but he demonstrated it by a series of inoculations.[1] It is true that this last procedure was inspired in him by the labors of Hunter, but he succeeded where Hunter had failed. The English author did not admit of the contagion of secondary lesions; the surgeon of l'Hôpital du Midi was wrong in defending this opinion. This was his greatest mistake, but it is meet to add that Ricord did not delay in recognizing the fact himself that he had followed the wrong path. It is to him,

[1] Ricord, Traité de l'inoculation. Paris, 1838. Treatise on Inoculation.

also, that is due the theory of the *larvated chancre* (*chancre larvé*). Hernandez had a glimpse of this, this is certain; but a great deal can be wagered that it would have been soon forgotten if Ricord had not made it his own matter, in a sort of way, by the developments he gave to the question.

At all events he was still ignorant, about 1850, of the chancroidal virus. Of course, the great syphilographer had not failed to note that chancres were not all followed by constitutional symptoms, but he believed at the beginning in the influence of the different soils upon which the disease developed itself. Later on he brought forward the hypothesis that the difference might well exist in the very essence of the two venereal lesions. One of his pupils, Bassereau, made researches in this direction and established, in 1852, by means of numerous observations, that there were two kinds of chancres,—the one *hard*, the other *soft*,—and that the consecutive symptoms observed in the former were totally wanting in the latter. He concluded in the existence of two distinct viruses. It is the theory of the *duality of the chancre*, which Ricord adopted and defended.

Later on, the School of Lyons (Diday, Rollet, and others) admitted the existence of the *mixed chancre*, which is explained by the inoculation of the soft chancre on the hard chancre. Ricord accepted this theory. To sum up, it may be said that Ricord entered the Hôpital du Midi at a time when confusion reigned in the domain of venereal pathology, and that he was the leader of a true revolution whose results have been confirmed.

Of course, the laws established by the master are attacked at the present hour and there is an attempt to overturn the universally-known division of syphilis into three periods,—primary, secondary, and tertiary. Certain authors, basing themselves upon pathological anatomy, and especially upon the fact that lesions of the tertiary period may manifest themselves prematurely during the secondary period, and that, conversely, certain secondary late symptoms sometimes show themselves during the tertiary phase,—these authors, we say, have desired to adopt another classification. It is thus that there exists a tendency to reduce the evolution of syphilis to two periods: (1) primary syphilis; (2) consecutive syphilis. *Primary syphilis* would comprise in itself two phases,—the *incubation* and the *morbid determination*. *Consecutive syphilis* would be divided into a *virulent* phase and into a *destructive* phase.

We would have more easily understood, if it be desired absolutely to be limited to two periods, that the virulence be taken as the line of demarkation, and would mark out a *contagious period* and an *organic period*. In fact, no matter the manner in which we look upon the syphilitic process, nor the number of years which are allowed, for virulence, to the symptoms called *secondary*, —five, six, or seven years,—it is none the less true that the phenomena known by every one by the name of *tertiary* are not contagious. This is one fact gained. The period called *transition*, imagined, if you will, to supply the needs of the case, were sufficient for us: why then seek to overturn the classification of Ricord, so simple and so easy to remember? Because it is false in theory? We will admit it; but, if it be good in practice, why not retain it? We humbly believe, for our part, that the proposed division, even the distinction into *resolutive* phenomena and *destructive* phenomena, can only lead to one immediate and even consecutive result, which is to confuse students whose minds are now already pretty well burdened with things to remember. It is evident, for instance, that if the characteristics of a destructive necrosis of the nasal bones or of the hard palate be easy to recognize, it is less easy in exostoses and in certain late cutaneous manifestations of syphilis. For this reason we believe it to be much more simple to abandon this quarrel over words, and to limit ourselves, until further orders, to the division of Ricord, which amply suffices for our scientific well-being.

We cannot go on without saying a few words on *syphilization*, a method imagined by Auzias Turenne, who was soon followed by Sperino, at Turin, and Boeck, at Christiania. This method[1] had the claim of being at once preventive and curative. It was proposed, on the one hand, to come to the point of obtaining an attenuated virus, a sort of vaccine, as a result of successive inoculations; on the other hand, a cure was believed possible when the organism became saturated with the virus. The only thing arrived at was in succeeding to communicate syphilis to those who did not have and who possibly might never have had it otherwise.

We here cease the examination of the works of our contemporaries, not having the intention of analyzing the works of authors who are still living, and this for several reasons. The first is that these works are in all the libraries and known by the majority; certain ones are even in every one's hands. The second is that we would fear being looked upon as prejudiced if we permitted ourself the slightest criticism. Now, as it would be impossible for us to compliment everybody, we will praise no one. Finally, the best reason is that a work, even historical in character, should have an end, and the reader's patience must not be imposed upon too much.

[1] Auzias Turenne, Cours de Syphilization. Toulouse, 1852.

It remains for us to examine a few epidemics, almost all modern, in which certain authors, among others Giraudeau de Saint-Gervais (1838), have recognized syphilis pure and simple. Rollet and Lancereaux—to mention distinguished men only—have upheld this way of looking upon the matter, which has nothing unreasonable about it. The majority of the symptoms described seem to be those of syphilis; and we think that, if these isolated epidemics cannot all be looked upon as solely venereal, they must at least have served as labels for a large number of cases of syphilis.

We will divide them, with M. Rollet, into three general classes. The first includes those cases in which the virus, accidentally brought in a locality, has first spread itself there, then has diminished and ended by disappearing. Of this number are the disease of Brünn, the disease of St. Euphémie, the pian of Nérac, and the disease of Chavanne-Lure.

The *disease of Brünn* was brought, in 1758, to the town of that name, in Moravia, by a barber who had made scarifications with a dirty razor. Thomas Jordan,[1] an author of the time, considers the epidemic which followed as having been of venereal nature. The patients were treated with mercury and sudorifics.

The *disease of St. Euphémie* was brought by a midwife, according to Jean Bayer.[2]

"In the month of May, 1727, a midwife of St. Euphémie was attacked, on the forefinger of the right hand, with a pustule, . . . and soon the body was covered with a universal eruption (*dartre*). . . .

"This woman, continuing to follow her profession,

[1] Brunno gallicus, seu luis novæ in Moravia exortæ descriptio. Francofurti, 1579. Description of the French or New Pox Arisen in Moravia. Frankfort, 1579.

[2] Acta. nat. cur., vol. iii.

communicated her disease to more than fifty pregnant women."

Au mois de mai 1727, une sage-femme de Sainte Euphémie fut attaquée, au doit index de la main droite, d'une pustule, . . . et bientôt le corps se couvrit d'une dartre universelle. . . .

Cette femme, continuant à exercer sa profession, communiqua sa maladie à plus de cinquante femmes enceintes.

Some lost their hair, had angina, and communicated the disease to their husbands. A surgeon who was consulted diagnosed "*syphilitic* herpes," on account of the resemblance, and not daring to say "syphilis"; why is not apparent, for it would have been much more simple.

The *pian of Nérac*, introduced in that place in 1752, was given this name by Joseph Raulin[1] because that author found points in common with the *pian* of negroes. The case was that of a nursling, infected by a nurse first employed, who contaminated other nurses. The children of the latter were infected in their turn, and probably the husbands also, since the entire locality suffered.

The *disease of Chavanne* (Haute-Saône) was observed in 1816. It was characterized by ulcers in the throat, aphonia, pustules on the body, crusts on the head; besides this, it was highly contagious. Taken altogether, the classical phenomena of syphilis.

In the second class are found drawn up the cases in which the disease, developed in one locality, has formed a focus which still exists. They are: the radesyge, the sibbens, the disease of St. Paul's Bay, the Falcadine, and the disease of Scherlievo.

The *radesyge* was brought from India into Scandinavia about 1709 by the crew of a Danish vessel. It is characterized by cutaneous eruptions, tubercles of the

[1] Observat. de médecine. Paris, 1754. Medical Observations.

skin, ulcers, caries of the bones, alopecia, and genital lesions. The greater part of Swedish physicians look upon it as syphilis.

The *sibbens*, or *siwin*, was observed in Scotland toward 1765; according to Gilchrist, it manifests itself under the form of ulcerations of the mouth and of the throat, of hoarseness, of an eruption at the commissure of the lips, of copper-colored macules on the skin, of crusts in the hair, of tumors, and of pustules on the limbs, etc.

The *disease of St. Paul's Bay* appeared in Canada in 1776: ulcers of the mouth, highly contagious; osteocopic pains; ganglionic swellings; eruptions; caries of the bones of the nose, of the hard palate, etc.; being communicable especially through coitus.

The *Falcadine*, observed in 1786 at Falcado, in Illyria, presents about the same symptoms; it is treated with mercury.

The *disease of Fiume* or of *Scherlievo*, also in Illyria, seems to be an extension, pure and simple, of the Falcadine; the symptomatology is the same, also the treatment.

Finally, the third class of M. Rollet includes the cases in which the disease, developed in certain climates upon a certain race of men, presents a few peculiar characteristics. Of this number are the Amboyne boils (*boutons d'Amboyne*), and especially frambœsia, yaws, and pian.

Amboyne boils were studied in 1718 in the Moluccas, and chiefly in the island of Amboyne. Bontius[1] states that the symptoms are exactly those of syphilis, with this difference: that the disease may be communicated *sine congressu venereo.* We now know that sexual relations are not indispensable for the propagation of

[1] Medicina Indorum. Medicine of the Indies.

syphilis. The author speaks of deep ulcers, of caries of the bones, and of tumors of the limbs which break open at last and permit the escape of a gummy matter, etc.

Frambœsia, *yaws*, and *pian*, according to Giraudeau de St. Gervais, are to be included in the same list. The physicians who have studied them—yaws on the coast of Guinea and at Jamaica, pian at Guadeloupe, at San Domingo, and in Brazil—look upon them as identical. Indeed, certain modern physicians of our navy seem to see in this a disease peculiar to the negro race. We will wait, to make a positive assertion on this last point, for more complete observations to be published by those who have the opportunities of studying these diseases in their localities.

To sum up, with the exception of pian, yaws, and frambœsia, whose history is not complete, all the diseases whose symptomatology we have summarized manifestly refer to syphilis.[1]

[1] We have ceased, at about the year 1855, the examination of the works on syphilis which have appeared, and whose authors no longer live. This does not mean that nothing more has been discovered in syphilography since that date. Let us not forget that, since the fifteenth century, tertiary syphilis was scarcely known; very little but its external manifestations had been observed,—gummata or exostoses. It required the remarkable labors of Virchow and of Lancereaux to establish, in some sort of a way, *visceral syphilis*, hardly suspected before 1858 or 1860.

CHAPTER V.

Treatment and Prophylaxis of Syphilis.

Review of the procedures employed in venereal therapeutics from the most remote times until the present day.—The medication of to-day.—The hypodermatic method.—Precautions taken against venereal patients in antiquity, in the Middle Ages, and in modern times.—The prophylactic measures in use at the present time; their value.—The hospitalization of prostitutes.—Sexual contagion; examination of the various preventive measures proposed up to the present time.—The simplest and most effective preservative.

We have stated, in the preceding chapter, that we did not desire to permit ourselves to judge the works of our colleagues; we repeat it, and bequeath this care to the historians of the twentieth century. At all events, we may examine the different therapeutic procedures in use at the present time without running the risk of being accused of malice, each one being left free to adopt or to reject any given formula.

We have seen, in the course of this history, that the treatment of venereal diseases varied markedly according to the epochs. Without going back as far as the Deluge, we will be content to recall the fact that therapeutics, in Pagan times, was reduced to prayers, and especially to hygiene. The Greeks added to these topical applications with a basis of oil or of wine; the Romans, more radical in their procedures, acted by means of the iron, fire, and caustics in general. In the Middle Ages—the epoch of superstition, if ever there was one!—fasting and prayers alternated with the most unnatural debauches, and pomades and lotions were seen to successively appear. Later on, thanks to alchemy, quicksilver entered into the composition of certain ointments; but this special mode of treatment hardly extended beyond the haunts of prostitution.

Then comes the epidemic of Naples. At the beginning all the patients succumb, or very nearly all. No one will take care of them. Then the empirics set things going; mercurial inunctions are used and abused and the ovens overheated. In 1533 appear the first mercurial pills. The lesions of stomatitis having soon become more terrible than those of syphilis itself, a reaction declares itself in the opposite direction about the middle of the sixteenth century. Mercury is completely abandoned and recourse is had to sudorific woods. The latter are dethroned in their turn, and mercury is restored to favor about 1560. It is then given in the form of liniments, ointments, fumigations, or lotions, without abandoning the inunctions for that reason.

In 1743 corrosive sublimate is made fashionable by Van Swieten, whose solution remains classic. At the end of the eighteenth century salivation is conclusively stricken off the list of therapeutic measures. Mercurials are then administered in the form of pills or of solutions.

We then enter upon the nineteenth century. Then we see, successively, Dupuytren praising the bichloride of mercury and giving it in the form of pills of one centigramme (gr. $\frac{1}{6}$) each; Biett, Cazenave, Ricord, using the protiodide also in the form of pills, and abuse of it a little, especially Ricord. Since then, treatment by inunctions—which is very good—has been restored to favor, principally among foreigners (not French).

In 1836 venereal therapeutics enriches itself with a most valuable remedy, the *iodide of potassium*, of whose value Wallace, of Dublin, gave the first intimation.

Brera, in 1822, had already employed it for the first time in Italy, but no one paid any attention to it. It was Ricord who, by his experiments, did the most to render common the use of the iodide in France and abroad.

This work not being a didactic treatise, we are not called upon to enter into the various details of the treatment of syphilis at the present day; besides, we have drawn its broad lines in our first volume. However, there is a method which has enjoyed a great popularity since a few years, and of which we cannot help saying a few words. We wish to speak of the *hypodermatic* method, which might, perhaps, become the medication of the future.

The first trials of the kind appear to have been made in 1854 by Professor Scarenzio,[1] of Pavia. The author injected beneath the skin from 20 to 30 centigrammes of sublimed calomel, held in suspension in 1 gramme of glycerin. One or two injections sufficed and the beneficial effects showed themselves a week or a fortnight after the injection; unfortunately there was sometimes the formation of abscess. Dr. Ambrosoli, of Milan, obtained about the same results, as also other Italian physicians.

In 1866, Berkeley Hill, in England, employed injections of corrosive sublimate in doses of 1 milligramme, which is but a small amount; above this dose there were local and general symptoms.

In Germany, Lewin (1868) injected from 5 to 10 milligrammes of sublimate to which was added morphine; the results were reported as magnificent. Nevertheless, Hardy and M. Diday, who tried this procedure, were

[1] As a matter of fact, Hunter and Hebra had attempted, before Scarenzio, to inject corrosive sublimate into the connective tissue; having failed along the whole line, they immediately gave up this procedure. Let us add that Scarenzio was ignorant of these attempts.

obliged to abandon it on account of the pain, abscesses, and eschars which the injections produced.

Finally, the biniodide, the albuminate, the cyanide, the perchloride, the thymolo-acetate of mercury, and other mercurial compounds were tried. Almost all of these methods have their advantages and inconveniences. The ammoniacal mercurial peptone employed by Martineau, our master, has never produced an abscess. It is known that it was Martineau who contributed the most —about twelve years ago—to bring about the adoption, in France, of the hypodermatic method in the treatment of syphilis. The results which we have witnessed and which we have ourself obtained are very encouraging.

Now, the preference is given—in a general sort of way, and when the kidneys are in good order—to insoluble preparations; this method has the advantage of acting rapidly and of rendering necessary but a very small number of injections. It goes without saying that the medicinal antisyphilitic injections can only be properly administered by a physician. Whatever interest may attach to this important subject, we cannot dilate upon it at further length, our subject being limited to the history only of syphilis. However, we propose to study thoroughly, in a future publication,[1] the treatment of contagious diseases of sexual origin.

We cannot close this long study without speaking of the prophylaxis of syphilis. This is divided into public hygiene and private hygiene.

Public hygiene comprises the totality of the measures which may be adopted by society to prevent the propagation of venereal diseases. From the most ancient

[1] F. Buret, Traitement des maladies contagieuses de l'appareil genito-urinaire. Treatment of the Contagious Diseases of the Genito-Urinary System. In preparation.

times efforts were made to curb debauchery, and precautions were taken to limit the consequences thereof, ofttimes terrible. In our study on antiquity we have seen that Moses was the first legislator known who occupied himself about venereal diseases. The means he recommended to limit the spread of gonorrhœa would not have been rejected by Ricord; at all events, he was quite radical at the time of the plague of Baal-Peor. To cause the death of twenty-four thousand men—not to count the women—to endeavor to arrest a venereal contagion is a procedure entirely too savage. And to say that that was not sufficient!

A thousand years later (594 B.C.), Solon, with the object of restraining prostitution, established the first brothels (*dicterions*). In A.D. 535, under the Emperor Constantine (Consulate of Belisarius), debauchery was also punished; then, during almost ten centuries, Europe became covered with those establishments, called *leper-houses*, in which were huddled, almost without food and certainly without care, all patients affected with diseases of the skin or of the generative organs. In 1162, in London, clandestine prostitutes were prosecuted, and those who gave them an asylum were fined one hundred shillings. At the same time there were, in Southwark, special hospitals in which women with venereal diseases were treated. In 1302 the Senate of Venice condemned to twenty cents' fine any individual convicted of having transmitted the venereal disease then known as the *vermocana*.

Then comes the epidemic of Naples. The venereal individuals are at first compelled to leave Paris under penalty of being hung or thrown into the Seine. Then it is only the strangers who must leave, and they are given an indemnity of four cents for traveling expenses.

Very soon patients of the city are placed in Bicêtre, where they are treated by fasting and flogging: this state of affairs lasted until 1787.

In the East venereal patients were bastinadoed until 1833; Namich Pasha alone was able to abolish this cruel and absurd measure. We should not come to an end if we had to relate all which these unfortunate beings, victims of ignorance, had to suffer in the different parts of Europe. Fanaticism, which is never behindhand when it is a question of persecution, also made itself a party to the affair; it was soon a charitable deed to tyrannize over these unfortunate beings, in whom are more particularly seen guilty persons. Well might one ask of such persons as those who then made it a practice to outrage nature under the pretext of chastity the simple pity which is due to a patient, if it is averred that this patient obeyed physiological laws! If the Creator has provided the human being with genital organs, it is certainly not with the object of reducing His creature to a state of contemplation! But it appears that logic did not reside beneath the frock in the Middle Ages.

Accordingly, under the pretext that syphilis was a just punishment (?), patients were refused, for centuries, care and even food; they had the *shameful disease!* Nevertheless, in spite of the specious arguments of a certain sect, we shall not fear to ask which is the more despicable, in the sight of the child which inherits syphilis from its father, of the nurse, or of the mother who contracted it by the intermediary of the child; even of the poor young man who is contaminated at the beginning of his sexual life, or even of that honored old man, paralytic and wasted, who has worn out his spinal cord in the refinements of contemporaneous vice?

We will now inquire into the measures enforced at

this time. It is known in what, in France, the administrative measures regarding prostitutes consist. There are: (1) the daily examination of inscribed girls (*filles inscrites*),—that is to say, the unfortunates of the pavement,—all flanked by the unfailing bully, always a thief and often an assassin; (2) the arrest of a certain number of night-walkers from time to time; (3) the hospitalization of the contagious women at St. Lazare; and that is all. The remainder—that is to say, 99 per cent. of the army corps of Cythera—frequent balls, concerts, *brasseries* and *cafés*, and sow syphilis on their way. The three-fourths of these last also have their bullies, generally taken from the dregs of society, but raised one notch above the prowlers of the *barrière*. These do not wear the cap with the classic peak, the blouse of intact blue linen, without a trace of work, and the cravat of pink or green silk,—the rallying sign. No; they dress like everybody, and a few are even very well clad. They are assassins only accidentally, most often pickpockets, and play in dens in which the innocent are fleeced. Others become bookmakers on the turf; a few even have the semblance of a profession: amateur employés, intermittent hairdressers, promoters of unsavory business, etc. All these fine gentry swarm in public places and bully decent people under the very eyes of the impotent police. And yet, how willingly would we send them to be cooked, smothered in the open-air ovens of the gentle Kanakas! Add to this that they all have syphilis at some time, and that they do not scruple to transmit it during the entire duration of the lesions.

This is why the imprisonment of the diseased girls will never be more than a lure in regard to prophylaxis, so long as their men and, in a general way, all syphilitic men may freely circulate. Let us hasten to add that the legislator cannot adopt measures in regard to this without infringing upon the liberty of the individual. To succeed in wiping out syphilis it should be possible to place in hospital *all syphilitics* without distinction as to age, sex, or social condition. To mention such a proposition is to say, at the same time, that it is practically impossible to realize. The conclusion forces itself upon us: imprison no one.

This does not imply that some prophylactic precautions cannot be taken; all depends upon the manner in which they will be taken. If it be proven that violence does not give good results,—that is to say, does not interfere with the propagation of venereal diseases in an appreciable manner,—something else must be sought for, and good-will asked to do that which coercion does not succeed in obtaining. It is a simple matter of figures; preference is to be given to that system which is capable of withdrawing from circulation the largest number of contagious women, without inquiring whether the guardians of public morals (*police des mœurs*) can or can not continue their edifying exploits.

It is generally agreed to number as *one hundred thousand* the aggregation of women who give themselves up to prostitution [in Paris]. Now, of this number, forty thousand are *inscrites*,[1] and *two thousand* only come for examination. The number of girls examined decreases every year. Why? Because they are the affair of the police,[2] and the police, not being physicians, treat them as criminals, and not as patients. Despite the raids, the house of detention of Saint-Lazare never

[1] The women who are *inscrites* are those placed on the list of the police and kept under surveillance.—O-D.

[2] The *agents des mœurs* "make themselves, so to speak, their *official supporters*," declared Prof. Léon le Fort, at the Académie de médecine, in 1888.

contains more than *five hundred* venereal women. Those who succeed in hiding themselves in ordinary hospitals —where they are admitted with difficulty—complete the thousand, and there remain about four thousand who run the streets; for we estimate at five thousand the constant number of contagious women in Paris, but we are, perhaps, too modest. Police intervention, which re-assures M. Prudhomme, is, consequently, absolutely illusory.

Enumerations made abroad[1] have demonstrated—oh, irony!—that it is precisely in those countries in which coercive measures are in vigor that the proportion of current venereal diseases is most high. And almost everywhere they have given up a procedure which gave such miserable results; and syphilis is on the decrease in those countries in which the physician has replaced the police-officer.

Then let the doors of hospitals be thrown wide open, is our conclusion, with Professor Alfred Fournier; or, better still, let there be constructed, among the additions to each hospital, vast barracks *without special labels* and in which the venereal shall be treated. This is what we said already in 1890.[2] Let prostitutes not be permitted to go out until after the cure of their transmissible symptoms, and then let them be furnished with a little book officially certifying that they are healthy. At all events, there would be some interest in that this little book should contain not the name and address,—a useless thing,—but a *photograph*, such as is done in certain foreign cities. Could not public women go, as

[1] Malécot, Les vénériens et le droit commun. Paris, 1888. Venereals and Common Law.

[2] F. Buret, Les mesure répressives à l'égard des vénériens. Autrefois; aujourd'hui. Clermont (Oise), 1890. Repressive Measures in Respect to Venereal Patients. Formerly and to-day.

in Russia, to be examined, not at the health dispensary, but at the office of a physician designated for each quarter of the city? There, no ambulance, no policemen, no prison; a simple hospital-blank would replace absurd measures, uselessly vexatious and too often inhumane. And they would go to the hospital alone, you may be sure; I only want, for the proof of this, the constantly-increasing number of syphilitic patients who are daily refused admission in hospitals, sometimes as a matter of principle,—then so much the worse!—but most often for want of room. Police measures having always failed everywhere, it is time to try medical measures. Persecution never has and never will result in any good; accordingly, practice hygiene, but do so intelligently!

By the side of the public hygiene of syphilis the question of *private hygiene* ranges itself, and it is far from being a thing to be neglected. It should not, in fact, be passed over in silence, unless it be by virtue of a badly-understood professional dignity. Certainly, the only true method of escaping syphilis would be, as Ricord has said, not to expose one's self to it. It is the same as to avoid poisoning by mushrooms,—do not eat any; with such a principle one would never get in a railway-car, much less in a carriage, etc. But, as sexual relations will occur as long as there will be men and women, it is not a matter of indifference to examine into the different precautions which may be taken with the object of avoiding possible contamination.

The most elementary of these precautions consist in careful cleanliness and thorough washings. It would, at least, be also useful to take a look at the suspected parts and to beat a retreat at the least appearance of abnormal products; and the greater reason still is there to keep from the woman if she explicitly refuse to submit to an examination, this resistance hardly being attributable to offended modesty. It has been advised, in a general sort of way, after each coitus with a professional,—and especially with those who are intermittent,—to use lotions containing certain astringents and even slightly caustic. Parent-Duchâtelet informs us that in the houses of prostitution of Brussels these precautions are ordered by a regulation. Each boarder of said places must have in her room:—

1. A bottle containing a solution of caustic soda made according to the following formula:—

℞ Solut. natri caustic., 35°, ...	1 part.
Aquæ destillat., ...	20 parts.

2. A bottle of fresh oil. The whole legibly labeled.

The object is the following: the oil, by facilitating intercourse, prevents abrasions; the solution of soda, of which a certain quantity is poured in the wash-water, renders the cleansing as thorough as possible. Certain substances which should have the property of neutralizing the different venereal viruses have even been proposed. Such, for instance, is Rodet's lotion, which is to be applied after a complete washing:—

℞ Ferri perchloridi,	
Acidi hydrochlorici, ...	āā ʒj.
Aquæ destillatæ, ...	℥j.

All these procedures are good, but not one realizes absolute perfection; infection has taken place in certain cases in which this entire programme had been carried out to the letter. At all events, it is better than to do nothing at all and to trust to one's luck.

Another thing was imagined. The English physician Condom had the idea of making protectors with the membrane furnished by the ileo-cæcal appendix of certain herbivorous animals.[1] These little contrivances, employed more especially in bourgeois households, where a fear exists of the multiplication of mouths to feed, are too well known for us to dilate on them. We will only add that preservatives are also made of rubber. In addition to the inconvenience caused by these cuirasses, a tear may occur, and then all safety is gone.[2]

And we have asked ourself, for a long time already, if there is not a simple and practical way of avoiding, as far as this can be done, the terrible contagion. Oil, by a purely mechanical action, prevents tears, but it is rather a vehicle for septic products than a protection against them. So that two conditions must be fulfilled: (1) suppress the wearing off of the epithelium, and, as a consequence, the possible avenues of entrance for the virus; (2) to interpose between the mucous membrane and the virulent liquids an unctuous and impermeable varnish. Vaselin has seemed to us to answer these various requirements. It presents the mechanical advantages of fatty bodies without being composed of fat, and it is, consequently, incapable of becoming rancid. However thin the layer with which the hands, for instance, may be covered, it is seen that water does not penetrate. To make vaselin perfectly aseptic, we would

[1] A popular form in use in the United States is made of thin rubber tissue, there being several sizes on the market.—O-D.

[2] We cannot refrain from quoting the following from Ricord's "Letters on Syphilis." Boston, 1853. Letter xxii, p. 200. "There is a method which morality repudiates, and in which debauchees put much confidence, which doubtless often guarantees, but which, as a woman of much *esprit* has remarked, is a cuirass against pleasure and a cobweb against danger. This mediate agent is often rotten, or has already been made use of; it is frequently displaced; it performs the office of a bad umbrella which the storm may tear, and which under all circumstances, while it guarantees badly against the storm, does not prevent the feet from getting wet."

advise incorporating boric acid in the following proportions :—

℞ Acidi borici, ... ℈ij.
Vaselini, ... ℥j.

It will be found very useful, when applying this mixture, to introduce a little in the urinary meatus and to push it up as far as possible. Its use is infinitely preferable to that of cold-cream, and does not oblige the performance of a ceremony as grotesque as the *condom* of sheep-gut; this latter, however, is accepted by the most rigorous ladies; it is true that it is not syphilis which they fear, but maternity.

Our procedure does not exclude a thorough toilet at the time of the ablutions; and if it do not, theoretically, guarantee absolute security, it at least procures it often enough in practice to merit its being taken into consideration. All those to whom we have mentioned it for the past twelve years have derived benefit from it; we may even mention the case of a rash student whom an evident syphilis did not always deter. He ended, it is true, by contracting a syphilitic chancre, but, it must be added, that, a month previously, he had pursued an adventure, although he did not have his tube of vaselin with him. This neglect of one day had rendered nugatory years of precautions!

Such is the result of our researches and of our observations in regard to this important branch of medicine, which is called venereal pathology. We esteem ourself too happy if we have succeeded in interesting our readers and in having been useful to some.

SYPHILIS

IN ANCIENT AND PREHISTORIC TIMES.

VOLUME I.

AMS PRESS
NEW YORK

No. 12 IN THE PHYSICIANS' AND STUDENTS' READY-REFERENCE SERIES.

SYPHILIS

IN ANCIENT AND PREHISTORIC TIMES.

BY

DR. F. BURET,

PARIS, FRANCE.

TRANSLATED FROM THE FRENCH, WITH NOTES, BY

A. H. OHMANN-DUMESNIL, M.D.,

PROFESSOR OF DERMATOLOGY AND SYPHILOLOGY IN THE ST. LOUIS COLLEGE OF PHYSICIANS AND SURGEONS; CONSULTING DERMATOLOGIST TO THE ST. LOUIS CITY HOSPITAL; PHYSICIAN FOR CUTANEOUS DISEASES TO THE ALEXIAN BROTHERS' HOSPITAL; DERMATOLOGIST TO ST. MARGARET'S HOSPITAL, ETC., ETC.

"Syphilis To-Day and Among the Ancients." In Three Volumes.

VOLUME I.

"*Nihil sub sole novum.*"—ECCLES., i, 10.

PHILADELPHIA AND LONDON:

F. A. DAVIS, PUBLISHER,

1891.

Library of Congress Cataloging in Publication Data

Buret, Frédéric.
"Syphilis to-day and among the ancients."

Reprint of the 1891-95 ed. published by F. A. Davis, Philadelphia, which was issued as no. 12 and 15 of the Physicians' and students' ready-reference series.
CONTENTS: v. 1. Syphilis in ancient and prehistoric times.—v. 2-3. Syphilis in the Middle Ages and in modern times.
1. Syphilis—History. I. Title. II. Series: Physicians' and students' ready reference series; no. 12, 15.
RC201.4.B8713 1975 616.9'513 72-9627
ISBN 0-404-57422-X

Reprinted from an original copy in the collection of the University of Chicago Library

From the edition of 1891, Philadelphia and London
First AMS edition published in 1975
Manufactured in the United States of America

International Standard Book Number:
Complete Set: 0-404-57422-X
Volume I: 0-404-57423-8

AMS PRESS INC.
NEW YORK, N. Y. 10003

AUTHOR'S PREFACE.

Our object in writing this book has been to spare the reader a herculean task. It is hardly possible, in fact, no matter how willing one may be, to wade through a couple of thousand volumes, merely for the purpose of becoming acquainted with the history of a disease. Syphilis, since it must be called by its name, is one of those affections which interests everybody: in the first place, those who have it,—a very appreciative audience; and then those who are not affected by it; that is to say, those who run the risk of acquiring it. Do not protest; when you will have read this medico-literary study, if, perchance, you have the courage to go on to the end, you will not dare affirm that you will always be unscathed, for evil, like good, comes upon us while we sleep.

When we contemplate the interminable list of authors who have written upon this disease since the great epidemic of the fifteenth century, and the divergence in their opinions upon the origin and nature of it, one is, in a manner, dazed, and it is difficult to determine where to begin.

It would certainly have been more convenient for us to have first read modern authors, several of whom, such as Hunter, Ricord, Alfred Fournier, Lancereaux, Mauriac, Rollet, and others, have described syphilis in a masterly manner. We might also have remained content with merely reproducing, without confirming them, a number of Greek and Latin quotations, thrown pell-mell in a host of works of the eighteenth century,—a method which would have considerably lightened our labors. But we have scrupulously studied the text of the authors of antiquity, and with profit; we have been enabled, in this way, to eliminate numerous so-called proofs, which prove nothing, and re-establish in their integrity many of the verses of Martial and of Horace which had been mutilated and rendered unintelligible. Other reasons also influenced us to make our own researches: we have desired to acquire personal impressions from our readings, without being influenced by the opinions of others. Thus, we had scarcely analyzed thirty small works of the sixteenth century before we began to entertain doubts as to the nature of the epidemic of 1494, which the majority of authors look upon as the starting-point of syphilis. We were not loath to believe, at that time, already, that the famous epidemic was not concerned solely with the disease which occupies our attention, but that several venereal or cutaneous affections, without syphilitic virus, must have been described under the general term: *le Mal Français* (the French disease). Ricord, Lancereaux, and others, whose works we read later on, give the same opinion; and we feel happy to coincide with such competent authorities.

We adopted the plan of reading syphilographers in chronological order, from the fifteenth century to our epoch. Then we searched for the traces of syphilis in antiquity, and in this study we followed the degree of antiquity of the literary documents which we have inherited from the people of primitive times.

Our researches, which were commenced in 1887, have now ended; we have analyzed all the authors which we have been able to find in the various libraries of Paris.

In order not to interrupt the easy reading of the work, we have added translations, as exact as possible, but devoid of all pedantry, of all quotations which appear in foreign tongues, be they dead or living. We have also met with translations, and we have most often given the readings of the translators; but, whenever they seemed to us not to reproduce exactly the thoughts of authors, we have permitted ourself to make modifications.

We also desire to state that we have written in plain language, for we are addressing this as much to those interested in science and in letters as to physicians and patients. So that, in order to be understood by all, we have not employed technical terms, except in those instances where decency might be shocked, or for a want of sufficiently explanatory terms in our ordinary language.

To those professional brethren who, losing sight of the end we are aiming at, believe that they should pass severe judgment upon our work on account of the quotations taken from the lighter poetry of antiquity, we will recall the fact that we are sustaining a thesis upon a subject which has been much disputed; and, as a result of this, we have been forced to seek our proofs wherever we could find them. If we analyze Martial, Horace, Juvenal, and many others whose writings are licentious, as a compensation to be borne in mind we draw largely from the Bible, the Fathers of the Church, and the Lives of the Saints. Of course, we cannot ignore the fact that these works could scarcely be placed in the hands of young ladies until after careful expurgation. As proof, we need only the singular mode imagined by the Christian martyr, of whom Palladius speaks, to preserve her virginity despite her executioners.[1]

[1] Greek Patrology, vol. xxxiv. Palladius: Lausiaca historia. (See translation in the tenth chapter of this book.)

But the letter which Latour wrote to Ricord, in 1851, when the former was editor-in-chief of *l'Union Médicale*, does not deceive us as to what we are to expect, not having, like the great syphilographer of that time, a "heap" of former publications, nor long years of battling against a myriad of enemies who are continually endeavoring to depreciate the efforts of a man who tries to become marked; it appears as if he was trying to deprive others of something.

We will quote a few fragments from that letter, which precedes the work of Ricord entitled "Lettres sur la Syphilis."[1] We have purposely omitted the eulogistic remarks addressed to the author, in order that it might not be supposed for a moment that our intention is to compare ourself to the master.

Let us let Latour speak: he well knew that patient who, without taking into consideration university or hospital titles, judges a physician by his cravat, his social position, the brim of his hat, the gossip of servants and janitors, and other things, consecrating a man solely upon the manner he pontifies:—

"How happy you must be," says Latour, "not to be at your professional beginning! You would have died as a practitioner. . . . A physician who does not hesitate, miserable man, to relate anecdotes, and who does not fear, imprudent man, to make his reader smile, as is done by him. . . .

"You did well to begin with solid memoirs, by a large octavo, to elevate yourself up to the heavy folio full of beautiful pictures, before writing your letters. Without this respectable luggage, you risked very much not being regarded as a *serious man*. . . . Instead of putting your audience to sleep, you keep it continu-

[1] Paris, 1851.

ally awake. . . . But there are many persons who do not care to be disturbed in their slumbers."

There is but little to add to these observations, which are based upon the sad experience of facts. In spite of all our precautions, we will infallibly be blamed, either by those unfortunate minds who see morals in peril at the mention of syringe, or by the moralists *ad hoc*, who, returning from the boudoirs *à la mode*, will say that one should not write upon such a subject. But little reck we. Like Martial, we will say to the ones and to the others: "If any one is apt to be scandalized by the nudity of expressions (*lascivam verborum veritatem*),—whose faithful interpretation necessitates crudity,—let him limit himself to reading this introduction, or even be content with the title of the work (*potest epistolâ, vel potius titulo contentus esse*)."

DR. FRED. BURET.

PARIS, November, 1889.

AUTHOR'S LETTER TO TRANSLATOR.

Au Professeur Ohmann-Dumesnil:

Vous me faites savoir, mon cher confrère, que vous avez traduit mon histoire de la syphilis chez les anciens, et vous me demandez mon autorisation pour publier. Je vous la donne avec un double plaisir, au point de vue de la science d'abord et au point de vue personnel ensuite. En effet, l'auteur le plus modeste ne peut se défendre d'une certaine satisfaction intérieure lorsqu'il voit le fruit de ses travaux recevoir l'approbation éclairée d'un des savants les plus compétents. Quelle preuve d'estime scientifique plus éclatante est-il possible de donner? Vous avez apprécié les efforts, approuvé les conclusions et partagé l'opinion de l'auteur: alors vous avez voulu que vos compatriotes des Etats-Unis pussent tous constater par eux-mêmes que *l'antiquité de la syphilis est désormais un fait acquis.*

A Paris, cette opinion gagne du terrain tous les jours, et elle est adopté par presque tous les jeunes médecins qui pensent pour eux-

To Professor Ohmann-Dumesnil:

You have informed me, my dear colleague, that you had translated my history of syphilis among the ancients, and you ask for my authority to publish the translation. I give it to you with twofold pleasure,—first, from a scientific point of view, and, next, from a personal point of view. Indeed, the most modest author cannot refrain from a certain degree of self-satisfaction when he sees the fruit of his labors receive the intelligent approval of a most competent savant. What more brilliant proof of scientific esteem is it possible to furnish? You have appreciated the efforts, approved the conclusions, and shared the opinion of the author: then you desired that your American countrymen should be placed in a position to determine for themselves that *henceforward the antiquity of syphilis is an established fact.*

In Paris, this opinion is daily gaining ground, and it is adopted by nearly all the younger phymêmes. Quant à ceux qui règlent tous leurs gestes sur ceux du *maître*, cela dépend : si le maître choisi est partisan de l'origine américaine de la syphilis—légende encore très en houneur dans le public—ils ne veulent même pas discuter : *magister dixit !* Je constate toutefois que la presse médicale française a fort bien accueilli ce livre, car la plupart des comptes-rendus sont très bienveillants : maintenant ce sont les hommes de science de la plus grande république du monde qui vont exprimer leur avis.

Comme auteur et comme syphiliographe, j'accompagne de mes voeux les plus sincères l'œuvre de vulgarisation de mon distingué collègue le Professeur de Syphiliographie des Hôpitaux de St. Louis ; et, étant donnés la largeur d'idées, l'intelligence et l'esprit de progrès qui caractérisent la grande nation américaine, je ne doute pas que cette publication ne réussisse au-delâ de ses désirs.

DR. F. BURET.

PARIS, 1er Mai, 1891.

sicians who think for themselves. As to those who regulate all their movements by those of the *master*, it depends : if the chosen master be a partisan of the American origin of syphilis—a legend still held in great honor by the public—they do not even wish to discuss it : *magister dixit !* I have noticed, however, that the French medical press has received this book very well, for the majority of the reviews are very kind ; now, it is the scientific men of the greatest republic in the world who will express their opinions.

As author and as syphilographer, I contribute my best and most sincere wishes to the work of dissemination of my distinguished colleague, the Professor of Syphilography in St. Louis ; and, taking into consideration the breadth of ideas, the intelligence, and the talent which characterize the great American nation, I have no doubt that this publication will succeed beyond his expectations.

DR. F. BURET.

PARIS, May 1, 1891.

TRANSLATOR'S PREFACE.

IN offering this translation, the purpose has been a twofold one,—first, to afford those who are unable to read French an opportunity of enjoying a very interesting work; secondly, to show upon what proofs the antiquity of syphilis rests. Of a necessity, the proofs must be sparse, and, at the same time, of a rather weak nature. The very nature of things presupposes this. The interpretations which are placed upon many constitute the real proof; and those which appear the most reasonable should, of necessity, be adopted. A careful perusal of the contents of this volume will demonstrate the ingenuity of the author, as well as his painstaking efforts to obtain evidence. This herculean task occupied several years, and, in some cases, fortune seemed to have favored Dr. Buret in his efforts.

No assumption could possibly be made that the author's thesis has been *proven;* but the mass of evidence which he has gathered is of such a character as to induce an unprejudiced reader to incline very strongly to the view that syphilis is very ancient, and that its appearance in Europe did not date from the siege of Naples, but was most probably anterior to it, existing in such a form that but little attention was paid to it; and not until it constituted a large and fatal epidemic did physicians study it. Fortune-tellers, charlatans, prostitutes, *et id omne genus*, had, before that time, constituted the principal practitioners in the line of venereal diseases. As is pointed out by the author, another reason existed for this non-publication of any knowledge physicians might have acquired, in ancient times, at least. The reason was, that venereal diseases were looked upon as the results of the wrath of some offended deity, and to tamper with them would have been considered a sacrilege. Prayers and offerings to the deity, aided by simple remedies, constituted the treatment.

In addition to this, these diseases were considered "shameful" (*morbus indecens*), and, being located, for the most part, upon the "secret parts," were not to be exposed to the critical or inquiring gaze of strangers. Moreover, women were not permitted to expose themselves to any men but their husbands; so that it can be easily understood how the open debauchery could serve as a prolific means of spreading venereal disease. The migrations of Orientals, the invasions and returns of armies, all contributed to a further dissemination of the evil. In fact, it can be safely asserted that these diseases are as old as prostitution itself, and a necessary appanage of that pursuit.

A few words in regard to the description and treatment of syphilis given by the author. In the former, only the broad, salient lines are sketched. As regards therapeutics, we find a true reflection of one of the French schools; but every one who has had experience will differ more or less from the lines laid down, unless that experience has been gained in the same school. So that a criticism of the methods advocated would be superfluous, and each one is very apt to pursue that course which seems best to him from the results attained. Still, as a reflex of French methods, it cannot fail from being interesting.

So far as the translation is concerned, a close adherence to the text has been the main object.

Elegance of diction has been sacrificed to exact interpretation, and this has necessitated the occasional use of Gallicisms. That these faults may be overlooked by the indulgent reader is the earnest hope of

THE TRANSLATOR.

CONTENTS.

CHAPTER IV.

CHAPTER V.

CHAPTER VI.

CHAPTER VII.

CHAPTER VIII.

CHAPTER IX.

CHAPTER X.

CHAPTER XI.

CHAPTER XII.

SYPHILIS

TO-DAY AND AMONG THE ANCIENTS.[1]

CHAPTER I.

IN WHAT MODERN POX, THAT IS TO SAY, SYPHILIS, CONSISTS.

Syphilis ! à ce nom que, saisi de scrupule,
Un vulgaire lecteur s'épouvante et recule,
Qu'il inflige à mon œvre un pudibond mépris,
Qu'importe? Je m'adresse à ces graves ésprits
Dout l'œil philosophique embrasse pour domaine
Tout ce qui touche au sort de la nature humaine,
Ceux qui n'ont pas l'orgueil de croire au-dessous d'eux
Ce que le monde appelle effrayant ou hideux,
Et qui, de l'ignorance affrontant l'anathème,
Sèment au champ public la verité . . . quand même!

BARTHÉLEMY.[2]

FIRST of all, what is syphilis? Everybody talks about it, many have it, and very few know in what it consists. What heresies do we not daily hear retailed in regard to the subject! Some mistake it with blennorrhagia (flow), and with an appearance of reason. In fact, it is scarcely earlier than the beginning of this century that blennorrhagic urethritis was no longer considered as one of the initiatory symptoms of syphilis.

[1] This subject, too extensive to be included within the limits of a volume, will form the subject of several publications. After the appearance of the work on Syphilis Among the Ancients, will appear one on Syphilis in the Middle Ages.

[2] Syphilis, a poem in two cantos. Paris, 1841.

1 A

Besides, did not Grisolle say, not twenty-five years ago, "Following several blennorrhagias, diverse accidents of constitutional syphilis manifest themselves"?[1] This is what he calls *virulent* blennorrhagia, regarding as too exclusive the opinion of Ricord, who did not admit of syphilitic infection by blennorrhagia alone, without a chancre of the urethral canal. Other patients become re-assured when you diagnosticate syphilis, and they ask in what it differs from pox. Do not smile, for this question has been often asked of me.

I have promised a talk rather than a treatise, and I will take good care not to submit a didactic description of the disease with which we are concerned. I have no other object—and in this I am sincere—than to furnish the public with a number of facts which are almost unknown, and yet very curious. Those who desire a book which is purely scientific will have only the *embarras de choix:* there exist a few hundreds.[2] In a later publication, when we examine the modern opinions of syphilis, we will make it a point to call attention to the better works.

Let us end this digression, which has already been too long, and state in a few words what is to be understood by *syphilis* in the year of grace, 1889, and 1891 as well.

It is a complex disease, having an evolution characterized by three distinct periods: the first two, *contagious from their inception*, have their seat over all the integument,—the skin and mucous membranes; the third at-

[1] Traité de path. int. Paris, 1864. Treatise on Pathology.

[2] Charles Girtanner has devoted an entire volume to the critical bibliography of 1912 works on Syphilis, published from 1495 to 1794; that is to say, within a period of three hundred years. It may not be superfluous to add that a great number of authors, especially of the sixteenth century, copied each other.

tacks the subcutaneous connective tissue and the different organs,—the bones, the nerve-tissues, glands, viscera, etc.; beyond this it is *not contagious.*

First Period.—Limiting itself to a local accident, at the site of contact itself, it consists of one or sometimes several chancres: this is what has been, by consent, denominated the *primary lesion.* Let us remark at once that the term *chancre*, sanctioned by usage, is a misnomer so far as syphilis is concerned; at least, in the majority of cases. As a matter of fact, the primary lesion in no way corresponds with the conception of chancre, which might be rightfully entertained, if the only reason were its Latin derivation (*cancer*).[1] One immediately thinks of a sore that eats, and nothing is farther from the truth, as we shall see.

The *typical* syphilitic chancre, also called *infecting chancre* and *indurated chancre*,—due to the parchment sensation it gives, as a rule, upon attempting to bend it between the thumb and index,—is naught but a simple

[1] It may be objected that there are syphilitic chancres which are gan grenous, through *excess of inflammation*, according to Ricord; others, phagedenic, through *excess of induration;* others, again, are diphtheritic, etc. I will not deny this, but contend that they are pathological varieties; at least, to-day. Ricord, in his Atlas Iconographique, has illustrated a few marked cases, but he carefully chose them from thousands of cases. As for myself, since sixteen years that I have been examining patients, I have scarcely seen two or three such cases, and, be it understood, in a prolific field, which agrees perfectly with the theories of the illustrious master. I had an opportunity of observing a phagedenic chancre of syphilitic origin in 1873, at the hospital of Boulogne-sur-Mer; another at l'hôpital St. Sauveur of Lille, in the venereal division, to which I was attached as an externe during 1874; and the third, five or six years ago, in the service of Dr. Benjamin Auger, at Lariboisière. But, during the many months I passed at Lourcine, I did not have the good fortune of seeing a single one. And yet, in many cases of syphilitic chancres called phagedenic, I am not certain that they were not *mixed* chancres; that is to say, a sort of fusion of the two varieties of chancre. I cannot dilate any further upon this subject, for it would only be possible to discuss all the sides of this question in a didactic treatise.

erosion, an excoriation[1] if you wish, markedly superficial, which does not deepen, scooped out, with marked round contours, never suppurating, and exuding a colorless, transparent fluid, giving the ulcerated surface a varnished appearance. Its color is, in general, a brick-red, sometimes a lardaceous gray. Most often the syphilitic chancre is single; at times several exist, but they have all appeared at the same time and disappear together. And, as a last symptom, which is extremely important in the diagnosis, there is *no pain* elicited by pressure. Honestly, was that the conception you had formed, my dear reader, of the *syphilitic chancre?*

Now listen, for comparison, to the description of the *soft* chancre, also called the *simple chancre*, non-infecting, *flying* chancre, *which does not get into the blood*, as the popular expression goes. But this flying chancre, which annoys the patient without frightening him, may become phagedenic,[2] serpiginous, or even both at the same time; that is to say, which eats and advances.

The *soft chancre* rarely exists singly: often several chancres appear, simultaneously or successively, by auto-inoculation. We no longer deal with a simple excoriation, it is a true loss of substance: here the word *chancre* does not belie its etymology. The skin is destroyed, the edges are perpendicular, as if punched out, and slightly undermined. A slight serration is observed along the edges, which are red and terminating in a white line, having the form of a collarette. The bottom is grayish; suppuration is abundant and highly contagious. The slightest contact produces *acute pain.*

[1] Women will always tell you that they have *scratched* themselves with the finger-nail, in order to explain the presence of the *excoriation* which is so stubborn and which has not healed at the end of a month.

[2] In Greek, *φαγέδαινα*, a devouring hunger; in Latin, *phagedæna*, —the destructive ulcers described by Celsus. (See Chapter XI.)

In the phagedenic chancre, the ulcer increases peripherally or advances, eating right and left, almost in a zigzag. It penetrates into the connective tissue, which it destroys, and under the skin, which it perforates at various points. Sometimes one of the extremities cicatrizes as the chancre pursues its destructive march. Its invading and serpiginous course is rarely regular, and the disturbances are difficult to repair. They may even bring on death. I saw a case of this nature at Lourcine, when I was interne at that hospital, in 1881.

CASE I. (*Personal*).—A poor girl of 23, in the *salle* Fracastor (formerly St. Marie), had upon the internal portion of the right thigh a simple chancre, which had increased in depth and extent. At the time I saw the patient, the chancre formed a very regular circle 10 centimetres in diameter, without exaggeration; the skin and connective tissue were absolutely destroyed, as well as the sheath of the muscles, which latter appeared naked, admirably dissected. One would have said that the coverings had been removed with a punch, and that a part of the skin had been cut out with scissors and Scarpa's triangle[1] prepared for demonstration. The unfortunate died of exhaustion about eight months after the first appearance of the chancre. It is the only death from a venereal disease that I had an opportunity of witnessing during my stay at Lourcine, and yet I observed many patients in that hospital; it would be difficult to tell the exact number within a few hundreds.

So, one can die of a non-infecting chancre, for this woman was not syphilitic; but it must be admitted that this is rare, especially nowadays.

A last point to note, and I will have done with this parallel. The soft chancre is sometimes accompanied by an adenitis, that is, of an inflammation of a ganglion in the groin (one only, ordinarily), commonly called a *bubo* (*βουβών*, groin), or "*kernel*," which is always painful, and often suppurates. With the primary lesion of

[1] Scarpa's Triangle: An anatomical region which is dissected preparatory to examinations.

syphilis—indurated chancre, if you will—several ganglia are engorged, especially at first, in the neighborhood of the genitalia. This ganglion, which is sometimes as large as a walnut, is known, in hospital slang, under the name of *préfet of the groin.* This ganglionic pleiad, very hard to the touch, is *absolutely indolent* and *never suppurates.* It is not a bubo, then, to speak properly.

When these buboes suppurate, the syphilis is accompanied by gonorrhœa, soft chancre, or scrofula, or a neighboring wound; but that it could occur from the syphilitic process, I would almost regard as an impossibility. Thierry de Héry, lieutenant-general of the king (Henry II), knew already, in the sixteenth century, that there were chancres not followed by secondary accidents, and that the suppurating bubo did not belong to syphilis. He had then foreseen the duality of the chancre established in our days by Ricord in an irrefutable manner. "As often appears in many who have bad and malignant ulcers, which will be difficult to cure, because nature makes an effort to evacuate the said venom by those parts, and *if a bubo appears*, otherwise called a 'kernel,' which receives the said fluxion, the ulcer will be healed and cured in a short time, and *the patient will be free from pox.*"[1] Besides, we have stated that the indurated chancre itself does not suppurate, and we shall see shortly that the secondary accidents do not suppurate either, or very slightly, this second period being a vegetating phase rather than a destructive one.

[1] The following is the original: Comme souvent appert en plusieurs ayant ulcères cacoeths et malings, qui seront rébelles à curer, pour se que nature s'efforce d'évacuer ledict venin par icelles parties, et s'il survient un bubon, autrement dict poulain, qui reçoive la dicte fluxion, en brief l'ulcère sera curé et guary; et sera le patient exempt de la verolle. Thierry de Héry: La Méthode curative de la maladie vénérienne, vulgairement appelée grosse vérolle. Paris, 1552. The Curative Method of the Venereal Disease commonly called the Big Pox.

In addition, the soft chancre appears immediately, two or three days after the infecting intercourse, rarely after eight days, whilst the syphilitic virus gathers its forces, as it were, and it is only at the end of twenty-five days, or one month on an average, that it sends its first rocket, the indurated chancre.

Such are the principal characteristics, hastily sketched, which serve to distinguish between the *small excoriation*, more or less indurated, the prologue of syphilis, and the soft chancre which may, as we have seen above, not be at all *simple.* To be complete, it would be necessary to enter into many other details, and describe, for example, *mixed chancres*, which contain both elements, and put the physician on the wrong track, at least at the beginning; but we would overstep the bounds which we have set for ourselves.

This exposition of the subject, as will be seen, is already long enough, but we believe it indispensable to enable the reader, who is a stranger to the art of medicine, to appreciate the value of our arguments. We desire to prove, text in hand, that syphilis is as old as prostitution; and, the whole world is agreed in the recognition of the fact that the latter is not precisely young.

The indurated chancre lasts in the neighborhood of four to six weeks, sometimes less, rarely more, and heals spontaneously: this is why we seldom have an opportunity of seeing it in women. As it produces no pain, and it only has to choose some fold to conceal itself, it is only by accident that the unfortunate possessor of a chancre notices it. And then she must feel worried at the persistence of the *nail scratch* to determine to seek the advice of a physician; or she thinks herself cunning in cauterizing it, and the erosion becomes larger without healing any faster. It is infinitely preferable to apply morning and evening some inert powder, take internal treatment, and patiently await the secondary accidents, which will not fail to make their appearance in six weeks or two months.

According to certain authors, the chancre might be wanting and syphilis commence with the secondary period; this is what happens in the newborn who are syphilitic by heredity. But is this possible in ordinary cases of direct contagion? M. Lancereaux says yes; Ricord has always formally denied it. Which is right? Our authority is not sufficient to decide the question. It will be conceded, however, that the chancre is sometimes so small that it may pass unperceived, even in a man. Here is an illustrative example which to us appears conclusive:—

CASE II. (*Personal*).—M. G., aged 21, student in one of our faculties, applied for advice, June, 1886. He asked for advice concerning a *hernia*, which had come on some time since. I examined the affected part and recognized, at a glance, the presence of an enormous bubo, which the touch showed to be very hard and absolutely indolent.

"Sir," said I, "this is not a hernia; it is a ganglionic engorgement with special characteristics which enable me to state that you have syphilis."

"But I have nothing else; I can swear to it!"

"Pardon me; you must have a chancre. Where, I do not know yet; but you have one, necessarily, along the course of the lymphatics, which connect with the inguinal ganglia."

"But, I repeat it; that I haven't the least abrasion."

"Let us search for it together: are you willing?"

"Oh! as much as you please."

Not admitting at all the famous *bubon d'emblée*, at least in our climate, I examine the anus first, as the patient states that he has seen nothing, and I find nothing. Then, going to the penis, I uncover the glans; it is intact; nothing in the balano-preputial sulcus; nothing in the urethral canal; nothing upon the lower limbs; nothing, nothing. The situation was becoming painful. And yet there *is* one, thought I, paraphrasing the celebrated expression of Galileo. Finally, in sheer desperation, I exposed the small folds which exist on each side of the frenum, and I discovered, on the right, a small, superficial erosion of an angry, red color, of the size of an ordinary *pin's head*, and distinctly indurated.

"Here is your chancre."

"Is that all?"

"It is enough, believe me."

The young student, although not thoroughly convinced, still followed the treatment I counseled, and showed me, a few weeks later, a superb roseola, the confirmatory mark of the diagnosis.

"Cure me quickly," said he, "for in two months I get married."

"You would never do such a thing! Wait at least until you have passed the virulent period; and between now and a few years——"

"It is impossible, doctor."

"But your action is dishonorable!"

"We will occupy separate beds."

"For how many hours?"

"Well, if you insist, I will tell my intended; but I cannot back out."

"Then it is a different matter. If the girl accepts, I have nothing more to say."

Epilogue.—Six months later I saw my patient, accompanied by his lawful spouse, who had, upon her own testimony, been honestly forewarned. The continence which the young husband had proposed having never gone beyond an intention, I was called upon to cauterize the vulvar syphilides of the one and palatine vault of the other. They left last year (1888) to go abroad in a pretty satisfactory condition.

As we are considering proofs, let us continue. We have already stated that the primary lesion might last less than a month; here is a very marked case:—

CASE III. (*Personal*).—A young man of 22 years, M. Paul D., studying in a military school, came to see me, October, 1887, to consult me regarding a small abrasion of the size of a lentil, and which had lasted five days. He would have paid no attention to it, said he, had I not told him previously to beware of the least erosion of the genitals. The abrasion, as is the rule, was located on the prepuce, near the balano-preputial sulcus, close to the frenum, on the right side. Very marked induration, cartilaginous in character.

On a voyage to Algeria he had had, on his return, intimate relations with a public girl of Marseilles. From that time, about twenty-five days, he had not been able to get out of school; so that he was certain as to the impossibility of having acquired the lesion in some other locality at a later date. I did not hesitate to diagnose *syphilis*, despite the doubtful looks of the patient, who believed with difficulty that such a small thing could justify such a large word, but, nevertheless, commenced the mercurial treatment, which I promptly prescribed.

The chancre, simply powdered morning and evening, healed in *twelve days*, and the induration persisted, as is usual. A month later I saw my patient. Over the scar of the chancre there existed an ulcerous plaque, together with two or three others in the neighborhood. Upon the body, a discrete papular roseola, which rapidly disappeared under internal treatment and steam baths.

January, 1889.—I received a call from my patient, whom I had lost sight of for several months. He is as healthy as possible, with the exception of a few syphilides which appear from time to time upon his mucous membranes and rapidly disappear. He is continuing the intermittent treatment which I advised.

This case is interesting in two respects: First, because it demonstrates that the appearance of the chancre may be transitory, and, as a sequence, may sometimes be regarded as herpes when the induration is not distinct; secondly, because it shows that specific treatment, given from the beginning, does not retard, as has been contended, secondary symptoms to the extent of causing one to abandon the idea of syphilis.

Commence by first making your diagnoses well, you who contradict; give mercury immediately, which will be time gained by your patients, and spare us all those so-called discoveries and idle objections which facts disprove or reduce to nothing.

Second Period.—The local accident has healed or will heal, and the patient observes a light maculation about the waist or upon the chest; small, red spots, lenticular, with or without elevation, covered or not with epidermic scales. This is *roseola.* There exist a number of varieties; but as we cannot enter into details, we describe what ordinarily transpires.

This roseola may be wanting; but most often it is the first apparent symptom. Sometimes, but rarely, it is psoriasis, or else pustulo-crustaceous syphilides; that is to say, large crusts, resembling pretty much, except in color, macaroons on a piece of paper. But these cases are almost pathological varieties now. They are observed, in general, but much smaller, upon the scalp (crusts of the head), in the beard and eyebrows.

Roseola may be abundant or discrete; its color is of a delicate rose at the beginning, rapidly changing to a coppery red; often then the spots, whether papular or not, become surrounded with an epidermic collarette, which is very characteristic. At other times the roseola spreads itself *en masse* or in irregular islets; then it is styled *erythematous.* So much for the body; there are yet other varieties of which we will speak, if there be occasion to do so. This roseola may cover the entire trunk and limbs; it is rare in the face, and fortunately so. However, it may show itself upon the forehead as a diadem of papules,—the crown of Venus (*corona Veneris*). Roseola is cured by baths; we will speak of this under the head of treatment.

Nine times out of ten the hair falls out, but rarely in its entirety. This is the *alopecia.* The beard, the eyebrows, and eyelashes sometimes fall out, but more rarely. The only treatment for alopecia is the general treatment of syphilis.

In the mouth, on the lips, the internal surface of the cheeks, the tonsils, the palate, the tongue, are frequently found, in greater or less abundance, ulcerated papular syphilides, often surrounded by a bright-red areola, and covered with a whitish secretion, which is very characteristic. These lesions heal rapidly under cauterizations and gargles,—always with internal treatment,—but are numerous under the influence of alcohol and tobacco-smoke. The posterior cervical ganglia are engaged like those of the groin, but are equally indolent, and never suppurate.

About the anus, on the penis and vulva, are generally encountered papular or papulo-hypertrophic syphilides, also called *mucous patches*, and which heal under cauterizations and lotions.

The mucous patches, or, to be more exact, the syphilides, which have their seat on the genitalia, affect two principal forms, the ulcerative and the hypertrophic, with all the intermediary forms. The ulcerative form has a preference for the cicatrix of the primary lesion, which leads patients to suppose that their chancre has re-appeared. The hypertrophic form has for its sites of predilection the vulva and anus. This is easily understood; in the first there is more room than on the penis; secondly, those parts being symmetrical and in juxtaposition, reciprocally erode each other and retain the acrid and irritating secretion, thus forming the most favorable soil for the production of vegetating syphilides. As a matter of fact, other things being equal, and the question of soil being left apart, we see vulvar syphilides less frequently in those women who have regular habits of cleanliness, and they diminish in a marked manner, without any treatment, in filthy girls by the sole use of baths.[1]

The papules sometimes form, especially upon the internal surface of the labia majora and buttocks, elevations 1 centimetre in height, more or less large, constituting a true ridge, and ulcerated on the free surface. The liquid which oozes is not pus, in the strict acceptation of the term; it is a sort of yellowish serum, with

[1] This may be daily observed at l'hôpital de Lourcine.

leucocytes, if you wish; very fetid, having a characteristic odor, which is more marked in inverse proportion to the woman's cleanliness.

All these lesions vary considerably, according as the soil is scrofulous or healthy, according to the age of the syphilitic infection, or the physiological condition and habits of temperance or excesses of the subject.

I have seen, at Lourcine, poor girls come to the *consultation* armed with a syphilis which they had nursed with jealous care for six or eight months, and fed with torrents of alcohol and an incalculable number of cigarettes. Add to that loss of sleep and its consequences, picture to yourselves the daily assaults of foul patrons, whom nothing could defile, either physically or morally, —walking masses of rottenness,—and you may have an idea of their state upon their arrival at the hospital.

As soon as they step into the room, a peculiar odor makes you retch; the diagnosis is already made. It would be difficult to describe the sight which presents itself to the physician. The genitalia, hidden by the syphilides, sometimes no longer present a human form.

All this heals rapidly, and *without leaving any traces*, under specific (mercurial) treatment, baths, lotions, and cauterizations. In cases like the above it generally requires three or four months to *bleach* the patients. Under ordinary circumstances, if the patient be tractable, the cleaning-up may be done in two months, sometimes in six weeks or less. All depends upon the extent of the havoc.

I will only mention, for the purpose of a reminder, the interdigital mucous patches found upon the feet, and syphilitic onychia, a special affection of the matrix of the nail. I have also seen in one of my patients, in 1883, a group of papulo-hypertrophic syphilides in the right axilla; a number of physicians of Brussels (she was a Belgian) were unable to give this affection a name, although it had lasted over a year, if we are to believe her. It is true that she presented no other lesion. I placed her under constitutional treatment, and lightly cauterized. Everything disappeared in less than a month, the disease first and the patient next.

Next, covering all, we have a special anæmia, which yields to mercury and tonics. For mercury, which was abused in the sixteenth century, but so unjustly condemned in our times, when we know how to give it, cures the anæmia of the syphilitic, in whom it attacks the syphilis, and not the constitution.

This does not mean that all this procession of physical ornaments may not relapse. Let the patient, who believes himself cured at the first truce, completely abandon internal treatment, take to strong liquors, and be a little too valiant in the *tête-à-tête*,[1] and before two months everything will have returned. It follows, then, that one must be temperate, well-nourished, avoid excesses of all kinds, and follow the intermittent treatment for the required number of years, if there never appeared the slightest sore. Do not forget, you who are syphilitic, that the sword of Damocles is continually suspended over your heads during the secondary period, and that, because you fail to follow the advice of a well-informed physician—specialist or other, so long as he knows syphilis—you expose yourself to bitter regrets, if not remorse. "*Maxima debetur puero reverentia*,"[2] says Juvenal; I would add, in a different train of

[1] The results of recent observations of M. Diday (of Lyons) show that venereal excesses paralyze the good effects of antisyphilitic treatment.

[2] The greatest respect is due to the child.

thought, *even before conception.* To those who understand, I salute.

There are still other symptoms less prominent, which I will merely mention. First, the *syphilitic fever*, which certain authors of the sixteenth century, Ulrich von Hutten,[1] for example, have perfectly recognized; so that it is not a recent discovery, in spite of what has been said. Next, the *nocturnal cephalalgia*, a sort of headache, giving the sensation of a band of iron pressing more especially on the occiput, and commencing in the evening, only to cease in the morning. The authors of the sixteenth century give, upon this subject, rather curious explanations, which we will publish in due course of time in our third volume. There has been a great deal of discussion upon the causes of this cephalalgia, which certain modern syphilographers imagine they have invented; it has been regarded as the consequence of precocious tertiary lesions of the skull, but it seems to be simply due to a general heat, and that of the bed in particular. If this was the true explanation, we could easily understand why this cephalalgia is, above all, nocturnal. This symptom, whose duration is ordinarily very short (eight to fifteen days), is generally observed, when it exists, at the beginning of the secondary period. We propose to take up this question later on.

Lesions affecting the eyes (keratitis, iritis, etc.) are also seen, but not very frequently; finally, articular pains, and even true arthritis, which have been well described by my colleague, Dr. de Fontaine,[2] surgeon-in-chief of the factories of Creusot.

[1] Ulrich von Hutten: De guaiaci medicina et morbo gallico. Moguntiæ, MDXIX. The French Disease and its Treatment by Guaïac. Mainz, 1519.

[2] Léon de Fontaine: De la syphilis articulaire (on articular syphilis), Thèse de Paris, 1883.

I will not dwell upon the distinction of the syphilides into *pustular*, *vesicular*, *bullous*, *tubercular*, etc.; let it suffice to know that they appear upon the skin; and when you observe anything abnormal upon your *external tegument*, consult your physician first. But beware of those healers of urinals, who have received their diplomas from the bill-posters, and who have received decorations most often in the police court. Advice costs nothing, it is true; but the medicines (!!!) which must be taken are rated according to the *face* of the patient, from twenty francs up to the infinite.

Before passing to the tertiary period, let us devote a few lines to the period called the *transition* stage. We first have iritis, a late secondary accident, but most often a transition lesion: it is not grave, providing that treatment is taken. Then, certain lesions of the skin, and especially of the cellular tissue, notably of the tongue.[1] These lesions of the cellular tissue properly belong to the tertiary period; but as they are coincident, at the time of their appearance, with certain late secondary eruptions of the skin (*palmar* and *plantar* syphilides, for example),[2] the patient is said to be going through the period of transition, and he is given the mixed treatment (mercuric salts combined with iodides). Sometimes sarcocele is also noticed, but this is rather observable at the tertiary period. [The author fails to mention the fact that iritis is frequently an early secondary symptom, as well as the squamous syphilides of the palms and soles.]

[1] Ulcerations; exfoliative dermatitis in segments of circles, or epithelial glossitis, etc.

[2] These desquamative syphilides, whose site of predilection is the palm of the hand and sole of the foot, follow the same course as the epithelial glossitis. Each is a circle, at first small, which goes on increasing, and whose circumference consists of a series of segments of circles.

Third Period.—Let us now approach that famous tertiary period in which the disease is no longer dangerous except to the syphilitic himself. Up to the present it was relatively nothing but roses; the danger existed only for others. Let me hasten to add, however, that in a patient who has treated himself well, and who *watches*, tertiary accidents, as a rule, are reduced to but a small thing, and often never appear at all; for they are then postponed to such an extent that the patient, before their appearance, has the time to attain the age at which death comes, no matter from what cause. Life being something relative, it is plain that if, for example, we prolong the life of a consumptive to the age of eighty in such a manner that he dies of apoplexy or syncope, we may consider him as having been cured of his bacilli (with or without *commas*).

We have already stated that the third and last period was, above all, directed to the connective tissue. Besides, the syphilitic virus, in a general way, is characterized by a proliferation of connective tissue. This is why alcoholic beverages are harmful to syphilitics. In addition to this, drunkards are predisposed to a host of other diseases which owe their origin to proliferation with condensation of the connective or cellular tissue. I will first mention cirrhosis of the liver, always mortal; then, cardiac lesions. As a matter of fact, the poor valves are continually bathed in a blood saturated with rum, and shrivel and become insufficient, from which an impediment in the circulation of the blood ensues. It is a recognized fact that the heart is a suction- and force-pump, the valves acting as movable valves. Try, in watering your garden, to use a pump whose valves are not large enough, and you will see, while doing double the amount of labor, how much water you have drawn at the end of the day. It is the same thing with the heart; disciples of Bacchus, think of your valves! The brain-substance, the spinal cord, the nerves, all yield to the pernicious influence of alcohol. Add to this a syphilis treated with contempt, and contemplate the result!

I would not put it down as a rule that drunkards are the only ones who can have serious tertiary lesions. It must not be forgotten that there are certain unfortunate cases in which, outside of alcoholism, syphilis produces deep ravages. But it is exceedingly rare when patients have faithfully followed out treatment. Let me say, *en passant*, that a certain number of patients, fortunately in the minority, have had dealings either with quacks who repudiate mercury[1] and treat their patients in a fantastic manner, or with homœopaths who gave them candy and clear water. Alas! these mountebanks are not the only ones who boast of not using mercury. I could mention a hospital service in Paris in which the liquid metal has been banished. If the quacks, the charlatans, the homœopaths, abuse their patients, either by their infernal drugs, which are worse than the disease, or by their inoffensive confectionery, which does not stop the invading march of the trouble, what matters it to

[1] All can see, not without pain, if they are physicians, the flaring advertisements posted in certain monuments (urinals): they are ornamented with colored pictures, in which a conjunctivitis is given as a consequence of injections or strictures!!! Another one of these horripilators bears the legend: *Effects of Mercury—Cancer of the Tongue; Amputation.* This is the flower: an injection in the urinary canal, causing an inflammation of the ocular serosa, was a dream; but mercury causing cancer is rather stiff! There are some more ignorant or boldly dishonest, but they are under the protection of the laws. When will the authorities, if they do not wish to defend the interests of the medical fraternity against the progressive invasion of certain rascals, with or without diplomas, protect at least the patient by regulating the bill-posting? Of course, it is only a matter of the public health (1889).

you, say you? Why do they go to them? This is true; but when a man of talent, and so situated as to make pupils, is concerned, the consequences are serious. At l'hôpital St. Louis one can see at one's leisure the consequences in the miserable patients suffering from serious tertiary manifestations.

A few lines of contemporaneous history will furnish an idea of the good faith of the celebrities of dead walls. In 1882, while I was an interne at l'hôpital de Bicêtre, one of our colleagues in the same institution conceived the idea of calling upon one of these fustians of drugging disguised as doctors.[1] He penetrates the blind office, where one enters *without speaking to the janitor*, and finds himself face to face with the preponent. Our friend relates a fictitious case. After the semblance of an examination, the seller gives him some product guaranteed to be *vegetable*, *without mercury*, in accordance with the handbill. A chemist, entrusted with the analysis of the pills which constituted the basis of treatment, found them composed solely of *protiodide of mercury!* Knowing that mercury is the only specific, after having maligned the poor metal in order to attract easily frightened persons, he gives it, right or wrong, under another label. If he only gave it to syphilitics alone! But no; each one is provided with his *little package.* This is logical: where would the profit be in *free* consultations if the patient did not carry off fifteen or twenty francs' worth of drugs, either useful or not? Let us return to our subject.

It may be objected that syphilis is a disease of well-defined cycles, that it has its three distinct periods, and that, no matter what is done, the patient will get well

[1] Many are only *officiers de santé*; a few convictions, which were published, have shown that certain ones had no diplomas of any description.

of his chancre, of his mucous or cutaneous syphilides, and will enter upon the tertiary phase without retaining any traces of his anterior lesions. Granted; but it is precisely from the point of view of this tertiary period that we are discussing the subject. The first two never did constitute any source of anxiety to us; they are disagreeable and inconvenient, but rarely painful. Mercury, administered according to the classical rules, helps nature in her reparative work; it eliminates itself by way of the secretions, after having hastened the resorption of that proliferated cellular tissue, whose exuberance manifests itself in a manner as varied as it is complex. When the tertiary period arrives,—if it comes on at all,—one-half of the work is done and iodine is sufficient. The paradoxical master, to whom we have alluded, gives the iodides in conjunction with bark; but, in my humble opinion, it is insufficient. I will even say more: I have observed at Lourcine, in 1878, several syphilitic women to whom iodide of potassium had been given immediately upon the appearance of the chancre; the secondary lesions presented themselves to an unusual amount. Was it a simple coincidence? I will not decide the question. At all events, one of our teachers, to whom I mentioned it the following year, stated that he had observed the same thing. This would open up an interesting field for investigation from a therapeutical point of view. We may, perhaps, some day have an opportunity of returning to this subject, which, in our historical study, we cannot consider in a manner which would prove satisfactory.

I have stated that the syphilitic virus, in the tertiary period, attacks the cellular (connective) tissue. The most common lesions, though late, are the masses, in the form of agglomerated tubercles, which are deposited in the connective tissue. They are *gummata*, so named on account of the gummy appearance of the products they contain at the period of their softening. These accidents show themselves at the end of eight, ten, fifteen, or twenty years; sometimes later, but rarely during the first few years of infection. At first they are hard tumors, *painful* to the touch, which soften, open, give exit to an ichorous liquid, similar to a solution of gum, and suppurating a little. When all this matter has escaped, cicatrization begins.

These gummata may occur in the brain, from which arise temporary paralyses, epileptiform attacks of an evanescent character, etc.; or, in the connective tissue of the glands, muscles, etc., from which arise various functional troubles whose description would make us lose sight of our objective point Let us note, in passing, syphilitic *sarcocele*, characterized by fibrous bands which traverse the testicle, changing it in a short time into a hard, elongated form, characteristic in appearance, and rendering it unsuited for fecundation. Sarcocele is sometimes a transition lesion, but it is most often observed during the tertiary period.

I will merely mention the lesions of the muscles and tendons, infrequent accidents in syphilis, as well as sarcocele, I may add. We will now pass on to the lesions of the bones and periosteum, which are more important: yet we can only describe them hastily.

First, we have *ostitis*, that is to say, inflammation of the bone, attacking preferably the superficial bones. The same is true of *caries* and *necrosis*, results of ostitis; it is, above all, the bones of the face which are attacked.

There is also observed swelling of the periosteum, without any lesion of the bone, constituting *periostosis.*

When it forms a tumor between the bone and periosteum, the periostosis is called gummatous; sometimes it becomes phlegmonous, but most often it gives rise to a plastic effusion, which may be the point of origin of bony tumors, known as *exostoses*, and which will now occupy our attention.

Exostoses, generally late accidents, but rather frequent in tertiary syphilis, are of two kinds—partial exostoses or *true exostoses*, and generalized exostoses, or *hyperostoses*. Partial exostoses are tumors developed upon any part of a bone; hyperostoses consist of a swelling *en masse* of a portion of a bone,—a hypertrophy, in fact. The former have the appearance of tumors stuck upon a bone, or developed in its thickness, if it be a flat bone; while hyperostoses, which are most often seen on long bones, are exostoses in which the body of the bone itself forms the tumor; it is no longer a simple swelling; it is the entire bony mass doubled or trebled. These morbid products are the more interesting to us, as they will serve us soon to prove the existence of syphilis at a prehistoric era.

Exostoses frequently cause characteristic pains, called the *osteocopic pains*. The sites of predilection of these tumors are: the middle portion of the *tibia*, the bones of the *skull*, the *clavicle*, the *ulna*, the lower part of the *radius*, the extremities of the *fibula* and the *sternum*.

Exostoses are not always attended by osteocopic pains; the bony swelling is frequently the first symptom which attracts the patients' attention, for they believe themselves cured long since. Here is a very interesting example of untreated syphilis, having gone through its course, and manifesting itself by rather benign symptoms in the tertiary period.

Case IV. (*Personal*).—A young woman, one of my patients, Mrs. N., came to my office in June, 1886. She was then thirty years old, and was a dressmaker,—an occupation she permanently retained after having had quite an exciting career.

"Doctor," said she, "there has grown, within the past few days, a swelling on my right elbow; I do not feel any pain, but it worries me. What do you think it can be?"

Without immediately answering, I felt the wonderful tumor, which could be plainly perceived through the satin sleeve. At the other elbow there was an enlargement of the same kind, but less distinct, and which the patient had not yet noticed. Suspecting an old syphilis, I asked her if she had not felt analogous tumors in other places, more especially the legs.

"No; but if you wish to see——"

"Willingly."

On each tibia, a little below the anterior tuberosity, was found a fine exostosis. I was certain. However, being desirous of having more light, I bluntly asked her this question:

"At what time did you have syphilis?"

Somewhat surprised, my patient hesitated a few moments; then, reflecting, like an intelligent woman, that a feint would be useless, if not harmful, she answered, plainly:

"Seven years ago."

"Very good. And did you treat yourself?"

"Certainly. I followed a *thorough* course for three years; it is Doctor X. [I have forgotten the name of this illustrious unknown] who undertook my case."

* * * * * * * * * * *

"Why yes, you must know him—a homœopathic physician."

"Ah! Well, it will be necessary to begin treating you."

"Commence?"

"Yes, madam; for seven years you have seen the successive symptoms of your syphilis, while eating sugar-pills; now you will have it treated with medicine."

"Very well."

I immediately prescribed mixed treatment, and had the satisfaction of learning from the patient herself, whom I frequently saw after this, that the exostoses had entirely disappeared in three months. Since that time she has been in the best of health; but it must be acknowledged that she follows treatment very conscientiously.

White syphilitic tumors have been described, but such things do not exist. There is here a mistake in terms, and this is due to the fact that the majority have misunderstood the memoir of M. Richet[1] on white tumors. As de Fontaine[2] very aptly states, "At the time of the publication of M. Richet's memoir, the name white tumor was used in the sense of arthritis, or even of chronic joint disease, while to-day it is only applied to scrofulo-tuberculous joint diseases. M. Richet, to avoid coining a new word, described as a simple variety a condition which he would have been justified to create, or perhaps should have created, a new disease. To-day he certainly would not act in the same manner. The cause is understood. We find synovites, ostites, syphilitic joint troubles, but never white tumors outside of scrofula.

On the part of the nervous system we find, more particularly, paralyses and certain sensory troubles, to which we will merely allude. Then we arrive at the visceral lesions. Let us note syphilitic affections of the liver (pseudo-cirrhoses), of the urinary apparatus, and of the respiratory passages (gummata of the lung), of the thymus, of the spleen, etc. Those of our readers desirous of entering into details upon these subjects are referred to special works upon the subject. Finally, we will mention the *cachexia*, since the term has been adopted; but, as Follin[3] very justly remarks, it is "less a symptom of syphilis than a complication of this disease." This weakness, which is not peculiar to lues, is found in patients who have been forced to suffer physiological poverty and have a broken-down constitution, caused either by bad hygiene or by an improperly applied and

[1] Mémoires de l'Académie de Médecine. Paris, t. xvii.

[2] *Loc. cit.*

[3] Traité élément. de path. ext. Paris, 1874. Elementary Treatise on Pathological Anatomy.

badly understood mercurial treatment, and in all cases badly carried out.

Tertiary lesions may be precocious and appear during the early months of syphilitic infection, but this rarely occurs. Let us also note the tertiary ulcerations of the genitalia, which may pass for soft chancres; the touch-stone is the treatment by iodides. I saw a very fine example of this in 1881, at Lourcine, in *salle* Astruc (formerly St. Clêments). M. Gouguenheim, then my chief of service, had a wax cast taken, and this is still in the small museum of Lourcine. Last year (1889), I again had the opportunity of seeing an analogous case which led to an incorrect diagnosis.

CASE V. (*Personal*).—One of my patients, a young woman, Clémence M., by occupation a concert-hall singer, had me called, in October, 1888, to have my opinion in regard to a small erosion which existed at the point of intersection of the labia majora, at the base of the clitoris. This erosion was very superficial and painful, not at all indurated, and existed since three or four days. Was it ulcerated herpes? I was satisfied to order a white precipitate ointment, advising the patient to watch the lesion and return in case it got worse. In fact, it was expectant treatment.

I saw her a month later: she had purposely come from a sea-port on the Channel, where a physician, taking it for a soft chancre, had made numerous cauterizations. This interference, as energetic as it was uncalled for, had transformed the erosion into a deep ulcer, as large as a silver half-dollar and very painful. A liquid of a lemon-yellow and looking like mucilage was discharging: considerable œdema of the whole region existed. The patient, questioned upon this matter, assured me that she never had syphilis, which, at all events, excluded any idea of former treatment. However, she remembered having, five or six months previously, spots on the body,—what she thought was "eczema," and to which she paid no attention.

I did not hesitate to prescribe iodide of potassium in large doses (3, then 4, grammes daily [45 to 60 grains]), and, for local treatment, I contented myself with starch poultices to relieve the tension of the œdematous tissues, followed by cocaine ointment, which removed the pain.

At the end of a week the ulcer was a third smaller; it was reduced one-half in a fortnight, and the œdema had disappeared. At the end of a month, healing was complete. At present she is taking a general treatment, convinced, and with reason, that she is syphilitic.

Let us state, in conclusion, that syphilis is acquired but once; the two or three cases of re-infection, reported by Follin, are too indefinite to admit of the matter without contesting it.

It is time to call a halt. Volumes could be written upon the manifestations of syphilis, and such is not my intention: the works of this character have already reached a number sufficient to constitute a chaos. Nevertheless, I have regarded it as indispensable to give a *résumé* of the leading symptoms which characterize syphilis. We show the thorns before the roses, so that the reader, if he has had the courage to read all of this sketch, will know, in the first place, that pox is a disease which must be treated; but that it is not, as certain patients imagine, a rotting away, which takes off an arm or a leg, or cripples one for life. Next, he will understand the terms which will recur upon every page of this historical study. He may even take interest in knowing the *entire* history of a virus which attacks all, young or old, learned or illiterate, smart or simple, innocent or guilty, *lascivious* or *prudish.*[1]

[1] We have found this idea expressed by Barthélemy in his poem on syphilis:—

"Nulle digue qui puisse arreter ce torrent;
Il saisit à la fois le docte et l'ignorant.
Le riche en son hôtel, le pauvre en sa cabanc,
L'impie et l'homme saint qu'abrite la soutane,
Le vieillard, l'enfant même, atteint souvent d'un mal
Dont il n'est pas lavé par le flot baptismal;
Et peut-être anjourd'hui, parmi l'espèce humaine,
Il n'est pas un seul homme, et dans l'homme une veine
Où, quoique bien souvent, encore non révélé,
Le virus destructeur ne soit inoculé."

CHAPTER II.

ORIGIN OF THE WORD SYPHILIS.

"Syphilidemque ab eo labem dixêre coloni."—FRACASTOR.
[The inhabitants of the country called it the disease of Syphilis.]

EVERY author who writes a work more or less connected with venereal diseases commences by giving some attention to the origin of the word *syphilis*. As to us, we will be very brief; for, to enter into many details as to the innumerable appellations which the *universal evil* received before a definite term was devoted to it would be to anticipate the most important chapter of our next publication. However, we may say, without further commentary, that this name was introduced by Fracastor in his Latin poem, which has deservedly remained a celebrated one.[1] The Italian physician, inspired by heroic epochs, places before us the divinities of Paganism, and supposes that a shepherd, whom he calls *Syphilus*, had addressed words offensive to Apollo, and had deserted his altars. The god, to punish him, sent him a disease of the genitals, "which the inhabitants of the country called the *disease of Syphilus*." From this incident, and from this *syphilis*, was derived:

"Syphilidemque ab eo labem dixêre coloni."

We will recur to the work of Fracastor when we study the authors of the sixteenth century.

But, from what source did Fracastor obtain this name? Opinions are divided. Let us immediately quote, to reject it completely, the opinion of Bosquillon, who proposes the orthography *siphilis*, which is inexact,

[1] Hieronymi Fracastorii: Syphilis, sive morbus gallicus. Veronæ, 1530. Jerome Fracastor: Syphilis, or the French Disease.

and derives this word from σιφλός, *reprehensible*, which is very vague. Others, like Swediaur,[1] seeing in this disease the result of bestial relations, find in it the two words σῦς, *hog*, and φιλεῖν, *to love*. Where has syphilis been seen to originate in the hog? As this theory is not mentioned by Fracastor, and as we must look not whence the name might come, but whence the physician of Verona obtained it, we will hold ourselves to the following explanation, which seems to us the simplest and most admissible. The word *syphilis* descends in a direct line (Rejes, Fallopius, Castel) from σύν, *with*, and φιλία, *love*, the companion of love; which means, in plain language, that the pox is a contagious disease, transmitted more especially by intimate relations. It is plain, then, that it is not necessary to incriminate the companion of St. Anthony; nor is it incumbent upon us to find out whether the poor devil who has had ill luck should be congratulated or despised. Every one is not so situated as to be able to have a harem guarded by eunuchs!

Before Fracastor, the current expression was *morbus gallicus;* it was also called the *Neapolitan disease*, the *disease of the Germans*, the *disease of the Poles*, *of the Spaniards*, *of the Turks*, etc; the *disease of the holy man Job*, of *St. Sementius*, of *St. Mevius*, of *St. Roch*, and others. All nations have received credit for it, as well as all the saints. But, of all these names, the one most generally employed in the sixteenth century was that of the *French disease*, or, rather, *morbus gallicus*, as that Latin was the scientific language of the times. There is no agreement in regard to the origin of this expression. Certain authors, starting out with the principle that pox also received the name of the *bad*

[1] F. Swediaur: Practical Observations on Venereal Complaints. Edinburgh, 1784.

itch (*mauvaise galle*), have seen in the word *gallicus* an adjective designating the kind of disease. Others have found a nationality in it,—*gallicus*, *Gaul;* otherwise, *French.* They base themselves upon the refutable fact that the French were the first ones contaminated at the siege of Naples. We will allude, later on, to this great discussion. The fact to remember, for the time being, is that the expression *morbus gallicus* was that currently used by authors in the fifteenth and sixteenth centuries, as well in France as in all the rest of Europe. This is clearly brought out in a passage of Ulrich von Hutten,[1] where this author states that, if he has used the expression *French disease* in his book, it is solely to conform to a usage which has become prevalent; and "certes not," adds he, "by reason of hatred against a celebrated nation, and one which is, perhaps, the most civilized and hospitable of our times; but because I would fear not to be sufficiently understood by every one if I employed another term to designate this disease." We are happy to note this declaration from a foreigner, although it dates from the sixteenth century; and, coming from a German knight, it has still more value.

Later on, as a few points of resemblance (especially at the end of the variolous eruption) between the pustules of syphilis and those of variola (Latin *variola*), which was first called *variole*, then *vérole*, were noted, the *morbus gallicus* became the *grosse vérole* (big pox), and, in order to avoid confusion, variola was given the name of *petite vérole* (small pox),—a name which it still retains. Syphilis has also been called *gorrhe*, *grand gorrhe*, etc.; each people gave it a special name. The enemy of the time being was employed as an appropriate sponsor. That is why the Turks called it the *Christian*

[1] *Loc. cit.*

disease; the Spaniards, the *disease of the Turks;* the Italians, the *French disease;* the French, the *Neapolitan disease*, etc. At last, the expression *lues venerea*, or simply *lues*, or *venereal disease*, or *venereal evil*, placed everybody in accord; then the word *pox* (*vérole*) prevailed, and was designated by a capital V,[1] or written out in full, in almost all the works of the eighteenth century treating of this matter. The term *syphilis*, forgotten since the poem of Fracastor, was adopted by the authors of the nineteenth century, and received the sanction of science. Our prudish epoch hides its face before the word *pox*. Our contemporaries mention it only in a whisper, seeming to find in it a flavor of obscenity. This false idea has regrettable consequences. "Syphilis," says Patton,[2] "receives a bad character from the prejudices which exist in the world; the idea which has made it considered as baneful, no matter what its origin, has especially tended to render it such. It is not the disease which is shameful, but the libertinage which gives birth to it." It is very plain that, the origin of syphilis being the same in all planes of society, syphilis may attack the "steady" man, who simply obeys physiological laws, as well as the vicious one, given over to all forms of debauchery. To classify the former as in the same category as the latter would be a crying shame and injustice, for chance alone, in this case, can be blamed. Let us bury that word *pox*, if you wish it, as it recalls a terrible hydra, terribly exaggerated; but let us, at least, print the word syphilis, for we have no other one with which to scientifically designate the *cosmopolitan evil!*

[1] We would say with a large P.

[2] De la Prostitution et de la Syphilis dans les grandes villes. Lyon, 1842. Prostitution and Syphilis in Large Cities.

CHAPTER III.

THE AGE OF SYPHILIS.

"Faire l'histoire de la syphilis, cést pour anisi dire tracer celle de l'humanité."—PHILIPPE ALBERT.[1]

"Je croirai avec Guy Patin que non seulement Job, David, Salomon, et Adam avoient la Vérole, mais qu'elle étoit dans le cahos avant la création."—DE LA METTRIE.[2]

THE date of the birth of syphilis—here is a controverted question! Torrents of ink of *all virtues* have been spread, some wishing to prove that syphilis was born in 1494—theseare the fierce ones; others, to establish that it existed in all antiquity—these latter comprising the minority. Between these well-defined theories are found intermediate opinions—the mean terms. Among the former, at least in the sixteenth century, how many ignoramuses copied each other! How many empirics! How many charlatans! And the reasons invoked! There is sufficient material for several volumes. This is what will be found condensed in a subsequent publication.

Nowadays, there is more and more of a tendency to declare America innocent; let us say right here that it took more than twenty years for the authors, who were more or less contemporaneous of the epidemic, to think of finding the origin in San Domingo. Christopher Columbus himself never suspected it; at all events, he

[1] To write the history of syphilis is, so to speak, to trace that of humanity. Mémoires sur les malad. vénér. Bordeaux, 1836. Memoir on Venereal Diseases.

[2] I am inclined to believe, with Guy Patin, that not only Job, David, Solomon, and Adam had the pox, but that it was in chaos before the creation. Saint Cosme vengé (St. Cosmos avenged), an anonymous work attributed to de la Mettrie by Barbier. Strasburg, 1744.

does not mention a word of it in his letters, even after several voyages; and it required an individual who was not very reliable—Fernandez y Oviédo—to accuse the natives of the Antilles, nearly *twenty-five years* after their discovery, to have this tale come to us. The best proof of the falsity of this assertion is in the multitude of names given to syphilis at the time of the great epidemic of the fifteenth century. If the disease, supposed to have been unknown up to that time, had really been brought from America, would it not have immediately received the name of the *American evil*, a name which it certainly would have retained? And Christopher Columbus would have gone to his eternal sleep without ever having suspected that the country discovered by him was the focus of a new virus! It would be very strange. However, we will give Oviédo his proper deserts later on.

The legend of the American origin of syphilis, still in great favor with the public, is actually no longer defended, except by a very small number of authors.[1] A few find another origin for it—Africa; others concede that it may have shown itself in the middle ages; but the majority attest its birth, for Europe, to Naples, during the siege of that city by Charles VIII, in the year 1494. The truth is, that syphilis is and was everywhere, but not as intense in all countries and at all times, and, above all, but little known, not to say unrecognized.

We have already said that we considered this disease as old as the world; now we are going to prove it. We propose to quote and elucidate the ancient texts already noted by our predecessors, who have endeavored to support the same theory. The arguments, good as well as

[1] In this connection the reader is referred to "A Study of Pre-Columbian Syphilis in America," by Jas. Nevins Hyde, A.M., M.D., in Am. Jour. Med. Sci., August, 1891.

bad, will be analyzed. We will add others, and bring out other quotations which we have not found cited before anywhere. We will thus arrive, from age to age, to the epidemic of the fifteenth century, which will constitute the subject of our second volume, together with an analysis of the most interesting authors of the middle ages.

For instance, it is well understood that our first volume is entirely devoted to the proofs of the existence of syphilis from the creation of the world to the middle ages. Let those who doubt this ancient origin read *Nuei-King*, a medical treatise edited after the traditions and secular documents of China, by the Emperor *Hoang-ty*, who lived 2637 B.C. When they are sufficiently edified by this, I would recommend them to visit the Musée d'Histoire Naturelle and the Musée d'Anthropologie; they will see prehistoric human bones bearing the undeniable evidence of tertiary lesions. We will now guide the reader in these interesting researches.

CHAPTER IV.

SYPHILIS IN PREHISTORIC TIMES.

"La syphilis heréditaire déforme le crane d'une maniére typique."—J. PARROT.[1]

"Anjourd'hui l'anthropologie a douné son puissant appui aux partisans de l'origine ancienne en montrant sur des squelettes préhistoriques des traces indéniables d'altérations syphilitiques."—P. HAMONIC.[2]

IT is necessary, to begin with, to be agreed as to the significance of the word *prehistoric.* You may say it is very simple: præ, *before;* historia, *history;* that is, that which appertains to a period anterior to history. While this may be good enough, it is, nevertheless, useful to give more ample explanations; for a number of persons regard the word *prehistoric* as synonymous with *antediluvian.* This is too absolute; many peoples, in fact,—were it only the French, without going any further,—are ignorant of their history during the first three or four thousand years which followed what it has been agreed to call the deluge: this is the prehistoric period of Gaul. A nation, such as China, for example, had its history thirty-two centuries before Christ, and knew that one of its emperors, *Chinnong*, lived three thousand two hundred and sixteen years before our era; whilst all the other countries, with the possible exception of India, Chaldea, Egypt, and Judea, were yet, at

[1] Hereditary syphilis deforms the skull in a typical manner.

[2] To-day anthropology has given its weighty support to the partisans of the ancient origin by showing the undeniable traces of syphilitic alterations on prehistoric skeletons. Des maladies vénériénnes chez les Hébreux à l'époque biblique. Paris, 1887. On the Venereal Diseases Among the Hebrews in Biblical Times.

that time, at their prehistoric period. Without going so far back, at the time of Hippocrates,—that is to say, in the fifth century before Christ,—history, among the Gauls, was limited to obscure legends or traditions, and there existed as yet no dynasty known or recognized among these bands of barbarians with their cannibalistic tendencies. The human bones half burnt, found in caves, leave no doubt in this respect.[1] From this it may be seen that it is impossible to stop at the same date to begin the period called prehistoric; since, at the same epoch, we find certain peoples cultivating the sciences, having treatises on medicine written through the means of the carefulness of their rulers, while others were still in the fullness of barbarism, not to say savagery. It is true that the former have remained stationary, and still travel in palanquins, while the latter get into the *express* and speak with their transoceanic friends by means of the telephone.

Astonishment may be expressed at seeing us give as our first proofs those drawn from anthropological discoveries. It is very plain that Chinese manuscripts, which date back more than forty centuries, are much anterior to certain Gaulish sepulchres in which have been found bones bearing pathological lesions. I will only cite as an example the skull of the cemetery of Brény (Aisne), which belongs to the Merovingian epoch. The contradiction is only apparent, however. As a matter of fact, the bones discovered in France, or in South America, might as well date from the deluge; and, as long as they do not date from an epoch in which the nation from which they are derived had a history, at home or among its neighbors, they are prehistoric.

[1] Conf. Le Baron : Lésions osseuses de l'homme préhistorique. Thèse de Paris, 1881. Osseous Lesions of Prehistoric Man.

It is for the purpose of disposing of the bones that we speak of the skull of the Frankish period, a historical epoch; we may then consider the written documents, and thus avoid repetition.

This being determined, let us desecrate the ancient sepulchres; let us draw from the clays, from the conglomerates containing bones, from the caves or Celtic dolmans, the remains of prehistoric man spared by the great cataclysm! Let us evoke the spirits of these first representatives of our species, from whom five or six thousand years separate us; then, perhaps, their skeletons, ranged in the cases of our museums, lifting up their skulls studded with osteophytes, and brandishing their tibiæ swelled with exostoses, will cry to their descendants of the nineteenth century: "Yes, we escaped the universal deluge; we are those human beings you dominate prehistoric, and whose flight upon the elevated ridges of the continents of those times inspired the symbolic ark of Noah. The race of the mammoth is forever lost: it sleeps in the midst of the polar ices which have served as its winding sheet. The mastodon and the dinotherium giganteum repose between the layers and strata of the tertiary period; they are lost in sands or locked up in the centre of the rocks which were their tombs; the species is extinct! We, your ancestors, we have survived where these colossi perished; and we had syphilis. Know then that it is with it that our race has traversed the centuries!"

It was the heritage of the antediluvian man: that one has come to us intact.

My colleague and friend, P. Hamonic, in a very interesting monograph, of which we will speak later on, thus sums up his opinion on the proofs, I would almost denominate *fossil*, of syphilis: "At this day anthropology has lent its powerful support to the partisans of the ancient origin by demonstrating upon prehistoric skeletons the undeniable traces of syphilitic alterations. This is an irrefutable demonstration. It is true that the nature of the lesions found in the majority of specimens may be discussed. A few, however, are so typical that it is *impossible* not to admit them."

With prehistoric syphilis is connected the name of J. Parrot, the late lamented Professor of the Faculty of Medicine of Paris. He was the first who dared demonstrate that venereal disease existed in the Stone Age. Born in the immense caves or in the shade of the pines and of the gigantic trees, syphilis now rules, the world over, after having passed through royal alcoves.

Without permitting himself to be daunted by the incredulous smiles of some, or the lively sallies of others, Parrot maintained his position before and against all, and, thanks to him, prehistoric syphilis has left no doubts except in the minds of the intractable. It is really painful to see the convictions of thirty or forty years overthrown by material proofs which are not as easy to refute as more or less obscure tests. Few minds, even of a superior order, consent to burn their idols, and, for want of arguments, they quibble, but do not surrender. We will pass on.

We will first consider the discovery of Solutré, which has excited anthropologists so much. Solutré is a locality in the department of Saône-et-Loire; we find here a prehistoric site. In the different excavations made since 1867 have been found the bones of reindeer and of horses, cut flints and remains belonging to the Gallo-Roman and Merovingian epochs. The human *débris* of Solutré appear to belong to a race coming from Asia. In 1872, the Abbé Ducrost, having undertaken some excavations, found a female skeleton lying in a direction from east to west, and surrounded by defaced stones; these remains, according to the opinion of anthropologists of the best authority (Broca, Parrot, and others), could be referred to the Stone Age, the period of the reindeer and of primitive man. The two tibiæ of this woman, according to the scientific reports, are the seat of *exostoses* manifestly *syphilitic.* The right one, especially, shows three elevations which are particularly characteristic. One is situated at the middle part, on the crest of the bone, from which it extends half-way to the internal and half-way to the external surface. Below, at a distance of two centimetres, a similar one exists, situated upon the crest of the tibia and upon the free border which forms its continuation; it also extends to the internal and external surface of the bone. Finally, a third exostosis is located upon the internal surface of the upper third of the bone. Examined by Broca, Ollier, Parrot, and Virchow, these exostoses were, by common consent, pronounced syphilitic.[1] M. Rollet, who upon several occasions examined these valuable relics, remains convinced that the exostoses of the skeleton of Solutré are to be considered as "more certain indications of syphilis than the cranial deformities" described by Parrot, and with which we will occupy our attention.

Professor Parrot gave his first lectures on prehistoric syphilis, at l'Hôpital des Enfants-Assistés, in 1877. It was upon an occasion when a few skulls of children, upon which lesions existed, were presented before the Société d'Anthropologie, that Parrot asserted that they were due

[1] We have derived this information from the Bulletin de la Société d'anthropologie, the Dictionnaire de médecine et de chirurgie pratiques, the Traité des maladies vénériennes (Treatise on Venereal Diseases) of M. Jullien, and the Dictionnaire encyclopédique des sciences médicales.

to hereditary syphilis. His opinion was shared in by Broca, whose high authority in anthropological matters no one could deny, as well as by other savants whom we will have occasion to quote. Parrot repeated what he said at the Enfants-Assistés to the Havre Congress and to the Anthropological Society the same year; and it is from the report of the meeting of the congress that we cull what follows.[1]

The Professor begins by describing, from his daily observations in his service at the Enfants-Assistés, the lesions produced on the skulls of infants by hereditary syphilis. As we are not giving lectures on syphilography, we cannot go into details. The important fact to remember is that, as a result of syphilis in the parents, the children present, especially at the superciliary ridges, thick and *persisting osteophytes.* These bony productions, due to the syphilitic process, are characteristic, and cannot be confounded with any other lesion. If the presence of these persistent lesions is noted upon the skulls of children found in the diluvian or other formations, they certainly cannot be attributed to whooping-cough. We will now let the Professor speak:—

> The Anthropological Institute possesses five Peruvian skulls of children; three are from Arica, and were sent by Dr. Bourrut; the other two were donated by M. Destruges. With the exception of one of the former, they are all pathological, and show the *undeniable traces of hereditary syphilis.*

It may be immediately objected that, Peru being in America, no one ever thought of denying the ancient existence of syphilis on the new continent. I will answer that, first, I am writing the history of syphilis from the traces it has left, and it has left them every-

[1] J. Parrot: les Déformaitions craniennes causées par la syphilis héréditaire (in Associat. franç. pour l'avancem. des Scienc. Congrés du Havre, 1877). The Cranial Deformities Caused by Hereditary Syphilis.

where, without distinction as to country; and, furthermore, that if patience be taken to read this entire chapter, there will be found, further on, identical descriptions of European bones, which may be compared with the descriptions that precede them. In 1887 there existed four syphilitic skulls in the Musée Broca. As we might be accused of making too vague or incomplete a quotation, we will give the proceedings *in extenso*:—

This is, in a few words, what is observed: In *No. 5*, *Case XI*, from a child which had six teeth, the fontanelle is large and the orbital arches are covered by a thick and porous *osteophyte*. Within, the bregmatic region of the frontal and the cavities of the parietals present a thin layer of a very porous morbid tissue, full of vascular furrows.

In *No. 6 of the same case*, the fontanelle is somewhat smaller than in the preceding, and presents externally, upon the frontal and upon the parietals, around the bregma, *four ossified ridges*, of oval form, with numerous porosities and furrows directed from in front backward. The glabella is covered by a similar plaque. Some portions of the internal surface are involved, even to a feeble degree, and at points which do not correspond to the external lesions. One of the skulls of M. Destruges, whose fontanelle is largely open, has at its periphery, in the bregmatic angle of each frontal, an *osteophyte* of circular form, 40 millimetres in diameter by 3 in thickness, porous and traversed by numerous furrows. There exists another, more extensive and presenting the same structure in a marked degree, on the left parietal, near the lambdoid suture.

The last, very incomplete, is *altered*, the same as the preceding, at the *orbital arches*.

All these skulls are of an undoubted antiquity. . . .

A study of these skulls of children teaches us two things: (1) that syphilis existed in Peru before the Spaniards discovered America; (2) that this disease was frequent there, since the greater number of the skulls of children which come from there bear traces of it. . . .

Thanks to the kindness of Professor de Quatrefages, and with the assistance of Dr. Ern. Hamey, I have discovered in the collection of the muséum *two skulls*, no less ancient than those of M. Destruges, *which present the typical lesions of hereditary syphilis.*

One of the two, donated by M. Ducroy, is that of an adult Peruvian of Arica. It bears no trace of artificial deformity, is slightly natiform, and an epactal bone 55 millimetres in height is visible. Along the sagittal suture, for a length of 70 millimetres, the parietals are symmetrically covered with a *porous layer*, having numerous deep *vascular furrows*. The frontal has the same lesions as are found in the neighborhood of the bregma. The alteration is much more marked on the right one, and extends to the fronto-parietal suture of that side, where a rather extensive *synostosis* is apparent.

The other skull is of a more striking form, the *characteristic lesions being very marked*. It is catalogued as No. 9 of the Champeaux collection (muséum). The teeth of the upper jaw are worn. It is very brachycephalous, and there can be seen a double epactal bone, surrounded by a few Wormian bones. The coronal and sagittal sutures are completely obliterated. It is natiform to a marked degree, and presents, in addition, *two bosses* on the frontal. The *prominences of the parietals*, exceedingly prominent, are separated by a deep furrow. They are *porous* and *furrowed* by irregular *vessels*. Those of the frontals, much less marked, are pyriform, while that which is slender terminates at the glabella. The bregmatic region is a sort of a quadrangular space, prominent more especially at its centre.

The thickening of the skull-walls in the diseased portions is considerable. At one point of the parietals it is 38 millimetres thick, and at the temporals 27, while that of the unaltered portions does not exceed 10 millimetres. This enormous thickening of a rather extensive portion of the skull accounts for its excessive weight, which amounts to 1340 grammes, while the average weight of the skulls of the same derivation, which are unaltered, does not exceed 800 grammes.

Here it may be necessary to make an observation, as American skulls are under consideration. The syphilitic deformity recalls the well-known one of the trilobe skulls of Ancona. But the resemblance between them is only apparent, while there are profound differences. I will content myself in mentioning the principal one, which consists in the absence of porous and furrowed osteophytes on the skulls of Ancona.[1] . . .

The *exposé* which I have just given may be summed up as follows:

1. *Hereditary syphilis* deforms the skull in a *typical* manner.
2. Syphilis existed in Peru before the Spanish Conquest.

At the same meeting, M. de Quatrefages quoted the work of M. Jourdanet, reciting the history of syphilis in Mexico before the Conquest, and recalled the opinion

[1] We ask the indulgence of our readers for giving these rather abstruse descriptions, but they are indispensable for a proper understanding of the rest of this long chapter.

of Captain Cook on the pre-existence of this disease in Oceanica,—an opinion confirmed by different authors. M. Bertillon said that another work, emanating from a Spanish monk and translated by M. Jourdanet, also admits that among the number of diseases to which the Mexicans were subject is found syphilis. Finally, M. Broca concluded with these words: "I take the opportunity of making a note of the proofs which have been given of the existence of syphilis in the New World before the advent of the Europeans. There is nothing astonishing, taking everything into consideration, that the same diseases should attack the majority of humanity; what is important to note is, that the appearance of syphilis in the human race is much anterior to the Middle Ages."

All that precedes refers solely to America, but forms a part of the entirety of the documents which prove that syphilis existed everywhere, at all times, and these bony lesions serve as types for the study of the skulls discovered in Africa and in Europe.

As we have already said, Parrot had occasion, at a previous meeting of the Société d'Anthropologie, of speaking on prehistoric syphilis. It was concerning the skull of a young Indian of Pernambuco, which M. Thulié presented. This skull presented the typical lesions of hereditary syphilis. We give the proceedings of that meeting,[1] which took place in July preceding the Havre Congress:—

M. Parrot called attention to the fact that hereditary cranial syphilis takes on two distinct modes of evolution. It proceeds either by erosion, which is not the case in the present instance, or by hyperostosis. Osteophytes then develop, which choose as their sites of election the orbit, the frontal, and the parietal bones, and have the double effect of increasing the thickness of the central wall of the bone and

[1] Bulletin de la Société d'anthropologie, 1877.

of inducing a deformity of the vault of the skull. He submitted a number of specimens of these lesions to the society, derived from subjects in whom *the diagnosis had been confirmed by a knowledge of the pathological state of the parents*. . . .

It appears demonstrated that syphilis existed in Peru before the Conquest. The museum possesses several Peruvian skulls bearing lesions of an osteophytic character, which are unequivocal. Upon one of them, as in the skull described by M. Thulié, the lesion has the orbit for its site. *The identity of site confirms the identity of diagnosis*, and at the same time the opinion that syphilis, in Peru, preceded the arrival of Europeans.

"This conclusion," says M. Broca, "is a very important one, and I feel very much inclined to accept it, without admitting, on that account, that the syphilis of Europe is of American origin; for that disease may, like many others, have taken its origin at several points on our globe. The existence of syphilis in Europe before the discovery of America is, if not absolutely demonstrated, at least rendered very probable by a large number of documents."

In 1880 the Musée d'Anthropolgie was enriched by a new specimen, proving the existence of syphilis at a prehistoric epoch. This was the fragment of a skull belonging to a race which had disappeared before the fifteenth century, and it would be a difficult matter to say exactly at what epoch the man lived from whom this bony fragment was derived. We will give a short *résumé* of the meeting at which it was examined[1]:—

Meeting of July 1st.—M. Moreno presented two skulls from the old burial grounds of the Rio Negro; they are representatives of races anterior to the Spanish Conquest and extinct before it. The one[2] which presents pathological characteristics was at a depth of about four metres, in a sandy, argillaceous layer similar to the quartenary loam of the pampas. Not far from there, in the same stratum, were a few fragments of the carapace of a glyptodon. The other skull is more modern, although quite ancient. It was at a depth of two metres, in dunes which are to-day solidified. It is deformed after the manner of the Aymaras.

M. Moreno called attention to the fact, in connection with the subject, that his discoveries were related to several forms of skulls con-

[1] Bulletin de la Société d'anthropologie, 1880. [2] A calvarium.

nected with different races. The oldest, represented by the calvarium, should have existed in the glacial periods of Patagonia; which are known to be later than the glacial epoch of Europe. . . .

M. Bordier called attention to the *lesion, undoubtedly syphilitic,* of one of the skulls presented by M. Moreno. . . .

M. Bertillon drew attention to the fact that the second skull presented the marked remains of an ostitis of long duration, "and," added he, "*I only see syphilis as the cause which could have produced it.*"

M. Broca concurred in this opinion. "The ostitis," said he, "appears to be neither tuberculous nor traumatic; *tertiary syphilis alone could have produced it.* This specimen is still more demonstrative than the skulls of the Peruvian children, upon which were demonstrated lesions attributable to the same cause."

This proves more than sufficiently that syphilis existed in Peru and in Patagonia at a time when the Europeans still ignored the use of iron. We will now investigate the skeletons of the wandering tribes of a cannibal nature who peopled the Gauls in the Stone Age, and in druidical times before the Frankish dynasties. Syphilis, as we shall see, reigned supreme, and spared no more the tibias of the Celts than it did the skulls of the Peruvians whom an ocean separated from them. We have found, in a very interesting thesis, some valuable information[1]: we will examine the different descriptions given by the author. But all are not searching, to the same degree, for the cause we are defending: so that, after quoting the text and giving the explanations necessary to facilitate their understanding, we will limit ourselves to stating the ideas set forth. The reader may draw his own conclusions.

In Chap. II, Sec. 1, these descriptions, of some interest, are found :—

No. 65. Fragment of the frontal bone from a tumulus of Meloissy (Côte-d'Or). Musée Broca, Case XXIII.

The lower surface of this bone has *two exostoses* to the left of the corneal crest. The one measures 1 centimetre in length, 6 millimetres

[1] Le Baron : Thèse de Paris, 1881.

in breadth, and 3 millimetres in thickness. The other is 8 millimetres long, 5 wide, and 2 thick. To the right of the same crest there is a third exostosis somewhat smaller. The surface of all of these bony growths is irregular. . . .

Was the subject under the influence of a scrofulous or *syphilitic* diathesis?

We will simply observe that these exostoses correspond to the superciliary arches, and Parrot has shown us that this was the site of election of osteophytes in hereditary syphilis.

No. 66. Skull from Grottos of Bray-sur-Seine (Seine-et-Harne). Musée Broca.

This was presented to the Société d'Anthropologie, in 1881, by Professor Parrot, who expressed the hypothesis of syphilis, but did not venture to sustain it.

It presents, as a matter of fact, nothing but simple depressions. Le Baron sees in this lesions due to atrophy, which seems quite probable to us; and we have mentioned this skull merely for the sake of the truth, in view of the hypothesis advanced by Parrot. The third description furnishes material for controversy.

No. 85. Skull of Liby (Ardèche). Musée Broca, No. 3.

Upon a few teeth of this skull, there exists a remarkable lesion, misinterpreted a few years ago, and with which Drs. Parrot and Magitot have been particularly occupied,—I mean the dental erosion. It is characterized by *transverse striations*, which are single or multiple and correspond each one to an arrest of development. M. Parrot attributes these furrows to *syphilis*, and M. Magitot sees in them the indelible traces of convulsions which have occurred in childhood. Upon which side is the truth?

Without wishing to contradict M. Magitot, we will say that we have observed, upon many occasions, the transverse striations upon the teeth of children whose parents were syphilitic, notably at Lille, and at the dispensary of the Société Philanthropique, at La Villette. This does not mean, however, that convulsions may not sometimes bring about an identical result, but perhaps not as characteristic. Let us concede to M. Magitot that one should not indistinctly trace syphilis in every prehistoric tooth that bears transverse furrows, but let that skillful practitioner permit us to partake of the opinion of Parrot in the majority of cases.[1]

Le Baron quotes, in addition, a large number of cases of exostoses, but without giving any description nor explaining their origin. In section two, he describes a specimen which, for him, is a typical syphilitic hyperostosis :—

No. 89. Fragment of the right tibia, from the dolmen of Léry (Eure). Muséum.

Near the middle of the crest of this tibia there exists *a considerable hyperostosis* of the anterior half of the diaphysis. As a result the anterior border presents a very marked curve, with an anterior convexity. This hypertrophy has an elongated, ovoid form, and its surface is as smooth as the rest of the bone. It extends to a length of 85 millimetres. In this locality, the tibia is 24 millimetres thick. A longitudinal section, made through the tumor, shows that it is composed of compact tissue. The medullary canal has preserved its normal dimensions.

Should this hypertrophy be attributed to a varicose or other ulcer? I think not, on account of the polished surface of the tumor. I prefer seeing in it a *syphilitic* alteration of the bone. Besides, it is one of the localities where syphilis preferably evidences its ravages.

We do not see anything to add to these conclusions.

No. 90. Tibia of the dolmen of Maintenon (Eure-et-Loire). Musée Broca.

This bone has multiple lesions in all its length. Near the centre of the crest of the tibia there is a *nummular exostosis* about 3 centimetres in diameter and 7 to 8 millimetres thick at its middle portion. The surface, almost smooth, is riddled with a multitude of small holes. Within and below, it is detached from the rest of the bone, and at that point forms a sharp border, which is free. Without and downward, on the contrary, it merges into the rest of the diaphysis. . . .

[1] See further on an article by Parrot concerning the lesions produced in the teeth by hereditary syphilis.

The internal border, at its upper half, is studded with *numerous* regular *exostoses* several centimetres in height. . . .

Finally, *multiple* and irregular *exostoses* are seen at the inferior peroneo-tibial articulation. . . .

In order to determine the nature of this lesion, I thought that I could not do better than compare it with the diseased tibias of the Musée Dupuytren. There I found, in No. 415, an identical specimen, bearing the diagnosis of *hyperostosis*. M. Houël, in his catalogue, adds that there probably existed an ulcer at the site of the tumor, which is observed upon the crest of the bone.

To this cause was there not probably superadded some scrofulous element,—I dare not say *syphilitic ?*

Perhaps both were united; the hyperostosis may have been produced under an ulcerated gumma; this hypothesis is probable, on account of the smooth appearance of the bony tumor.

The author terminates his work with the following observations:—

Syphilis, relatively rare in ancient times, has become a common disease since steam has rendered the mingling of people so easy. Many tribes of Oceanica, still exempt from this disease at the beginning of this century, are to-day the subjects of pox. . . .

Do the eight teeth which I found marked with erosions prove that he (the primitive man) had syphilis? M. Parrot would answer affirmatively. M. Magitot, on the contrary, would conclude that they had convulsions.

I have found no other proof of prehistoric syphilis than the hyperostosis of the tibia of Léry. If it be well proven that this tibia is syphilitic, *and such is my opinion*, prehistoric syphilis is no more a matter of doubt. But it must be confessed that it is rare.

Le Baron, while thoroughly convinced, does not dare advance too much. Let us not forget that the author was sustaining his thesis for the doctorate, and contemporaneous history has shown us that to advance opinions which might not be shared in by a majority of the judges is not always unattended with danger.

Let us now give a final extract from the proceedings of the Société d'Anthropologie:—

Meeting of Nov. 18, 1880.—M. de Mortillet presented a skull and a jaw-bone obtained from the cemetery of Brêny (Aisne). The skull, taken from a Merovingian sepulchre, presents all the characteristics of the Frank race. The jaw is that of a child, all of the teeth being crossed by ***horizontal furrows***. There is present a sort of arrest of development, an erosion which M. Magitot believes is due to some convulsive disease, but which M. Parrot regards as a mark of *infantile syphilis*.[1]

We have already expressed our opinion upon these lesions of infantile syphilis, which M. Magitot refuses to admit for prehistoric times. For us, this proof, like others of a similar nature, has no real value, except as confirming or adding force to the first ones which we gave, and which seem to us irrefutable.

Such were the materials of anthropological origin which we were able to obtain at the beginning of our researches. But, in running over French and foreign medical journals which have appeared for the past thirty years, we found, among other valuable articles, one by Parrot, published in the *Revue Scientifique*, in 1882. It had for title, "Une Maladie préhistorique,"[2] and in it the author adduces new facts in favor of the theory he sustains. We will analyze this lecture of the Professor by letting him speak as much as possible. Parrot thus begins:—

Quite recently, Professor Rollet, of the Faculty of Medicine of Lyons, published, in the *Annales de Dermatologie*, two articles upon the ancient foci of syphilis, in which may be found a choice erudition, and an argument full of method and of proof. This study commands attention, and disposes one to the views of the author.

He thinks that this disease is very ancient in humanity; that India, from the documentary evidence found in the Vedas, is one of

[1] Later on will be found, in an article by Parrot, which we will analyze, a detailed description of the teeth of this jaw of the Frank epoch.

[2] "A Prehistoric Disease." This article of the Revue Scientifique is reproduced in its entirety in the works of Parrot, published under the care of Dr. Troisier, in 1886.

the most ancient foci; that China, as has been proven by Commander Dabry, has known it from time immemorial; that the *yaws* of Africa is identical with syphilis, but that nothing demonstrates that the latter was not carried by the Mohammedans and Jews whom Ferdinand and Isabella drove out of Spain; that it existed in America before the arrival of the Europeans, as related by Oviedo; that the companions of Christopher Columbus introduced it. . . .

Europe alone, according to M. Rollet, did not know syphilis before the end of the fifteenth century, no written document mentioning its existence. And he adds that the excavations made in alluvial soils and in old burial grounds, while they have brought to light many skulls which go back to prehistoric times,—that is, to the most remote periods of our history,—do not demonstrate upon any of them the characteristic lesions of syphilis. The female skeleton found at Solutie shows upon the tibias, and especially upon the right one, *syphilitic exostoses* (Broca, Ollier, Parrot, Virchow); but the Abbé Ducrost, to whom this discovery is due, raises doubts as to the epoch to which this sepulchre should be referred.

I here put myself down as opposed to this last portion of the thesis sustained by my learned colleague of Lyons, for I am convinced that syphilis manifested itself, long before the discovery of America, at several points of that part of Europe which to-day constitutes France.

Letting aside the texts, with the interpretations and commentaries which have been made, I will merely produce, to support my view, *material, visible, tangible proofs;* specimens analogous to, and even identical with, those which pathological anatomy permits us to gather every day.

The author next considers the pathological anatomy of hereditary syphilis:—

The bones and the teeth are the only parts of the organism which, in certain conditions, resist destruction, and which, at times, from a morphological point of view, remain for several centuries in the state in which death surprised them. And for this reason, when the pathology of remote periods is studied, it is only from their examination that data of any real value can be derived.

I made this inquiry in regard to syphilis, and it has furnished me with valuable memoranda; but, before making them known, and to show their great importance, I will describe briefly the bone and dental lesions of hereditary syphilis, such as pathological anatomy has taught us, leaving aside all those which might not prove useful to my end.

Remains of skulls being the only bone specimens which I have had an opportunity of examining, I must limit myself, in the study of lesions, to this part of the skeleton. They appear under two aspects, widely different and even opposite. Some consist in a normal loss of substance, sometimes worn to perforation; while others are like small tubercles, which thicken, to a considerable extent, certain portions of the parietes.

These two pathological conditions are generally found in the same skull, but not in the same region. The first one was described in 1843, by Elsässer, under the name of *cranio-tabes*. It is on the internal face of the calvarium that it begins and that its different degrees may be noted. It only appears externally at its last period. At first depressions are seen, a sort of cup-shaped excavations, excavated in the walls of the skull, which is rugous at their site, thinned to a great extent, and even perforated.

I have shown that there are two varieties of cranio-tabes, having each one a distinct site and etiology. The one almost always symmetrical affects the frontal and parietal bones around the bregma and along the sagittal suture. It is developed during intra-uterine life, by means of a perversion of nutrition, as is proven by the weakly condition of children affected by it. I have qualified it by the epithet *congenital peribregmatic*. The other occupies, without exception, the portions which slope downward in the dorsal decubitus; that is to say, the parietal bones, behind the occipital, at the cerebral and cerebellar fossæ. It is always produced after birth, recognizes hereditary syphilis as a cause, and belongs to the rachitic period. Skulls involved in this manner lose in specific gravity; they are porous, fragile, and look as if they would crumble at the slightest touch.

The cranial alterations of the second variety, instead of being atrophic and destructive, appear, on the contrary, as exuberant vegetations upon the most elevated portions of the calvarium, and externally. They are flattened, circular elevations, sharply defined from the healthy portions by their elevation, porosity, and, in the fresh state, by their red or violaceous color. Primarily but little spread, they sometimes invade the larger portion of the external table. The walls are here notably thickened, and may be 10, 15, 20, and even 40 millimetres thick. Their tissue consists of large, vasculo-medullary spaces, limited by bony trabeculæ, perpendicular to the cranial surface. At first spongy, elastic, and soaked with a large quantity of liquids, it ends by acquiring considerable hardness. Very frequently the skulls affected with osteophytes present a typical deformity, which I have qualified as natiform.

So much for the bones; let us now see what the indelible traces are which hereditary syphilis leaves upon the teeth:—

Upon the teeth, the imprints of hereditary syphilis are *tenacious* and *characteristic*. They often preserve their original appearance, not only during the life of the individual, but after death, *during long centuries*.

According to Parrot, these impressions affect both dentitions and follow physiological development in a regular manner. It is an atrophy, of which he recognizes five varieties. The first, the beginning of the others, consists in small, rounded depressions around the crown; he calls it *cupuliform*. The second, which is derived from the first, is represented by a furrow, due to the approximation of the cup-shaped depressions; this has the name of *sulciform*. The third, *cuspidian atrophy*, has its site of preference in the canines and premolars; the crown appears to be divided into two unequal parts. The free portion seems to be driven in like a peg into that which is nearer the gum, and apparently healthy. The *hatchet* atrophy is seen in the four upper incisors only, during the first dentition; it is a consecutive caries. In the form described by Hutchinson there exists, upon the cutting edges of the incisors, a notch of variable depth, triangular or crescent-shaped.

Such is a rapid sketch of the bone and dental lesions caused by hereditary syphilis. "*No other disease*," says Parrot, "*can produce them*; so much so that their very existence justifies us in affirming that the subject we observe affected with such remains was a syphilitic."

The author then goes on to speak of two skulls at the Anthropological Institute, donated by M. Destruges, and which come from Guyaquil (Ecuador). They are the skulls of two children, a description of which by Parrot, at the Congress at Havre in 1877, has been given, as also of that which follows it, of which we will recall the principal lesions, and add new details. This third skull is at the museum (No. 9 of the Collection Champeaux); it was found near Lima, in the valleys of Chancai. It is an adult skull, natiform to a marked degree, and having *four* peribregmatic *osteophytes.* At a few diseased points its walls are 38 millimetres thick, and it weighs 1340 grammes, instead of 800, the average weight of unaltered skulls of the same origin. The objects found in connection with the bones (vases, jewelry, cloths) in no wise point to the Spanish occupation. Syphilis, then, existed in Peru and in Ecuador before the advent of the Spaniards,—a fact which no one doubts. In order to show its presence in Europe before the return of Columbus, Parrot also relies upon anatomical specimens.

He first describes the lower jaw of a young Frank of the Merovingian epoch, found in the cemetery of Brény, whose discovery we have already mentioned. Of the fourteen teeth in this jaw, eight are affected,—the four incisors, the two canines, and the two premolars; the others are intact, as is always observed, since their evolution only takes place after the period of activity of hereditary syphilis. It is the *sulciform atrophy* which predominates: two clearly-defined horizontal furrows are to be seen. *Hereditary syphilis alone* can produce such lesions; hence, it existed in France at an undetermined period, "but certainly *before the seventh century.*"

These times are still within the domain of history. Let us look at prehistoric times. Parrot bases himself upon the fragments of skulls of children and a few teeth found by Dr. Prunières, of Marvejols, in the dolmens and caverns of Lozère:—

One of these fragments comes from the dolmen of Cauquenos. It is a portion of the right half of the occipital bone. Its length is 47 millimetres and its width 36. There exist two perforations identical with those produced by syphilitic cranio tabes, 3 millimetres in diameter and corresponding to the occipital fossæ. Around them the internal table is slightly porous, as is usually found in rachitics.

A second specimen, much more significant, is the remains of the posterior half of the parietal bone of a child; it comes from an excavation made in a dolmen of Boujassac. Upon one of its borders are seen numerous serrations, corresponding to the sagittal suture. It is 74 millimetres long and 53 wide. Its internal surface is perfectly smooth. Externally may be seen a pathological layer, having irregular contours, from 3 to 5 centimetres in diameter and 2 to 3 millimetres thick. There are numerous openings and canaliculi, slightly oblique in reference to the surface of the bone. All these peculiar features can leave no doubt as to the *syphilitic* origin of this osteophyte.

Another fragment, more curious than the preceding, on account of the clearness of its characteristics, is that of a child's parietal bone, found, like those of which I have been speaking, in a dolmen of Lozère. Of a length of 55 millimetres and 44 wide, of an irregular triangular shape, its internal surface is normal; over almost the entire extent of the external table there exists a hard, porous, morbid layer, identical with the osteophytes, which are generally found on the skulls of children affected with hereditary syphilis. At those points where it is in a state of preservation the border is rounded off, and contrasts sharply with the sound parts. Its thickness varies from 2 to 3 millimetres. The small openings which cover its surface are pretty regularly distributed. It is formed of trabeculæ, which are perpendicular or slightly oblique to the surface of the parietal bone. This lesion, really specific when it is attentively studied, leaves no more doubt as to *its syphilitic nature* than those of the skulls of Chancai and Guyaquil.

In addition, there have been found, in the sepulchres of which we have just been speaking, teeth affected with syphilitic lesions. Parrot adds that he has found *sulciform atrophy* in the teeth that M. Magitot had sent him. The latter, as we have already said, attributed these lesions of the teeth to convulsions of childhood; but, remarks Parrot, this way of viewing the matter is losing each day "the credit it owed to the talent and to the legitimate force of its author."

Those who have studied pathological anatomy will appreciate all the importance of these proofs brought forward "to support the high antiquity of syphilis," as Parrot says. Since the epoch of the dolmens, there have not been produced in the human organism such changes that we cannot regard as identical the bony lesions of those times with those of to-day. These same lesions, in our modern skeletons, being due to hereditary syphilis alone, we are forced to conclude that the bony remains, almost fossil, which we have just examined, belonged to human beings whose parents were syphilitic.

"How much these proofs are superior in certainty," says Parrot, "to those derived from written documents! To simple presumptions, to discussions of texts, to the interpretation of terms, to assertions, to the accounts of authors, I oppose the fact itself, the disease in action. It is the *delictum flagrans* which forces conviction with its irresistible power. Syphilis existed, then, in Europe at times which preceded history; and if, as everything would lead us to suppose, it existed equally in other parts of the world, we are justified in considering it as one of the most ancient, and, perhaps, as *the most ancient* disease of man."

The question which arises is, if it has not exercised some influence upon the genesis of other diseases. This is, perhaps, going too far; syphilis of itself is already sufficiently complex, and has manifestations sufficiently numerous to dispense with the accusation that it is the parent of every virus. Let us attest that it existed in quarternary man; but let us not make it the reservoir of all the microbes, on that account.

In conclusion, let us reproach Parrot with one false theory: there is no man so great but may commit an error. According to him, all the bony deformities which we know as rachitic have for their origin hereditary syphilis; and, what is more grave, he goes so far as to write that rickets, in children, is solely due to the syphilis of their parents. Now, we daily see improper alimentation bring on rickets; very few children who are young can resist the food termed strengthening, consisting of bouillons, soups, eggs, meat, etc.; those that do not die of gastro-enteritis become rickety—all, or very nearly all. I do not hesitate to affirm that bouillon alone kills ten times as many newborn infants as syphilis, whose murderous reputation has been exaggerated. We cannot dilate to any greater length, not having rickets to describe here. Nevertheless, with the exception of this inexact opinion of the Professor, the lectures of Parrot on the bones of quarternary man are none the less in conformity with scientific observation; and his conclusions concerning prehistoric syphilis have received the approval of such men as Broca, Ollier, Rollet himself, Virchow, and others, whose authority and competence are universally recognized.

How much osteology! the unfortunate reader who is a stranger to the medical art, and consequently unfamiliar with these gruesome investigations, will say. Let us definitely leave the museums, those catacombs of science, and explore secular literature.

CHAPTER V.

TCHOANG.

Syphilis Among the Chinese Five Thousand Years Ago.

"Pour expulser du sang le virus syphilitique, ils (les chinois) se servaient du mercure bien des siécles avant la découverte de l'Amerique."—L. Soubeiran.

[In order to expell the syphilitic virus from the blood, they (the Chinese) employed mercury many centuries before the discovery of America.]

In 1863, Captain Dabry, consul at Hang-Keou, published a very complete work on China, from a medical point of view.[1] This *litterateur*, who was thoroughly acquainted with the Chinese language, had, fortunately for science, the idea[2] of translating the secular manuscripts which escaped the holocaust ordered by the Emperor *Tsin-che-houang*.[3] And these manuscripts, as Soubeiran will inform us soon, treat of nothing but medicine, and are curious in more than one respect. Objection will not be wanting that checking is not easy, and that there is no proof that these manuscripts are not of recent manufacture. We will content ourselves with answering that Captain Dabry, not being a physician, had no interest whatever in upholding the antiquity of

[1] P. Dabry: la Médecine chez les Chinois. Paris, 1863. Medicine Among the Chinese.

[2] He thus exceeded the expectations of M. Rollet, who had simply requested him to answer a few written questions on the venereal diseases of the ancient Chinese. Dabry returned with a large volume, a valuable document for retrospective science.

[3] Anglicé, Tsin-che-Hoang.

the diseases considered among us as modern; that the Chinese, ignorant of the old quarrel which has divided the medical world of Europe for three centuries in respect to syphilis, would not have amused themselves manufacturing mountains of manuscript to favor one opinion to the detriment of the other; that few persons, among Europeans, are, even now, able to commit such forgeries, and, above all, in a position to place them in the archives or analogous building in Pekin; finally, that Dabry, far from defending a thesis, has simply translated a collection of manuscripts, and that these had the characteristics of age sufficiently marked not to be considered as recent. Besides, each one of these manuscripts has its history, and they are certainly kept in a secure place. We are not far from believing that, even in his position as consul, Dabry had considerable difficulty in obtaining access to them. To those who might be inclined to express a doubt as to the literary good faith of the translator, we think it sufficient to remind them that Dabry was an officer and represented France.

Here we will make a digression. The above paragraph had already been written several months when we had occasion to peruse a work of the eighteenth century, in which was stated, among other details, that Astruc had a knowledge of Chinese manuscripts treating of syphilis. It is not neccssary to feel much surprised by this fact, which, at first sight, may seem strange. As a matter of fact, Astruc, who would have rejected the same evidence in his efforts to uphold before and against all that syphilis did not appear in Europe until 1494, admitted willingly that it might have existed from time immemorial in other parts of the world. The best proof is in a passage in "Jourdan de

Pellerin,"[1] which we will quote entire. This document is the more valuable as the information emanates from Astruc himself, and confirms the authenticity of the manuscripts with which we will occupy ourselves in this chapter. The following is the passage in question:—

We owe to the indefatigable, fortunate, and useful care of M. Astruc, an account of China, which informs us—

1. That, in that empire, venereal diseases are spread in the same manner as in Europe.

2. That Chinese physicians believe that it has been spread *from all time.*

3. That the medical books which are regarded as the oldest, far from speaking of the beginning of the disease, speak of it only as a *very ancient disease.*

4. Finally, that the remedies for these diseases are particularly *mercury.* . . .

Comments are unnecessary. The forgery of documents, already very difficult in 1864, would have been impossible in 1740. We shall see, later on, that Astruc did not stop here, but furnished himself, without suspecting it, all the material necessary for his own refutation without any possible answer.

A year after its appearance, the work of Dabry was quoted by a physician of Florence, Dr. Galligo, who has devoted a very interesting chapter to this history of syphilis, in his work on venereal diseases.[2] Ten years later, M. Lancereaux, in his excellent work, also gave several extracts.[3] With the exception of these authors and a few others, who have analyzed it in articles for dictionaries or in medical journals,[4] I do not know that

[1] Traité sur les maladies vénériennes. Paris, 1749. Treatise on Venereal Diseases.

[2] J. Galligo: Trattato teoretico-pratico sulle malattie veneree. Firenze, 1884, Theoretical and Practical Treatise on Venereal Diseases.

[3] Lancereaux: Traité historique et pratique de la syphilis. Paris, 1873. Historical and Practical Treatise on Syphilis.

[4] M. Verneuil, in the Archives de Médecine (1863), gave an account of the work at the time of its appearance.

the book of Dabry has been given that attention which it deserves. We will examine it a little more in detail, leaving the author speak as often as possible.

We learn from the researches of the captain, in the historical documents of China, that the most ancient emperor, whose name has come down to us, is *Chin-nong*, who lived three thousand two hundred and sixteen years before Christ; then, among prominent names, we find *Hoang-ty*, about a thousand years later; and the entire dynasty of *Tchou*, which began in 1222 B.C.

At a time which exactly corresponds to the year 2637 B.C., the Emperor Hoang-ty, solicitous of the health of his people, caused all the documents on medicine to be collected, and carefully reduced to writing on parchment all the traditions in regard to therapeutics. Europeans, at that time, were still frightful savages who devoured their captives, as shown by the researches of Le Baron on the diseases of prehistoric man, of which we have spoken. As a matter of fact, the majority of the remains found in the bone caves, of human or animal origin, bore the traces of the action of fire. Among the long bones, some were half calcined and others split in half by a flint instrument, but all in the same manner. The author, agreeing in this respect with the most celebrated anthropologists (Broca, Parrot, etc.), concludes that these vertical incisions had for their object the extraction of the marrow of the bone after it was cooked.[1] The sons of Noah and their descendants—that is to say, our ancestors of the diluvian formation—were then horrible anthropophagi! This is flattering to our species! As for me, I limit myself to the statement that we have nothing with which to reproach the savages of America, not even syphilis.

[1] Le Baron, *loc. cit.*

Hoang-ty, armed with all these documents,—having all his notes, as we would say nowadays,—wrote or caused to be written the celebrated treatise which bears his name, *Hoang-ty-mi-king;* that is to say, the medical treatise of Hoang-ty. "This work" (*Nuei-king*), says Subeiran, in his preface to Dabry's book, "is certainly the most curious one in existence from a point of view of the history of medicine. As medical books were excepted from the edict of proscription of *Tsin-che-hoang*, the *burner of books*, we cannot doubt that China possesses the most valued secrets of antiquity. What lessons may not be expected, especially when we consider that forty centuries of experiments and observations have enlarged this treasure with an infinity of discoveries religiously transmitted from age to age!"

A little further on, in showing the knowledge of the Chinese in therapeutics at an epoch nearer to the deluge than ours, Soubeiran adds: "From time immemorial, they add to their remedies carbonate of soda, sulphate of iron, . . . sulphur, with which they cured the itch, known for more than four thousand years under the name of *tchong-kai* (words which signify *pustules formed by a worm*); . . . *mercury* to expell the syphilitic virus from the blood, and which they employed many centuries before the discovery of America." . . .

Even supposing the manuscript to be recent, the word *tchong-kai* is not: as soon as the Chinese knew the itch they found the *acarus*, as the Chinese name implies, and they understood that sulphur, in killing the sarcoptes, cured the cutaneous affection caused by it. How many cases of itch in Europe, how much syphilis, eczemas, and cutaneous affections, in fact, were held up to public horror in the Middle Ages under the convenient name of *leprosy!* How many unfortunates were incarcerated or hounded, in whom a little sulphur ointment or some mercury would have sufficed to cure them!

The medical treatise of Hoang-ty is divided in about the same manner as that of Hippocrates. General principles are piled up pell-mell; then are found several chapters dealing with particular diseases. When we arrive at that one treating of venereal diseases we are stupefied. The numbers 2637 added to 1889 give us 4526: so that it is forty-five centuries ago that the emperor Hoang-ty caused all the documents on the diseases of his time in China to be collected. Venereal diseases were better known than at the time Astruc wrote (1742), or even before Ricord. One would not expect to find a complete treatise; the symptoms are certainly described in a succinct manner, but one is forced to acknowledge that the Chinese, more than twenty centuries before Christ, knew the duality of the chancre established in our days by Ricord, and knew that gonorrhœa had nothing in common with syphilis, of which they were not yet certain at the beginning of this century. We may well be possessed of a legitimate stupefaction in recognizing the astonishing precocity of this people, who seem to have been slumbering for a long time. Let us remember that they had invented gunpowder when Europe was still using ballistæ and cross-guns. And it is presumable that syphilis, which was described by the Chinese, together with its treatment by mercury, four thousand five hundred and twenty-six years ago, was known long before the appearance of the *Hoang-ty-mi-king*, which is nothing but a collection of secular traditions upon the art of healing. Everything leads to the idea that the *Sons of Heaven* observed and treated their syphilides since and perhaps before the deluge.

Without wishing to anticipate one of our future publications, we may say that a somewhat similar phenomenon produced itself in the fifteenth century. The remedies relating to syphilis existed in a traditional state, but among a certain class only, and the physicians of the time proceeded in the same manner as Hoang-ty: on the whole, they merely reduced to writing the empirical formulæ transmitted orally for centuries. As is positively stated by a contemporary of the epidemic, Gaspard Torella,[1] and thirty years later Jacques de Béthencourt,[2] physicians never penetrated into the quarters of the prostitutes, did not treat them, and ignored the diseases endemic to the Cour des Miracles[3] and other analogous localities. The remedies were in the hands of quacks, and of courtesans, even. "Venus ill had to be taken care of by Venus well," says M. Netter, in a humorous article.[4] The physicians, understanding nothing of this complex epidemic, at first refused to attend the sick; these then applied to healers of all kinds, people of the worst sort, vagabonds, jugglers, procuresses, and prostitutes (Torella). And what proves that venereal diseases and their treatment were known in places of debauchery is, that a certain John Bale, writing, in a manuscript of the sixteenth century, of a certain Hugh Weston, a doctor of divinity and dean of Windsor in 1556, says that this debauchee was "more expert in the art of healing *burning* than all the whores of the stews."

These healers of one or of the other sex had marvelous successes, especially with their mercurial rubbings,

[1] Tractatus cum consiliis contra pudendagram. . . . Romæ, 1497. Treatise with Advice for the Diseases of the Pudenda (Shameful Parts).

[2] Nouveau Carême de pénitence et purgatoire du mal vénérien. Rome, 1527. New Lent of Penance and Purgatory of the Venereal Disease.

[3] An old quarter in Paris, somewhat similar to Whitechapel, London.

[4] Gazette des Hôpitaux, 1872.

which was their favorite remedy (Béthencourt). There is nothing surprising in this, for quicksilver, which played an important rôle in alchemy in the middle ages, must have been tried very early by beggars and ribalds. Whatever it was, such was the source from which the first physicians, who wished to make therapeutic rules for the disease which was new to them, derived their inspiration. It required the expedition of Naples, and the movements of troops consequent upon it, for syphilis to leave the domain of prostitution, where it was in a certain measure confined, and spread itself to all classes of European society.

M. Netter, in his interesting study of which we have spoken, is astonished, with reason, that a disease dating back but thirty years at the time Béthencourt wrote, could have been suddenly described with all its symptoms, even the most exceptional, and particularly that the specific remedy should have been immediately found. "Nothing seems to have been forgotten," he exclaims, "neither the initial contagion, nor the cutaneous eruption, nor the nocturnal pains, nor the exostoses, nor the caries, nor the cirrhosis of the liver, nor even the terminal consumption, so rare!" He concludes that Béthencourt and companions did nothing but appropriate the medical knowledge of one-quarter of the people of the time. This is the secret of many discoveries; but everybody does not possess the scientific honesty of that great physician, who sincerely confesses that it was solely to verify a popular tradition that he occupied himself with vaccination. "Sarah Portock," says he, among other things, "was convinced that she was protected from small-pox, because *twenty years before* she had been infected by *cow-pox*." The English physician wanted to have his mind clear on that point. As he was an investigator, he substituted for an accident his lancet dipped in the liquid of the pustules of a heifer. The same result. The same immunity; vaccination had been found. Thus, one of the greatest conquests of the medical art of modern times owed its origin to the gossip of a milk-maid! It is true that of those who heard it, only one understood; this man was Edward Jenner. Is this not another case of repeating: *Nihil sub sole novum?*

Vaccination for syphilis has also been tried. The success of Jenner would naturally lead to such experiments; but the vaccine was not forthcoming. We will recur to this subject at the proper time. Up to this time, it is on man himself that this vaccine has been looked for, but uselessly. Who knows but that it will some day be found upon one of our domestic animals? It is, perhaps, at Maisons-Alfort[1] that the key to the problem exists. We have wandered somewhat from our Chinese manuscripts; let us hasten to return to them.

Hoang-ty first describes gonorrhœa (*pe-teho*) as it would be in 1889. He distinguishes the simple burning, whose duration is relatively short, the *virulent* discharge of which he details the symptoms. Then he comes to chancres. The first paragraph is devoted to the soft chancre, the eroding chancre, the one "which develops from the *third to the ninth day*," and which may cause considerable loss of substance. The author then speaks of the resultant bubo, and of the vegetations which may occur upon the generative organs.

In the following paragraph, we find the description of an entirely different species of chancre. This second chancre is produced by a virus of a peculiar nature (*kan-tou*), and is communicable by contact. "It may

[1] The principal veterinary college of France is situated in this place.

happen," says the Chinese text, "that a woman meets a man whose vitiated blood develops the virus of which we have been speaking. This virus will cause an *ulcer*, and will *spread itself throughout the entire volume of the blood.*" An analogous passage, longer and more obscure, is found in the *Ayurveda*, a Hindoo medical treatise (see chapter ix), written by a royal prince. Hoang-ty recurs to the eroding chancre, which is *painful*, has *worm-eaten edges*, and shows the difference existing between this one and the second variety. "The latter," he adds, "is accompanied very frequently by tumors (*hiue-san-chan-on-pien-jong*)." These tumors might be ganglionic engorgements, or papulo-hypertrophic syphilides, but the text does not give their location. As treatment, is advised *mercurial frictions*, aided by an oily mixture and a powder composed of mercury (*choui-yn*).

So much for the primary lesion; let us now examine the secondary period. We leave the Chinese monarch speak:—

It sometimes happens that, several months after the cure of a venereal trouble, the patient suddenly experiences *headache* with *fever*, *pains in the bones*, and vertigo; shortly after there appear on the forehead small spots of a coppery red (*tan-hong*), which increase little by little. The face swells, and principally the nose; speech is difficult; there is pain and itching in the throat. . . . These spots are changed into violaceous pimples of the size of a pea, allowing a thick liquid of a fetid odor to escape, the body is soon covered with spots and pimples of a like nature; mucosities run from the nose; the breath is insupportable. The pimples, once excoriated, increase in size. . . . Sometimes the pains are only felt *at night*.

Here is a whole paragraph devoted to syphilitic affections of the mouth and throat:—

Section 6. *Keou-yay-tou* (poison of the mouth and throat). It sometimes happens, as a lesion consecutive to a chancre, after a period of time more or less long, that an ulceration forms in one of the two glands found at the entrance of the throat,[1] or on the membrane which covers the palate near the throat, or, finally, in the throat itself at a certain depth. This ulceration is *white;* the edges are straight and of a coppery red (*tan-hong*) ; the surrounding parts are violaceous, similar to corrupt skin (*py-lan*). . . . The breath is burning and fetid ; the ulcerated part bleeds as soon as the patient becomes angry.

This is what occurs nowadays, when children, who have mucous plaques of the lips with fissures at the commissures, begin to cry: a tear, with a slight hæmorrhage, is produced. Hoang-ty adds that the ulcer appears most often at the base of the tongue, that sometimes, also, that organ is suddenly covered with *white patches*, and that small *gray pustules*, which become excoriated, suddenly show themselves upon the *edges and tip*. He again says:—

It sometimes happens that, following an imperfectly healed chancre, there forms around the anus (*kong-men*) red or white spots, which are extremely small, and often painful and pruriginous. . . . Sometimes the edges of the anus are excoriated; at other times the body is covered with small red pustules, which disappear under pressure.

Section 7 is unimportant for our purpose; in the following one is found the description of syphilitic, papulo-hypertrophic, ulcerative patches of the margin of the anus. The author mentions, incidentally, the pigmentary syphilide of the neck:—

Section 8. *Che-kong-tou* (moist poison around the anus). Small spots, as large as millet-seed, of a coppery red, appear in variable numbers upon the perineum, scrotum, buttocks, and the superior and internal surface of the thighs. Little by little they become large, moist, exhale an odor of fetid sweat, and produce a slight itching. . . .

It sometimes happens that, thirty or forty days after the lesion derived from an impure connection, plaques, very small spots, either white or of a coppery red, surrounded by a red areola (*tche-pe-yeou-fong*), appear upon several parts of the body. . . .

[1] Evidently referring to the tonsils.

Sometimes there suddenly appears, after a venereal lesion, patches of *white spots* spread *under the neck.* Very shortly after, the whole body is covered with violaceous, red, or yellow spots.

The author also speaks of *tan-tou* (*red poison*) and of *tien-ho-tchoang* (ulcer, fire of heaven). "This disease," he says, "is sometimes *transmissible to children* who are new-born." He then describes syphilitic coryza under the name of nasal chancre (*py-ting*). In cases called *py-ynen* the symptoms are the same, but the bones drop out (caries and necrosis). Finally, it is the *yang-mey-tchoang* (ulcer in the form of raspberry), which may be compared to the modern *frambœsia*, of which we will speak later on. In conclusion, he gives a very exact description of the ulcerated papulo-hypertrophic syphilides, with their ichorous and fetid discharge.

We could make many more quotations; but they would not prove anything additional, and would lead to repetitions. The treatise of Hoang-ty will certainly be accused of being somewhat prolix, and of being far from didactic in construction. What matters it? The main teaching, which develops itself from these documents contemporaneous with the great-grand-nephews of Noah, is that syphilis was a current disease among the Chinese at this epoch, and its nature better known than among the Europeans at the beginning of the nineteenth century.

CHAPTER VI.

KASA.

SYPHILIS IN JAPAN, OBSERVED AT THE BEGINNING OF THE NINTH CENTURY.[1]

"Le mot *kasa*, en japonais ancien comme en japonais moderne, sert à désigner les affections contagieuses qui surviennent après les relations sexuelles et qu'on connaît très bien aujourd'hui au Japon."—DUPOUY.

[The word *kasa* in ancient Japanese, as in the modern, serves to designate the contagious diseases which supervene after sexual relations, and which are to-day very well known in Japan.]

AFTER having consulted a number of works regarding medicine in Japan (Ardoin,[2] Elridge,[3] and others), we began to despair of finding the least document regarding the antiquity of syphilis in that country, when, in reading the *Archiv für Pathologische Anatomie* of Virchow, we found an article by Dr. Scheube,[4] which made us give a sigh of relief. A few days later, in scanning the recent work of Dr. Dupouy,[5] we found, reproduced

[1] Although the information we have been able to obtain in regard to Japan does not date any earlier than the ninth century of our era, a period which corresponds with that which historians have called the Middle Ages for Europe and Africa, we have deemed it best to place this study after that which we have just made on China. Besides, these two peoples have the same origin: it is well known that the islands which constitute the present Empire of Japan were occupied by an Asiatic colony, probably from China, at a time which it is difficult to determine, but certainly after the dynasty of Tcheou (1222 B.C.). In fact, the first historical date of Japan, according the researches of Dr. Michéa, was six hundred and sixty years before the Christian era.

[2] Aperçu sur l'histoire de la médecine au Japon. Paris, 1884. Synopsis of the History of Medicine in Japan.

[3] "Syphilis in Japan," in New York Medical Journal, 1882.

[4] Archiv für Pathologische Anatomie (März, 1883, Capit. XXIV).

[5] La Prostitution dans l'antiquité. Paris, 1887. Prostitution in Antiquity.

in French, the principal passages of Dr. Scheube's article. M. G. Tissot, a pharmacist of the first class, kindly assisted us in completing the translation; so that we are enabled to furnish full information.

The article in the German medical journal concerns a Japanese manuscript dating A.D. 808. This valuable document has for title: *Dai-do-rui-shiu-ho*, which means: *A collection of formulas arranged in classes, of the period of Dai-do.* At that time, the emperor, Heizei-Tenno, seeing his country more and more invaded by Chinese sciences, thought of the same project as the emperor of China, Hoang-ty, although thirty-five centuries later; that is to say, he formed the resolution of gathering in one book all the elements concerning medicine, such as it was then practiced in Japan. He confided this work to his two physicians, A-be-ma-nao and Idzu-mo Hiro-sada. But the manuscript was soon lost or stolen, we do not exactly know: suffice it to say, that for more than a thousand years no one heard of it. At all events, in 1827, a shop-keeper of the province of Bungo (island of Kiushiu) found a well-preserved manuscript, in a pagoda of that country; it was the medical treatise of Heizei-Tenno, which the honest tradesman hurried to return to the proper authorities. Since that time, it has been published a number of times as a very curious work.

This work, which is similar to the most ancient writings of Japan, is written in old Japanese, which renders its translation very difficult, for the Japanese themselves have much difficulty in understanding the meaning. It was then almost unknown to the learned world of the extreme East, when Dr. Kayama, a physician of Kioto (Japan), who had studied in Leipzig, studied this document with care, and established the meaning of many obscure passages. In the course of this work he became aware that certain paragraphs, which had not yet attracted the attention of the medical world of his country, evidently treated of venereal diseases, and notably of syphilis. Immediately, with that spirit of disseminating science which is no longer surprising in a people with ideas as broad and advancing as rapidly on the road of progress, Dr. Kayama translated the principal passages into German and sent them to Dr. Scheubc, his former teacher, with a note in regard to the manuscript. So far as interpretation is concerned the professor of Kioto may be depended upon, for this physician applied for aid, in elucidating the difficult portions, to learned Japanese, his countrymen.

The work is divided into one hundred chapters; the first thirteen are long lists of medicines and methods of using remedies. The rest of the manuscript relates to diseases; the authors recognize one hundred and twenty-two; but these are rather groups of symptoms enumerated without order than descriptions of diseases properly so called. The confusion which is present in all the paragraphs should not be surprising in a work which is nearly eleven centuries old. Thus may be found under the same title symptoms belonging to very dissimilar affections. For instance, constipation is given in conjunction with syphilitic arthritis, and osteocopic pains as an accident of the second phase of a disease which affects the penis. Beyond these errors, which are almost fatal, it does not require very close attention to discover in the midst of the physical signs, described *grosso modo*, the course of syphilis very clearly mapped out. The three periods are described in their natural order and with their principal signs. However, the reader will be able to judge.

All the paragraphs relating to genital affections bear the heading KASA (literally: *eruption*), which serves as well to designate a chancre of the penis as a suppurating inguinal bubo, or syphilitic angina. Two chapters are devoted to venereal diseases. In Chapter XCIV, under the title *Kata-shine-kata* (eruption of one of the groins), is found a very clear description of suppurating adenitis. The paragraph which follows treats of the *chancre* in general, and more especially the soft chancre. As there is no special description of the indurated chancre, everything would lead to think that, as it does not pain and does not burrow, the latter was considered an attenuation of the ordinary type:—

Section 2. *Mara-kasa-yami* (eruptive disease of the penis).—In the beginning, a swelling as large as a millet-seed, with pain. After a few days, *ulceration* and a flow of pus.

Here comes, under the head *Fuse-kasa*, the œdema of the prepuce which so often accompanies the infecting chancre, and the consequent temporary phimosis:—

Section 3. The skin of the penis, the seat of the eruption, contains water. . . . The penis is swelled and much increased in volume. The swelling extends to the entire penis, and the glans cannot be seen from the outside. Pus flows from the skin.

The description which then follows is that of the *phagedenic chancre*, which has become serpiginous. The authors state that this trouble begins like the simple chancre:—

Section 4. *Schiri-mara-kasa* (other form of eruption of the penis).—In the beginning an eruption like the preceding one shows itself. Then come on ulceration and pain. At the end of a few days the ulceration extends and the glans drops off. Then the ulceration goes backward some, the penis falls off entire, and the testicles are similarly invaded by the ulceration.

So much for the local venereal symptoms, among which is concealed the primary lesion, no doubt considered as amounting to very little by the Japanese of the ninth century; however, before Ricord, Europe did not suspect the duality of the chancre to any greater extent. We will now observe the second period,—that is to say, the disease becoming general; the osteocopic pains of tertiary processes of the face are equally noted:

Section 5. *Hashiri-kasa* (running eruption).—The *poison*[1] of the penis rises, and the eruption becomes invading. Heat and cold declare themselves, and the *bones* of the extremities become *painful*. After a few months, a small eruption, without pain or itching, appears upon the back and face. . . . Still later, the face is attacked by *caries*, spreads a fetid odor, and runs pus.

Chapter XCV, or at least the extract published by Dr. Kayama, is particularly devoted to the tertiary lesions of syphilis. What confusion! What gropings! How many repetitions! Let us be indulgent with the authors, for we shall soon see that, after the year 1000, our *leeches*[2] described all the venereal diseases, even gonorrhœa, under the name of *leprosy!*

This second chapter begins with the lesions of the second period,—fever, ostitis, and syphilitic arthritis; besides, osteocopic pains are spoken of. The authors do not fail to notice the relations existing between these phenomena and the ulceration of the penis which has cicatrized long before.

Section 1. *Hone-no-hari-kasa* (eruption and swelling of the bones).—*After the cure of the eruption of the penis*, the *joints* of the limbs become *painful*, in such a way that they cannot be extended nor flexed. There exists in general a *fever*. Then the poison rises, and different disagreeable phenomena come on. The bones are *painful*. . . . Constipation is present. . . .

The virus has not completed its work; we are going to see it attack the throat, first, as a *syphilitic angina;*

[1] To-day we say *virus*.

[2] [The author uses the word *mire*, signifying the physician of the Middle Ages.]

later, it will be tertiary ulcerations, with caries of the bones of the face, and even of the skull. These lesions, says the Japanese text, require years to heal, when they do heal.

Section 2. *Nondo-fui-kasa* (eruption of the throat).—The rest of the poison of the eruption of the penis *extends to the upper regions;* the mucous membrane of the throat is swollen and painful. At the end of a few days there is a sanious discharge and a general rotting, which, after many years, is not yet cured. . . . The poison eats the skin of the head, the flesh, and the bones. . . .

Then follow some rather vague details, in which, however, the tertiary period always recurs:—

Then occur the ear diseases, or the nasal eruptions, and the *nose drops off;* or, again, it is the *ophthalmias.* . . . The poison attacks the entire economy; the testicles are covered with *eruptions* and *ulcerate.* . . . The entire surface of the body is attacked.

Section 3 has its title only, *Ana-kasa;* that is to say, *eruption of the anus* (*Lochausschlag* [eruption of the hole], in the German journal). Could the Japanese word *ana* and the Latin *anus* have the same origin?

Section 4, entitled *Mimi-no-hi-kasa* (eruption of the ears), is concerning auditory troubles following otorrhœas.

It is here that the valuable communication of Dr. Kayama, on "Syphilis in Japan in the Year 808," ceases. This learned practitioner adds that he can teach us nothing in particular in respect to treatment, as many of the passages of the manuscript are unintelligible. The text speaks of a few plants of no therapeutic importance. We will state, in conclusion, that in the "world," at Yeddo, the disease is designated by such appellations as *bai-doku* (mushroom-virus), or *so-doku* (virus of eruptive form). But among the people it has preserved its ten-centuried name of KASA. Similarly, in France, educated persons employ the word *syphilis*, but the people still say the *disease*, or the *pox*, like the physicians of the sixteenth, seventeenth, and eighteenth centuries [or, as many of the English-speaking people say, the *bad disease*].

CHAPTER VII.

Syphilis Among the Ancient Egyptians at the Time of the Pharaohs (Fourteenth Century B.C.).

"Ne faut douter qu'un tel mal (*la peste d'Egypte*) ne fust nostre verole d'apresent."—Guillaumet.[1]

[There is no doubt but that such a disease (the Egyptian plague) was our pox of to-day.]

The information furnished by Egypt from the point of view now occupying us is of very small importance. We hasten to recognize this, and we only give it as a matter of archæological curiosity. Besides, it can be understood how difficult it is, in a pictured language as old as that of the Egyptians,—and of which there only remains inscriptions on granite, or shreds of phrases traced on papyri,—to find descriptions referable to syphilis. At all events, if we do not lose sight of the fact that Egypt, in common with Syria and Chaldea,[2] was for a long time the centre of all debaucheries, we cannot see why this nation, with its worship of the phallus, should have been spared. If the Egyptian temples possessed the ancestor of our *bœuf gras*[3] (which has disappeared since 1870), the *bull Apis*, whose rôle was purely decorative, in revenge, they inclosed the goat *Mendes*, who was destined to satisfy the most monstrous lubricity. The nymphomaniacs of Egypt, we are led to believe, were locked up in the temples with this monstrous beast, and submitted to his assaults (Villemont). Of what

[1] Traité de la cristalline. Lyon, 1611.

[2] We will merely recall the fact that Chaldea had for its capital Babylon, whose reputation is well known.

[3] The *bœuf gras* was a bull forming the central attraction of an annual procession in Paris.

orgies were they not capable, these enervated beings, whom the most stupefying mental aberration led up to bestiality! And syphilis should have gone through such a nation without acquiring the freedom of citizenship? It is hardly admissible.

The hieroglyphics which we see upon monuments deal with historical events; the accounts found upon the papyri preserved in France, Germany, at Turin, at London, and at Athens relate to domestic robberies, to the flight of a slave, etc.; or else they are precepts, maxims,—the *Maxims of Ani*, for example. Upon others are found details in regard to the interior police of the kingdom of the time of the Pharaohs, or to the laws of the times. Up to the present but two papyri have been found relating to medicine,—one, the *Medical Papyrus*, forms part of the collection of the Berlin Museum; M. Chabas, one of our learned Egyptologists, gave a detailed analysis of it in 1867.[1] The other, known as the *Ebers Papyrus*,[2] was bought from a Copt at Luxor by Professor Ebers, who published it in 1875. M. Chabas has given us the substance of it in a notice which appeared the following year in his journal, *l'Egyptologie*.[3]

The *Medical Papyrus*, of Berlin, was commenced by King Thoth, as the text shows; and after his death it was continued by King Snat. It is not even a nomenclature of receipts; it is a collection of remedies (?) for different diseases, which are, on the whole, very obscurely designated. All that can be concluded is that ophthalmias were quite frequent among the Egyptians, for the greater part of these more or less scientific receipts refer

[1] Mélanges Egyptologiques, vol. i. Chalon-sur-Saône, 1867.
[2] Ebers' Papyrus. Leipzig, 1875.
[3] F. Chabas: l'Egyptologie, vol. i. Chalon-sur-Saône, 1876.

to eye diseases which are not specified. Clysters were held in very high repute, which goes to show that the persecutors of M. de Pourceaugnac[1] did not have the merit of invention. But the most curious part of this small collection is undoubtedly that which discusses the methods of finding if a woman is capable of becoming pregnant, and even of telling beforehand of what sex the child will be. The procedure is original, but it is not cleanly; may its great age excuse it (four thousand years)! The royal author of the treatise on therapeutics (!) counsels placing in the *natural passage*[2] of the woman two small bags containing, one some wheat, the other barley, previously steeped in . . . the urine of the *candidate for maternity.* If the wheat sprouts, she will be delivered of a boy; if it is the barley, she will bear a girl; if there be no germination, the woman will remain sterile.[3] After giving a few procedures of a like import, the book terminates with a long list of reconstructive ingredients, injections. As may be seen, it would be a difficult matter to find any allusion to syphilis any more than to typhoid fever, of which no one, as far as I know, denies the antiquity.

This is not the case with the *Ebers Papyrus*, which goes into greater details and touches medicine properly so called. It seems to go back to the reign of Rameses II,—Maëamoun, otherwise known as Sesostris. If this be true, it is three thousand years old. The editing is not a little mixed, and it would not be an easy matter to make any diagnosis of all this hotch-potch of symptoms piled up without order or method. Nevertheless,

[1] Apothecaries, who formerly administered rectal injections.

[2] Chabas has substituted asterisks for thisexpression.

[3] We have found the same idea expressed in an old English work dating back three centuries.

if we are to believe the interpretation of Chabas, certain descriptions would seem to have reference to constitutional syphilis; the ancient Egyptians, it would seem, noticed the relations which exist between certain lesions, which may be referred to the secondary and to the tertiary periods. This papyrus includes a series of hieroglyphic groups, of which certain ones deserve to be mentioned.

"There is," says Chabas, "a group which designates a disease located upon the *belly*, in the *extremities*, in the *joints*, in the *eyes*, and in the teeth (*gums*), and which is sufficiently *frequent* to deserve particular mention among those things which are noxious. The treatment is very varied, according to its location (external applications, fumigations, injections [rectal], etc.). The trouble is sometimes sufficiently *grave* to require supernatural means, consisting of a mystical formula repeated four times, and spitting on the diseased parts."

"This same disorder sometimes has its seat also in the *mouth;* . . . it also attacks the *anus.*"

The author notes, under the head "Diseases of the Limbs," the *tophi* on the arms, the *sore of the leg.* "At one time," says the translator, "*inflammation of the arms* is placed in relationship with swelling (or *tumor?*) of the *legs.*" Receipts are also found to cure the disease of the tongue, ulcers of the gums, etc., but it is all too vague to make us halt.

Further on we read: "Clysters caused the disappearance of eruptions which caused crusts of the flesh." All this proves that affections of the skin of a pustulo-crustaceous form were known to the Egyptians, but it proves nothing more. Next comes a remedy for "boils with fetid suppuration;" then quite a number of topical applications for the sexual parts, notably "for the pimples in the vagina; for the pains in the lips; to cool the *inflamed vagina;* for the inflammatory *fissures* in the vagina, etc." What are these pimples of the vagina, or, rather, vulva? Perhaps vegetations; but why not papular syphilides? This inflammation of the vagina might be of gonorrhœal nature; as to the fissures, they may be attributed to whatever one pleases, as erosions may.

Chabas terminates his review with these words: "In the group describing skin diseases it is difficult to designate those which are especially applicable to tetters (*dartres*), to the itch, to chancres, etc. The study of the remedies employed may clear the path. There may be distinguished receipts for pruritus, for swellings or *tumors* in all the limbs, *especially the leg.*" It is to be regretted that Chabas did not designate those remedies which, according to him, might *clear the way;* it is also to be regretted that he was not a physician, for he could have derived authoritative conclusions from the Egyptian text. And while we are expressing regrets let us regret, above all, that our countryman, Mariette-Bey, could not transmit in dying his Egyptological science to the children of Boulogne-sur-Mèr. We could then have interpreted the *fac-simile* of the *Ebers Papyrus.*

At all events, the publication of Ebers is accompanied by an Egyptian-Coptic-Latin glossary, in which we have found these words:—

AXAT, morbus vulvæ; that is, *disease of the vulva.* (Which one?)

ASIT, morbus leprosus? that is, a *disease in the form of leprosy.* (The author is not sure!)

ANUT, plaga vel ulcus; that is, a *sore or ulcer.* (Of what nature?)

BENTET, that is, *vegetations of woman.* (Are they condylomata, properly so called, or other morbid products?)

SETET, that is, *bubo*. (It would be interesting to know whether it is a suppurating bubo or not.)

MEHES, ulcus quoddam; that is, *any ulcer*. (It is not much in the way of information.)

It is quite certain that we cannot form any induction from these obscure texts alone that syphilis existed among the ancient Egyptians; but when we consider that they had the Hebrews among them for a long time, the medical history of the latter of which we will study, there can exist no doubt. We will also see, in the next chapter, that Pharaoh contracted syphilis from Sarah, the wife of Abraham.

If it is admitted that this disease has existed among all peoples and at all times, one cannot help but see, as we do, secondary, tertiary, and, perhaps, primary lesions in the quotations we have given. On this account, we would counsel our readers to re-read this chapter on Egypt, after becoming acquainted with those dealing with the Greek and Roman nations. They will see that syphilis—designated by Martial, Horace, Juvenal, etc., under the different names of *figs* (*ficus*) or large figs (marisca[1]), of *Syrian tumors*, *Egyptian ulcers*, etc.—followed the march of invasion of Western people by the Orientals. It accompanied the Asiatic debauchery in Greece, in Rome, and among the Gauls.

[1] Also denominated *hæmorrhois*, *emerods*, *émeraudes*.

Syphilis Among the Ancient Assyrians and Babylonians, 700 B.C.[1]

On the Assyrio-Babylonian cuneiform inscription tablets in the British museum, derived from the royal library of Asurbanipalus (Sardanapalus), it is related that Istar, the goddess of sinful love, of fruitfulness, of war, etc., and the mother of gods and men, proposed to Izdubar (Nimrod) to become his wife,—a proposition which he very ungallantly refused. Istar demanded satisfaction for this insult from her father, Anu. As a result, the sacred bull was sent against Izdubar and his friend, Eabani. According to some ancient Babylonian seal-cylinders, the latter took hold of the animal by grasping one horn and the root of its tail, while Izdubar bored its heart with some illy-defined weapon. Istar uttered an awful curse, to which Eabani replied by tearing out the ibattu (penis) of the bull and throwing it in her face.

A new curse, whose nature may be readily surmised, was hurled by the goddess, and Eabani died, after twelve days' illness. Izdubar was attacked by a terrible, painful disease (by leprosy, according to another interpreter). He wandered about until he reached the infernal region, where he was given a "magic food" for his disease. This either had no effect or it was merely

[1] This subchapter is added as a súpplement to the preceding chapter, as not only bearing upon the subject, but on account of the similarity the story bears to the myths of other nations, explanatory of the origin of venereal diseases. I am indebted for this to an article published in Monatshefte fuer Praktische Dermatologie, May 1, 1891, by J. K. Proksch, who has laid under contribution the translations of Zahnpfund and Jeremias, the interpreters of the cuneiform inscriptions found on Babylonian bricks.—O-D.

preliminary, for Izdubar complained that the shadow of death lay on his genitals. Sît-napiôtim, the god of the infernal regions, took him to Ara-Ea, the ferryman, and bade him take the hero to the fountain of life, saying: "The man whom thou hast taken has his body covered with *pustules; scales* have altered the fairness of his body. Take him, Arad-Ea, to the *cleansing-place*, where he can wash his pustules clean with snow, and take off his *skins;* the sea will carry them off; his body will appear well. The *coverings of his head will be renewed*, as also the *covering of his shameful parts;* by the time he returns to his country there will be no folds; all will be new." Then follows, without interruption: "Arad-Ea then conducted him to the cleansing-place, washed his pustules in water like snow; he cast off his skins; the sea carried them off; his body appeared healthy. He renewed his head-coverings; the sheath which clothed his shameful parts was new when he reached his native land." The covering which invested his pudenda and "shall show no folds," "must be new," cannot be understood as meaning anything else than that the covering over or about his genitals must not become unclean through pathological secretions and become corroded or fold-like; it must be made new; *i.e.*, clean.

Eabani evidently had syphilis, for Izdubar says that he may not die like him. And Eabani had spent six days and seven nights dallying with the lalû of his beloved, Uchat. Among the ancient Orientals venereal diseases were the result either of exciting divine wrath or of sexual excesses. The name of the hierodulus—Uchat—points very plainly to the Uchet disease,—the uχedu or uχetu; that is, syphilis of the ancient Egyptians.

CHAPTER VIII.

Syphilis Among the Hebrews in Biblical Times.

"Cette maladie (*la syphilis*) a un origine de plus loin (*que le xve siécle*), comme nous en aurons de bons tesmoignages par les histoires sainctes et prophanes."—Guillaumet.[1]

[This disease (syphilis) has an origin going back further (than the xvth century), as we have good evidence in sacred and profane history.]

"Guéris-moi, Eternel, car mes os sont frappés. . . . La nuit, je n'ai point de repos. . . . Il n'y à rien de sain dans ma chair."—David, *Psalms*.

[Heal me, O Lord, for my bones are stricken. . . . At night, I have no rest. . . . There is nothing sound in my flesh.]

In order to write this chapter, we first studied the Bible carefully; then we absorbed the works of Rosenbaum, Astruc, Dufour, Villemont,[2] etc., and especially the excellent monograph of Dr. Hamonic, from which we will quote several extracts. Our friend will pardon us for limiting ourself to a few quotations from his work, which we would like to reproduce *in extenso;* but this first volume is already quite long. For that reason we refer the reader to his work, if he be desirous of becoming thoroughly acquainted with venereal diseases in Biblical times.[3]

The Bible contains a mass of allusions referring to venereal diseases, and especially to syphilis. Gonorrhœa, according to modern authors, is perfectly de-

[1] *Loc. cit.*

[2] Hist. des malad. vénér. Paris, 1882. History of Venereal Diseases.

[3] P. Hamonic: des Malad. vénér. chez les Hébreux. Paris, 1887. Venereal Diseases among the Hebrews.

scribed; but it must be acknowledged that this truth has been recognized by all only since it has been known that this inflammatory affection is not a symptom of the primary period of syphilis. Astruc believed the contrary; and it will be seen, in our second volume, what useless pains this author took to deny the antiquity of gonorrhœa,—a thing which has become a modern axiom. This is not the case with the disease we are considering. We will answer, however, the same thing, whether it concern the Bible, the Vedas, or the works of Celsus, or of Hippocrates. It is not found there under its modern name; look for it in the symptoms, and you will find it. What is the Bible? A collection of stories, songs, laws, dogmas, moral counsels, and aphorisms, the whole clothed in an allegorical or symbolical garb, which was in accord with the religious poetry of that time. Among the precepts, the most brilliant are the rules for scrupulous cleanliness of Moses, the great hygienist, who could not have had them adopted, as well as other things, if he had not invoked Jehovah upon all occasions, and especially upon difficult matters. So that it is only for the physician free from all bias that a search in this long, secular poem—that descriptions or allusions which may be referred to one of the three periods of syphilis—will prove profitable.

In the fifth book of Proverbs, attributed to Solomon, will be found a few words of advice which go to show that visiting the hetairæ of the time might be followed by painful remembrances, capable of lasting for years, and of gravely compromising the general health. Solomon counsels to beware of them; his lessons have profited but little since his death. We will give the Latin version of the Hebrew text, from the edition of 1715, in the "Bibliothèque Nationale," in order that the reader may see for himself that our interpretation has nothing in it of a fantastical nature :—

v. 3. Favus enim distillans labia meretricis. . . .	For the lips of the harlot distill honey. . . .
v. 4. Novissima autem illius amara quasi absynthum, et acuta quasi gladius biceps.	But the *consequences* are as *bitter* as worm-wood, and *sharp* as a double-edged sword.
v. 5. Pedes ejus descendunt in mortem. . . .	Her feet lead down to death. . . .
v. 8. Ne appropinques foribus domûs ejus. . . .	Do not draw near the gate of her house. . . .
v. 9. Ne des alienis honorem tuum et annos tuos crudeli.	Lest thou shouldst give up thy honor to strangers, and the *remainder of thy life* to something *cruel*.
v. 11. Et gemas in novissimis quando consumeris carnes tuos et corpus tuum.	And that thou mayst not groan *later*, when thy *flesh* and thy *body* will have been *destroyed* through thy fault.

This *something cruel* which can bring on corruption seems to me to be a disease; and this disease which infects the entire organism, as a result of converse with a *tradeswoman in love*, what can it be, if not syphilis? For my part, I must humbly confess that I know of no other that would warrant Solomon's description. Our opponents may merely see, in these, regrets of a purely moral nature. Let us allow the *burning remorse* of more than one bachelor, and pass on.

In Ecclesiastes, a collection of maxims and moral counsels also attributed to Solomon, and which certain authors have confounded with the Ecclesiast of Jesus Syrac, a few verses are found which may also be referred to the tertiary period :—

Cap. xix, v. 3. Qui se jungit fornicariis, erit nequam; putredo et vermes hereditabunt illum, et extolletur in exemplum majus. . . .	He who has relations with prostitutes will become unclean for everything; gangrene and worms will seize upon him, and he will serve as a terrifying example to others. . . .

The idea of the debauchee who will soon be *rotten* (putredo), and who will see the worms crawling in his ulcerated gummata, is found in another passage, in which it is said that the libertine can reap, as the price of his caresses, nothing but worms and other parasitic insects (*vermes et tineas pro mercede reportare*). It is truc that, at that time, the antiseptic method was unknown, and the smallest ulcer, no matter what its nature, was provided with a quantity of *grubs* that would make the dream of a fisherman. In our days, unless it be in a hospital on our left bank, where Lister is damned, the classic worms of which the Bible is so prodigal are unknown.

The following verses of Leviticus prove that there were ulcers whose scar was white, and others which preserved a brownish color, as in syphilis, for instance; but it proves nothing else. However, let us note that the Bible distinguishes between superficial ulcers, which only involve the skin, and deep ulcers, which arise in the thickness of the muscles:—

Cap. xiii, v. 18. Caro autem in carnis et cutis in quâ ulcus natum est et sanatum,	If an ulcer has arisen in the skin or *within the flesh*, and it has healed,
v. 19. et in loco ulceris cicatrix alba apparverit, sive subrusa . . .	and there appears, at the place where it existed, a scar, white or *somewhat reddish* . . .

All this is vague, it must be acknowledged; but these documents are not without some importance, as complementary proofs of the more conclusive arguments which Rome will soon furnish us.

Finally, in Chapter XV is found the famous verse quoted by all the authors who have desired to defend the antiquity of syphilis since the sixteenth century. Unfortunately, it demonstrates but one thing; that is, that the Hebrews of Moses, like the Christians of Leo XIII, had frequent gonorrhœas. The Hebrew word, *mizobo*, if we are to believe the anonymous collaborator of Hamonic, literally signifies a *flow*, and not an *ejaculation*,—a phenomenon distinguished in verse 16 by the word *chighboth*. Here is verse 2, after the Latin *Vulgate*, so well known and misinterpreted :—

v. 2. . . . Vir qui patitur fluxum [seminis], immundus erit.	. . . The man who has a flow [of semen] shall be deemed unclean.

We have included the word *seminis* in brackets as it is superfluous, the translator having depended upon the Greek version of the Septuagint, without concerning himself with the Hebrew. The expression, ῥεον γόνον (loss of seed, pollution), which is given for the word *mizobo*, is a contradiction ; for Moses declares as also impure the clothing, seats, cloths, etc., which are used by the subject, as being one with him. Listen to what follows :—

v. 13. Si sanatus fuerit qui hujusmodi sustinet passionem, numerabit septem dies post emundationem.	If he who has this disease is cured, he will count *seven days* after his liberation.
v. 16. Vir de quo egredietur semen coïtûs, lavabit aquâ corpus suum et immundus erit usque ad vesperum.	He who has a loss of seed will wash his whole body with water, and shall be deemed unclean *until evening*.

The patient suffering from *mizobo*, then, had to wait *seven days after his cure* before he could mingle with others ; while the man defined by the word *chighboth*, of verse 16, was declared impure until evening only. These are two very different cases : on the one hand, a contagious flow ; on the other, a simple pollution. Besides, the Talmud completes our information on this point.

There is nothing here referable to syphilis ; and

those authors who have copied their predecessors, one after the other, should have ceased to invoke this verse of Leviticus as soon as Ricord demonstrated that gonorrhœa was entirely independent of syphilis. To quote erroneously is to give arms to one's adversary; and we will not fail to reject, whenever we meet them, incorrect quotations of authors who are partisans of the ancient origin, whose zeal has obscured their sight. It is, perhaps, easier to compile than to look up proofs one's self and to discuss those found by others; but one is then liable to reproduce the errors and to publish texts which have not been understood.

Let us return to the Bible:—

The Hebrews were as much exposed as other peoples of Asia to contract venereal diseases, as they had the depraved habits of all the Asiatics. Without mentioning Sodom and Gomorrha, does not Moses forbid, in Leviticus, incest, bestiality, abnormal sexual relations, and even legal prostitution, which is the best proof that these vices existed? In spite of the most severe punishments, the Hebrews gave themselves up to these shameless excesses; and, as prostitution was forbidden in their camp, they visited strangers, particularly the Medianites and the daughters of Moab. These latter initiated them into the worship of Baal Peor, or Belphegor,—a sort of Priapus, whose temples were nothing but places of debauchery. These orgies in common were eminently favorable to the propagation of syphilis; and, as a matter of fact, it was rapidly propagated, and known as the *plague of Baal Peor*,—an epidemic which will arrest us a moment.

From the information furnished us by Rosenbaum,[1]

[1] Geschichte der Lustseuche in Alterthum. Halle, 1845. History of Syphilis in Antiquity.

the name "Baal Peor" signified among the Hebrews *the god Penis*, the Priapus of the Romans, of whom we shall have occasion to speak shortly. His temple was built on Mount Peor, and young girls repaired to it to prostitute themselves. This worship was analogous to that of the *Lingam* of India, and of the *Phallus* of the rest of Asia. We may still see to-day, in China, a phallus on a stone over the door of houses of prostitution [as it was in Pompeii]. Here are, according to the Old Testament, in the Book of Moses, which the Greeks have called the Pentateuch, the passages concerning the scourge which the Jews brought upon themselves by the worship of Baal (Numbers, chap. xxv):—

v. 1. Morabatur autem eo tempore Israël in Sittim, eo fornicatus est populus cum filiabus Moab.

However (after the exodus from Egypt), Israel had tarried at Sittim and inhabited there; it fell into fornication with the daughters of Moab.

In more symbolic terms, the Hebrews worshiped the gods of the daughters of the Moabites and devoted themselves to the worship of Baal Peor:—

v. 3. Initiatus est Israël Baal Peor.

Then the wrath of Jehovah made itself felt—always according to Moses—and manifested itself as an epidemic disease, which spread like a train of powder and decimated the Israelites. Moses, frightened, caused all those who had worshiped Baal to be killed; that is to say, all those who had had relations with the Moabite women; for they were all infected, or likely to be:—

v. 9. Et occisi sunt viginti quatuor millia hominum.

Twenty-four thousand men were thus killed by the steel.

A rather radical prophylaxis, but one of which Jehovah shouldered the entire responsibility. "In order

D²

to appease my anger," he is made to say, "let each chief of the tribes sacrifice those of his tribe who have gone over to Baal Peor." Later on, the Bible adds: "Thus the plague was averted, after having cost the lives of 24,000 men." Many commentators of the Hebrew text have departed from this to explain that the 24,000 men died of the disease, which is contradicted by the text itself. Besides, Philon and Josephus, Jewish historians, expressly state that this massacre was ordered by Moses. This occurred in the supposed year of the creation of the world, 2553, in 1451 B.C.; that is to say, forty years after the exodus from Egypt. At all events, this terrible execution did not prove sufficient to destroy the root of the evil; for Joshua, seventeen years later, reproaching the Hebrews for their debauchery, plainly says[1]:—

v. 17. An parvum vobis est quod peccatis in Baal Peor, et usque in præsentem diem macula hujus sceleris in nobis permanet . . . ?	Is it not enough for you to have committed the sin of following the worship of Baal Peor, a sin whose *sign exists unto this day* . . . ?

Nearly seven centuries later, in 810 B.C., the prophet Hosea again had occasion to rail against those who sacrificed to the altars of Baal Peor, and groaned over the results of this worship[2]:—

v. 10. Intraverunt ad Baal Peor, . . . et facti abominabiles sicut ea quæ dilexerunt.	They have been initiated in the mysteries of Baal Pecr, ... and they have become terrible like those things which they worshiped.

And still Moses had taken his precautions well; for, not content with killing the guilty, he declared war against the Midianites—always according to the com-

[1] Joshua, chap. xxii. [2] Hosea, chap. ix.

mands of Jehovah—because the women of that people had drawn the sons of Israel to the worship of Baal Peor. As a matter of fact, it was the principal focus of the scourge. The Hebrews marched against Prince Midian, defied him, killed all the men, and, after pillaging, *secundem artem*, brought back with the flocks the women and children. Moses became angered at the generals of the army because they had spared the women[1]:—

v. 15. Cur feminis reservatis.

As a matter of fact, it was scarcely worth while to have executed their own men, either diseased or suspected of being so, and then introduce in the midst of the Hebrew camp strange women who contained the virus. Moses had but one course to pursue,—kill them also. It was cruel, but logical. The great legislator proved that he was acquainted with logic before the birth of Aristotle. Let us listen to him :—

v. 16. Nonne istæ sunt quæ deceperunt filios Israël ad suggestionem Balaam, et prævaricari vos fecerunt in Domino super peccato Peor unde percussus est populus?	Are these not the women who have seduced the sons of Israel at the instigation of Balaam, and who have made you deny the Lord, your God, to make you sacrifice to *Peor*, *from whom is come the scourge which has stricken our people?*

The conclusion of this appropriate apostrophe is easily anticipated :—

v. 17. Ergo interficite quidquid est generis masculini, etiam in parvulis; et mulieres quæ noverunt virus in coïtu, jugulate; v. 18. puellas autem et omnes feminas virgines reservate vobis.	Therefore, kill all male children, even the newborn; and strangle the women who have known men carnally; but allow female children and young virgins to live.

[1] Numbers, chap. xxi.

This butchery, carried out, as we have said, 1451 years before our era, did not prevent the plague of Baal Peor from becoming one of the ornaments of our large capitals, after a lapse of more than thirty centuries. It is true that the sword of Moses is out of fashion, fortunately, and that in Paris, for example, the system of incarceration in St. Lazare is a very poor substitute. Treat them and cure them, but do not punish them. These patients are victims before necessity makes them criminals!

There is no doubt that the epidemic of which we have just been speaking was of venereal origin; for Flavius Josephus states that it was highly contagious, and was transmitted to different members of the same family,—no doubt, through toilet articles, vases, etc. Such, according to the Bible, is the legend of the disease of Baal Peor, of which several authors have spoken, chiefly Rosenbaum and Hamonic. We will here reproduce the conclusions of the latter, with which we fully agree[1]:—

"Do we ask what was the scourge of Baal Peor?

"We must, first of all, put aside leprosy. Moses knew its prognosis very well. He had it himself.[2]

"It was neither *gonorrhœa*, nor *balano-posthitis*, nor *genital herpes*, nor even *soft chancre*.

"These lesions, with the exception of the last, were frequent at that time, as I have pointed out in speaking of circumcision, and were, so to say, classical. They certainly would not have alarmed Moses to the pitch of adopting such a radical measure, even if they had multiplied, as a result of excessive coïtus and uncleanliness. Besides, they would not have perpetuated themselves in Israel.

[1] *Loc. cit.*

[2] Exodus, chap. iv, v. 6.

"The disease of Baal Peor was something more intense, more violent, and more dangerous for the public health; and, although the Bible does not furnish the clinical symptoms, it is plain that this disease constituted a grave social danger, which Moses endeavored to avoid by all possible means. *Certes* this legislator was too keen an observer of phenomena to make a gross error of diagnosis between diseases which already existed among his people and the new epidemic.

"The inevitable conclusion from what precedes is, that *the scourge of Baal Peor was syphilis.*"

Among the isolated verses which, outside of legendary or historical facts, deal with this affection, treat of this disease, a few are found in which *alopecia* is pointed out as a disease inherent to prostitution. Prostitutes and those who frequent them are to expect, according to the prophet Isaiah (785 B.C.), to see their skulls denuded and their bodies emanate a fetid odor[1]:—

v. 9. Agnitio vultûs eorum respondit eis: peccatum suum quasi Sodoma prædicaverunt, nec absconderunt. . . .	The appearance of their face speaks for them: like Sodom they publish their sin, nor do they dissimulate. . . .
v. 17. . . . decalvabit Dominus verticem filiarum Sion, et Dominus crinem earum nudabit.	. . . the Lord will render bald the vertex of the heads of the sons of Sion, the Lord will cause their *hair to fall.*
v. 24. Et erit pro suavi odore fœtor, . . . pro crispanti crine calvitium.	Instead of that pleasant perfume they will spread a stink, . . . instead of flowing hair, it will be *baldness.*

Was it the characteristic odor of vulvar syphilides? We do not know; it is possible, especially when we remember that this bad odor is coincident with alopecia.

In Deuteronomy, which is the second book of the

[1] Isaiah, chap. iii.

laws of Moses embraced in the Pentateuch, we see the legislator threatening his people with the *ulcer of Egypt* if they desert the Lord and refuse to hearken to his voice; that is to say, Moses himself, the forced intermediary (chapter xxviii):—

v. 17. Percutiat te Dominus ulcere Egypti, et partem corporis per quam stercora egrediuntur, scabie quoque et prurigine, ita ut curari nequeas.	The Lord will visit thee with the *ulcer of Egypt*, and that part of thy body by which the fæcal matters are evacuated will be the seat of itching *papules*, of which thou canst not free thyself.

So the Egyptian ulcer was accompanied by *folds*, *elevations* (scabies) about the *anus*, which caused the patient to experience tingling; and Moses knew that it took a long time to cure, at least. This description would apply very well to mucous patches of the anal region, without prejudice to the other manifestations alluded to in the verses which follow:—

v. 35. Percutiat te Dominus ulcere pessimo in genibus, in furis, sanarique non possis a planta pedis usque ad verticem tuum.	The Lord will cover thee with *bad ulcers* from the soles of the feet to the head, upon the knees, on the legs, and thou wilst not get well.

A generalized eruption with pustules and ulcerations. Let us continue:—

v. 59. Augebit Dominus plagas tuas et plagas seminis tui, plagas magnas et perseverantes infirmitates pessimas et perpetuas.	Thy sores will increase, by the will of God, as also those thou hast given to thy *progeny;* then they will be large and *persevering* sores, the worst and *most lasting* lesions.

Heredity is clearly indicated here, and it does not require a great stretch of the imagination to understand the medical meaning of these threats of Moses. Secondary accidents are numerous, succeed each other, and are rebellious to the primitive treatment of the Hebrew; the children born in these circumstances have syphilitic manifestations. Then come tertiary lesions,—ulcers which do not heal, necroses, and irreparable losses of substance. If we imagined this summary description deprived of its sententious and symbolic dress, we would think that we were reading one of those monographs of the fifteenth century treating of the *morbus gallicus.* This passage of Deuteronomy is one of the most interesting, especially as it informs us that the Egyptian ulcer was syphilis. Moses gave out these laws 1451 B.C.; that is to say, in the year of the plague of Baal Peor. These appellations, devoted to dissimilar symptoms of the same disease,—symptoms whose nosological bonds could not be suspected by the Hebrews,—were necessarily numerous, either on account of the seat of the lesions, or on account of the endemic or epidemic character which the disease might assume.

We will now go back still further,—to Genesis, which is lost in the twilight of time,—and relate the different excursions of Abram, who judged it better, later on, to call himself Abraham.

About the year 1921 B.C., if we are to believe the Bible, a Hebrew of the name of Abram, who dwelt between Bethel and Aï, was constrained to leave his country by the famine: he went down to Egypt, but, as his wife Saraï was beautiful, he made her pass herself off as his sister, "fearing," said he, "that the Egyptians might do him an evil turn by taking her from him." The beauty of Saraï gained him admission to the court of Pharaoh. The latter simply appropriated the beautiful Jewess to himself, and heaped her supposed brother with goods and presents. But the Lord, less satisfied with this amicable arrangement than Abram,—so the Bible states,

—"visited Pharaoh and his house with *great plagues*, on account of Saraï, the wife of Abram."[1]

v. 17. Flagellant autem Dominus Pharaonem plagis maximis et domum ejus, propter Saraï, uxorem Abram.

Which means that Pharaoh contracted from Saraï a venereal disease, which he transmitted to his other wives or to those of his officers, who gave it to others, etc. In short, the whole court was infected. Pharaoh, "like a true gentleman," as Hamonic says, after having reproached Abram for not having informed him that she was his wife, returned his goods to him, together with his dangerous mate, and dismissed him.

Later on, at Guerar, this accommodating husband played the same trick upon Abimelech, the king of that country. At that time he called himself Abraham and his wife Sarah. Same story of the sister, and the same foreseen taking away. But the Lord appeared to the king in a vision, and threatened him with death. Let us note, by the way, that the Lord was very indulgent with Abraham, and very severe to the kings who fell in the trap. M. de Montespan exhibited more pride than the Israelite patriarch; but divine wrath, no doubt, exhausted after thirty-five centuries of useless threats, or blunted by use, in no way troubled Louis XIV in the course of his adulterous exploits. Abimelech hastened to return Sarah to her husband, and loaded both with presents. He had, none the less, contracted the disease, which he transmitted to the queen and to his sewing-maids or concubines. But upon the prayer of Abraham —who could do no less for such a generous client—the Lord *cured* Abimelech, his wife and servants, and these could *bear children*.[2]

[1] Genesis, chap. xii. [2] Genesis, chap. xx.

v. 17. Orante autem Abraham sanavit Deus et uxorem, ancillasque ejus, et pepererunt.

v. 18. Concluserat enim Dominus omnem vulvam domûs Abimelech propter Saram, uxorem Abraham.	For the Lord *closed the womb* of all the women of the house of Abimelech on account of Sarah, the wife of Abraham.

This Sarah, while a source of profit to Abraham, was a danger to all those who allowed themselves to be captivated by her charms. Besides, the Bible informs us that she was for a long time sterile, and that all the women who were infected through her were also sterile. We will conclude, like Hamonic :—

"The disease transmitted by Sarah was always of genital origin.

"On account of its great transmissibility, its long period of virulence, and the relations which seemed to exist between it and sterility, it is not irrational to suppose that *syphilis* was concerned in this. It disappeared with age in Sarah, who became pregnant late, which is a good proof that her sterility was not due to an organic cause.

"Outside of syphilis, we cannot see any other disease of genital origin which could correspond with the foregoing facts."

This manner of interpreting the disease of Sarah is not new, although it is not expressed, as far as we know, by any author defending the antiquity of syphilis until 1887. A Spanish physician, a contemporary of the great epidemic of the fifteenth century, Francisco de Villalobos, wrote, in his youth (thirty-two years before Fracastor), a poem on syphilis, in which he relates in light verses that Pharaoh caught this disease from Sarah. This Villalobos became celebrated later on, and was successively physician to Ferdinand V, Charles V, and

Philip II. This is the passage: "On account of this sin," says Holy Writ, "King Pharaoh was attacked by it (the pox), because he could not resist the great beauty of Sarah." . . .

> Por este pecado en la sacra escritura,
> Al rey Faraon le hallamos tenella,
> Porque él fué vencido de gran hermosura
> De Sarra . . . [1]

In order to conclude with the Bible, we will examine the case of King David,—*Daoud*, according to the Hebrew text. Everybody knows his adventure with Bath-Sheba, that which our abridged sacred histories call Bethsabee; it may be seen, in these same abridgements, that David was punished:—

> Pleura quelque temps son péché,
> Mais garda toujours sa maîtresse. [2]

We will summarize, in a few lines, this authentic history, which proves that David, made king because he was a son-in-law, acted like a common assassin, and in a particularly disreputable manner. The syphilis which he reaped, to begin with, as we shall see, was really but a slight punishment, compared to the crime he committed. Pharaoh and Abimelech, more righteous, and certainly less cruel, were punished in the same manner, and yet Abraham was far from being as interesting as Uriah.

King David, the Bible relates, was enjoying the cool of the evening upon the terrace of his palace, when he saw a woman of rare beauty, who was washing herself in the brook. He made inquiries, and learned that she was the wife of one of his officers, one Uriah; he had

[1] Villalobos: Sumario de la medecina, en romance trovado, con un tratado sobre las pestiferas bubas. Salamanca, 1498. Summary of Medicine, in verse, with a Treatise on the Bubonic Plague.

[2] "Wept some time for his sin, but always kept his mistress." Parny: Les Galanteries de la Bible. Paris, 1831. The Galantries of the Bible.

her brought to him, said very little to her, and found her docile in every respect. The entertainment having terminated, Bath-Sheba very quietly returned home. It is not known whether she returned often to see the king, but it is probable; at all events, she became pregnant. Then David bethought him of getting rid of the husband, and found nothing better than to charge one of his generals, who was on a campaign, to place him in the most dangerous post, so that he might be killed,—which happened, as a matter of fact. A convenient method, in no way compromising, but not chivalric. Louis XV acted differently in respect to the gentlemen of his court, whose conjugal honor he damaged, if it was only *before the letter*. Other times, other manners.

Bath-Sheba put on mourning, and David married her. She was delivered. Up to that time, nothing was more simple. But our two lovers had reckoned without the Lord, who, having had enough time to think, declared himself angry, and sent, always according to the legend, a prophet to David, to rail at him and warn him that he would be punished where he had sinned. It is probable that tertiary accidents rapidly declared themselves in this lecherous king; besides, he may not have troubled himself about the two first periods; he may have had them in a light form, and, as he did not treat himself from the beginning, nine or ten months later, at the least,—since Bath-Sheba had time to arrive at term,—the symptoms of the tertiary period manifested themselves with a certain intensity: osteocopic pains, ulcerated gummata, and the rest. Nothing but what is very rational in the progress of the disease. But let us not anticipate our conclusions, and let us leave the Bible speak. The prophet Nathan brings to David the decision of Jehovah[1]:—

[1] Kings, chap. xii.

v. 11. Itaque hæc dicit Dominus : ecce ego suscitabos super te malum de domo tuâ. . . .	For the Lord has spoken thus : Behold, I will visit *evil* upon thee and upon thy house, . . .
v. 14. . . . filius qui natus est tibi, morte morietur.	. . . the son who is born to thee will die.

As a matter of fact, in spite of David praying to the Lord, fasting, lying upon the ground, etc., the child fell ill, and "died at the end of seven days."

v. 18. Accidit autem die septimâ ut moreretur infans.

This occurred 1034 B.C. Let us now listen to the lamentations of David, who will himself describe, with poetical metaphors, the symptoms of his disease (*Psalms*).

Chap. vi, v. 3. Miserere mei, Domine, quoniam infirmus sum : sana me, Domine, quoniam conturbata sunt ossa mea. . . .	Pity me, O Lord, for I am ill : cure me, O Lord, for *my bones are diseased*. . . .
v. 8. Inveteravi. . . .	I am become old. . . .
Chap. xxi, v. 7. Ego autem sum vermis, et non homo ; opprobrium hominum. . . .	I am a *worm*, and not a man : I am the opprobrium of men. . . .
v. 8. Omnes videntes me, deriserunt me. . . .	All those who have seen me have mocked me. . . .

David would have been pitied, instead of being mocked, if the origin and nature of his disease had not been known.

v. 15. Et dispersa sunt omnia ossa mea. . . .	All my *bones separate*.
v. 16. Aruit tanquam testa virtus mea, et lingua mea adhæsit faucibus meis. . . .	All my strength dries up like clay, and my tongue cleaves to my palate. . . .
Chap. xxx, v. 11. Ossa mea conturbata sunt.	My bones are diseased.
v. 12. . . . Sum opprobrium, . . . qui videbant forás, fugerunt a me. . . .	I am an opprobrium, . . . all those who have seen me abroad have run away from me. . . .

No one wished to come near him; it must have been known that his disease was contagious.

Chap. xxxi, v. 3. Inveteraverunt ossea mea. . . .	My bones have become old. . . . .

He recurs three times to the state of his bones; the bony frame was, without doubt, affected the most.

v. 4. Die ac nocte gravata est super me manus tua. . . .	Day and night thy hand weighs upon me. . . .

This was probably a nocturnal cephalalgia, as he did not even have sleep to forget his trouble.

Chap. xxxviii, v. 4. Non est sanitas in carne mea a facie iræ tuæ: non est pax ossibus meis a facie peccatorum mearum.	*There is nothing sound in my flesh* on account of thy wrath: my bones leave me no peace on account of my sins [transgressions (?)].

His bones always made him suffer; they were most probably osteocopic. This opinion is shared in by Galligo,[1] who says, in the beginning of his work, that "King David seems to have been the subject of syphilis, and to have suffered chiefly from *osteocopic pains* (*il Re David sembra che sia andato soggetto alla sifilide*, *e perfino ai dolori osteocopi*)."

v. 6. Putruerunt et corruptæ sunt cicatrices meæ a facie insipientiæ meæ. . . .	My ulcers are putrid and corrupt on account of my folly. . .

Ulcerated gummata, evidently treated in a primitive manner.

v. 8. Non est sanitas in carne meâ. . . .	There is nothing healthy in my flesh. . . .

He is forced to acknowledge a second time that he is not healthy. At that time the famous *alteratives*, vaunted with so much advertising to-day, were unknown.

v. 11. . . . et lumen oculorum meorum et ipsum non est mecum.	. . . and the light of my eyes is no more with me.

[1] *Loc. cit.*

Have we to deal with iritis, a common accident of the transition period?

v. 12. Qui juxta me erant, de longè steterunt.	Those who were near me now stand aloof.

For the second time he makes us understand that his disease had a contagious character, which was well known, as nobody trusted it. Finally, David beseeches the Lord to heal him completely. He doubtless knew that his disease could disappear without leaving any traces:—

Chap. 1, v. 9. Asperges me hyssopo, et mundabor . . . et super nivem dealdabor.	You will sprinkle me with hyssop and I will be purified . . . and I will become whiter than the snow.

This last phrase leads us involuntarily to think of the syphilitics of our century who, knowing that it takes several years to effect a complete cure, ask us to *bleach* them in the shortest possible time.

"Although somewhat vague," says Hamonic, "the symptoms mentioned in the Psalms of David have none the less a great value, especially if they are grouped and placed in relation to each other. Here is a man who contracted from a woman he rendered pregnant a disease of genital origin, whose symptoms are marked, since they are those upon which the patient especially insists, consisting in terrible *pains*, coming on chiefly at night, and in *alterations of the bones.* The bones are the seat of acute suffering. They disintegrate, *separate* (caries or necrosis). Purulent and chronic ulcers occur, and are probably related to the diseased bones. It must be through them that the fragments of bone escape.

"The patient loses his strength, and falls into a marked cachexia. His emaciation is extreme. His mouth (especially the tongue) is diseased. He is a disgusting object to everybody. The morbid symptoms, at first localized, become more and more general ("there is nothing healthy in my flesh"), and, what caps the climax, the eyes are implicated and the sight is obscured. Visceral symptoms appear at a given time, and this *terrible general disease* plunges the unfortunate David in a hypochondria and discouragement which it is easy to understand, in view of the chronicity of the lesions and of their resistance to the simple therapeutics directed against them.

"To what has preceded, let us add that the child borne by Bath-Sheba, who had transmitted her disease to David, died at the end of seven days,—a fact which, when added to the others, naturally leads us to make the diagnosis of syphilis. So I will conclude by saying that David, who, in his old age, required a young virgin to warm him,[1] is probably one of the most ancient *syphilitic* kings who ever lived."

We see nothing to add to the conclusions, which are a faithful reproduction of our way of seeing. We will merely say that, if syphilis is a just punishment, which is a debatable question, it was never, nor could it have been, better applied than in being grafted on the venerable David.

Let us now say a few words concerning the disease of Job. A certain number of authors, physicians, and others, such as Vatable, Cyprian, the Jesuit Jean de Pieda (or Pineda), the Capuchin monk Bolbuc (or Bolduc), Don Calmet, Ulrich von Hutten, Guy Patin, etc., saw syphilis in his disease; for others, it was leprosy. Hamonic, who is in accord with Bartholin and M. Rollet, holds it for scurvy. They base themselves upon the

[1] Kings, chap. iii, v. 1, 2, 3, 4.

fact that Lot had many children after his cure, and that his daughters were very beautiful. This is not an absolute reason, for all practitioners have had the opportunity of delivering syphilitic women, who were cured, and whose children have always remained handsome.[1] In addition, we will humbly observe that scurvy requires for its development physiological poverty, which is found everywhere; in the next place, the conditions of moisture, and especially of cold, are not present in all countries. It is plain that cold does not easily occur in Palestine.

At all events, the symptoms described by Job differ from those presented by David; and, with the exception of a few symptoms which are found in several diseases, and particularly in syphilis, we do not think that the story of Job presents arguments sufficient to permit this unfortunate man being dubbed the *patron of the poxy.*

Certain authors, M. Rollet, for instance, have seen syphilis in the sixth plague of Egypt (Exodus, chap. ix, v. 10 and 11). It is not impossible, but the Bible simply states that *ulcers* and *vesicular* (or pustular) *tumors* formed in men and in animals. This is very obscure, and we know that syphilis has never manifested itself in animals beyond the attempts at inoculation which succeeded. There was to be seen, in 1882, in the anteroom of the internes of Lourcine, a young monkey whom Martineau, our former teacher, had inoculated with syphilis, and who exhibited, for several months, very distinct mucous patches.

As to the *leprosy* of the Hebrews, a number of skin diseases may be recognized under this term, and it cor-

[1] We will return to this subject in our next volume, and adduce very convincing cases.

responds, in a great measure, to our expression *dartre* [tetter]. The leprosy of the Middle Ages was nothing else; to see in it true leprosy only, as we know it, or syphilis alone, is to be too exclusive. Many patients affected with benign or malignant affections of the skin, and occasionally syphilitics, were called lepers. We will soon see what part is to be assigned to leprosy proper, which became a pathological curiosity as soon as syphilis, rescued from the chaos in which it had been buried up to the end of the fifteenth century, occupied the place which properly belonged to it in nosology.

In the disease of Herod, in which there existed suppurating buboes and gangrene of the genital organs, like Apion the Blasphemer, if we are to believe Flavius Josephus,[1] the Jewish historian and writer, scarcely anything but a large phagedenic chancre can be seen. We will say the same of the case of the Emperor Galerius Maximus, related by Eusebius.[2] They might be regarded as ulcers of the tertiary period, but these are not, as a rule, complicated by gangrene. We are also aware of the fact that Ricord has described gangrenous syphilitic chancres; but such cases are extremely rare, as due to the syphilis itself; so rare that one is led to suspect some influence extraneous to the specific disease, and to give them their true name, perhaps,—that of mixed chancres. But we have already stated (chap. i) our opinion upon this subject, and this is not the place to enter upon a discussion which might lead us too far. We will close this study of syphilis in Biblical times by reproducing a few passages from a letter of Guy

[1] Flavius Josephus: Antiquitat judaic., lib. xvii, chap. viii (translated from the Greek).

[2] Histor. Ecclesiast., lib. viii, chap. xxviii (translated from the Greek into Latin).

Patin,—curious remains of the seventeenth century,—which we quote on account of its originality [1]:—

Lettre 370. A Monsieur F. C. M. D. R. [2]

Pour répondre à ce que vous me demandez, je vous dirai que Bolduc, Capucin, a écrit aussi bien que Pineda, Jesuite Espagnol, que Job avoit la vérole. Je croirois volontiers que David et Salomon l'avoient aussi. . . . M. Gaffendy m'a dit que la lèpre, dans la Bible, etoit la vérole. *Luis venereæ causa est scortatio turpis, vaga, promiscua, atque talis scortatio est ab omni ævo.* Ce serpent, dans la Genèse, disoit un libertin, étoit quelque jeune Dameret qui donna la vérole à Eve, et voilé le péché originel de nos Moines, ce nous disoit M. de Malherbe. Au moins est-ce chose certaine que la grosse vérole étoit bien fort connuë dans l'Europe devant que Charles VIII allât à la conquête du Royaume de Naples. . . .

De Paris, le 18 Septembre, 1665.

[1] Guy Patin: Nouveau recueil de lettres choisies. Rotterdam, 1725. New Collection of Selected Letters.

[2] Letter 370. To M. F. C. D. R.:—

In answer to your inquiry, I will state that Balduc, the Capuchin, has written, as well as Pineda, a Spanish Jesuit, that Job had the pox. I would willingly believe that David and Solomon also had it. . . . M. Gaffandy has told me that the leprosy in the Bible was the pox. *The cause of the venereal disease is a shameless libertinage, indulged in any where or with any one, and this prostitution has existed from all antiquity.* The serpent, in Genesis, said a libertine, was some young Lovelace who gave Eve the pox, and this is the original sin of our monks, M. Malherbe used to tell us. At least, it is certain that the big pox was very well known in Europe before Charles VIII went to the conquest of the Kingdom of Naples. . . .

From Paris, September 18, 1665.

CHAPTER IX.

UPADANSA.

SYPHILIS AMONG THE HINDOOS ONE THOUSAND YEARS BEFORE THE CHRISTIAN ERA.

" Un des plus anciens foyers de la syphilis est très probablement l'Inde, c'est-à-dire le pays qui a été le berceau du genre humain."—ROLLET.[1]

[One of the oldest foci of syphilis is most probably India; that is to say, the country which was the cradle of mankind.]

" Il est évident que le vocable *upadansa* désigne, en sanscrit, le *virus syphilitique:* tout le démontre, non seulement la description de la maladie, mais aussi les moyens thérapeutiques employés.[2]—HESSLER. (Latin translation of the *Ayurveda:* Notes on chapter xii of the *Pathology.*)

[It is very evident that the word *upadansa* designates, in Sanskrit, the *syphilitic virus:* everything shows this, not only the description of the disease, but also the therapeutic measures employed.]

THE origin of the documents, which are derived from antiquity on Asia in general, and India in particular, are of two kinds,—secular legends and Sanskrit literature. We will first examine the marvelous, to find, among the allegories, that which is referable to syphilis; then we will seek it in the Vedas,—a collection at once religious, literary, and scientific.[3]

[1] Dict. Encyclop. des sc. médic., article Syphilis.

[2] "Sanskritæ voci *upadansa* vim luis venereæ subjectum esse, non solum ex his allatis morbi causis, sed etiam ex hujus morbi curandi ratione cernitur." The expression *vim luis venereæ* means, literally, *the strength of venereal disease.* In the fifteenth and sixteenth centuries, the Latin expression which replaced that of *morbus gallicus* was *lues venerea.* In their writings, the authors of the sixteenth century who wrote in French call syphilis currently "la lues" [the lues]. For this reason, we believe that we have interpreted Hessler's idea exactly, by translating *vim luis venereæ* by *syphilitic virus.*

[3] This chapter should follow that which treats of prehistoric syphilis, as everyone is agreed in recognizing that India is the cradle of the human race, but we follow the chronological order of the written documents.

The Hebrews had the worship of Baal Peor; the Hindoos that of Lingam, based upon the same principles and including the same mysteries. A part of Chaldea, prostitution reigned like a mistress in all Asia; Babylon, the capital of Chaldea, then was the cradle of prostitution, and, consequently, of syphilis, its forced companion. Dufour, who has written the history of prostitution with much talent and learning, remarks that "this subject, at once delicate and questionable, connects itself on all sides with the history of religions, of laws, and of customs."[1] There are three forms which correspond to the three great periods of history: (1) hospitable prostitution, (2) religious prostitution, (3) legal or political prostitution. These details, which might, at first, appear tedious, are, nevertheless, of the greatest importance; for they will enable the reader to appreciate how venereal diseases could arise at a time when patriarchal customs existed, and to follow, step by step, the development and invading march of these diseases from the East to the West.

Legal prostitution is the traffic in charms deprecated by M. Prudhomme,[2] but authorized by the police and regulated by legal measures; it is the necessary evil, the safety-valve which protects the wife and daughters of even M. Prudhomme against bold attacks.

By the term *hospitable prostitution* must be understood that custom of the primitive peoples of Asia which consisted in putting a guest in the host's place, not only at table, but even in the latter's bed, and resigning to him his wife, according to the laws of hospitality.

[1] Dufour: Histoire de la prostitution chez tous les peuples du monde depuis l'antiquité la plus reculée jusqu' à nos jours. Paris, 1851. History of Prostitution among All Peoples of the World, from the Remotest Antiquity up to the Present Day.

[2] A character somewhat similar to the English Mrs. Grundy.

In this respect, Scotland was outdone; but it must be added that custom required the traveler to give a present to the wife of his host when he departed from the family, which he had sometimes helped to increase. There is no necessity of dwelling any further upon this; it can be easily understood with what facility contagious diseases of the genital organs could be transmitted, especially if the travelers made frequent stops.

By *religious prostitution* we are to understand the secret practices of the worship of the Lingam, of Baal, and later of Venus and of Priapus. At a still more remote period, it was not only the celebration of certain mysteries varying with the temples, but custom, which required young girls to offer their virginity to the divinity; and, as the idol could not descend from its pedestal, it accepted the gift by proxy. Imagine the officiating priest, subject to syphilis, and draw your own conclusions. It can also be seen, by the following passage, that there existed, in the Oriental manners of primitive times, other customs extremely favorable to the propagation of venereal diseases: "Among the ancient peoples of Asia," says Rosenbaum,[1] "the first fruits of everything had to be consecrated to the divinity; as a consequence, the virginity of women belonged to Venus. . . . In antiquity, like to-day among several savage nations, the menstrual blood, like that which flows as the result of defloration through the rupture of the hymen, and the act itself, were considered unclean. . . . The dwellers on the coast, who had more frequent relations with strangers, abandoned the act of defloration to the latter; in the interior, priests discharged this task for the people of quality."

[1] *Loc. cit.*

A remains of this custom may be seen in that well-known custom of feudal times known as the *droit du Seigneur*. According to Sonnerat,[1] the King of Calicut rewards his principal priest with five hundred ducats to "loosen the girdle" of his wives in the name of the divinity. This fact is confirmed by an English writer, Hamilton, in his "New Account of the East Indies." The same Sonnerat relates an Indian belief in regard to the worship of Siva, Brahma, and Vishnu, which is extremely interesting because it demonstrates that the origin of venereal diseases in India is lost in the darkness of ages. This is the legend, in brief:—

Penitents of the worship of Lingam, incensed against Siva for having obtained favors from their wives, made a terrible sacrifice directed against him. We must believe that it was very empyreumatic, for he overturned the whole Heaven of Vishnu, and, says the author, "the god himself could not bear it. It was like a *fire* which attacked the *generative parts* of Siva and separated them from his body." The god avenged himself by giving this disease to the women in such a manner as to "set the whole world on *fire*."[2]

This revenge is logical; but if the genital parts of Siva had fallen off, how did the god give his disease, unless it was by means of a lancet? However, legends

[1] Voyage aux Indes orientales et à la Chine, 1774. Journey to the East Indies and to China.

[2] There is a certain analogy between the maleficence of the Hindoo penitents and the Borbonessa tart of Panurge: this relates to a joke played against the theologians. "He made a Borbonessa tart (or filthy and slovenly compound), made of store of garlick, of asafœtida, of castoreum, of . . . which he steeped, tempered, and liquefied in the corrupt matter of pocky boils and pestiferous botches; and, very early in the morning, therewith anointed all the pavement in such sort that the devil could not have endured it, . . . and ten or twelve of them died of the plague, . . . and above seven and twenty had the *pox*. . . . Rabelais: Pantagenal, lib. ii, cap. xvi. Urquhart's trans., 1854.

are not so precise; the thing to bear in mind is the disease. Fortunately, continues the fable, Brahma and Vishnu stopped the conflagration, by persuading their colleague, Siva, to discontinue his inoculations. Siva permitted himself to be persuaded, on condition that men would render divine honors to his genital organs, which, in all probability, had grown back in their proper place. Rosenbaum is of the opinion that this *fire*, this contagious disease, was syphilis; it seems very probable. In the same way, the worship which limited its ravages must certainly have consisted in hygienic care and a little more continence on the part of the stricken people.

Such is the information furnished us by popular beliefs; it is the naked fact. Let us now examine the literary works, in which we shall find details given with more or less scientific precision.

The ancient books of India which have come to us are called the Vedas.[1] The Vedas, the Bible of the Hindoos, contain: some, secular poetry; others, historical facts, precepts, religious traditions, etc. One only is exclusively devoted to medicine; it is really a treatise upon medicine which Dr. Hessler, of Erlangen, has translated into Latin.[2] This book, the Ayurveda, contains several curious passages which we will examine.

Its title is: AYURVEDA. *Medical Precepts of the venerable D'Hanvantari, collated by his disciple Susruta.* According to Liétard,[3] this D'Hanvantari was the Indian

[1] Cf. Baudry (Fred.): Etude sur les Védas. Paris, 1855. Study of the Vedas. Royle: An Essay on the Antiquity of the Hindoo Medicine. . . . London, 1857.

[2] Ayurvedas, id est medicinæ Systema a venerabili D'Hanvantare demonstratum, a Susruta discipulo compositum. . . . Erlangæ, 1844-1850.

[3] Lettres historiques sur la médecine chez les Hindous. Paris, 1863. Historical Letters on Medicine Among the Hindoos.

god of medicine, an analogous being to the Greek centaur, Chiron. This author traces the origin of the Ayurveda to the beginning of our era. Hessler does not share this opinion; he assigns the appearance of this book to a more remote period, although he acknowledges that it would be difficult to name the exact year. At all events, he gives good reasons to support his opinion. It is mentioned in the Ayurveda, in several places, that Susruta is the son of King Visvamitra, whom the Rigveda mentions; and it is proven by old Hindoo traditions that Visvamitra lived at a very remote period of the heroic age of India. The heroic age of India comprises a very long period, "and," says Hessler, "the beginning of this period is lost in the immensity of time; but we know that it ended about one thousand years B.C."[1] Hessler is forced to conclude that the Ayurveda dates back at least three thousand years, for, adds he, "the name Susruta was celebrated among the Hindoos many centuries before our era. This much can be proven."[2] In conclusion, let us say that the Ayurveda forms part of the *At'harvaveda*, whose antiquity is undoubted. But as a few years more or less before Christ make but little difference in a question of antiquity, let us dismiss this matter of the origin, and let us analyze those portions of the Ayurveda which treat of diseases of the genital organs. To render an understanding of the text more easy, we will, as in the verses of the Bible, place the Latin and the translation in parallel columns, adding comments whenever they may be deemed necessary.

Under the heading, *Sutrast'hana* (matters in general),

[1] "Incipit enim illud ævum inde ab infinito temporis spatio et usque ad annum circiter millesimum ante Christum natum procedit."

[2] "Susruta nomen apud Hindos floruisse multis jam sæculis ante nostram æram; quæ conclusio certe potest probari."

we find in Chapter XXI, which treats of ulcers, the following sentences :—

Sic irritati humores morbos generant. Abdomen aggressi, urinæ difficultates, . . . gonorrhæam; penem aggressi, perversam expansionem, morbos venereos, seminis virilis vitia et ceteros morbos. . . .	Thus the irritated humors produce diseases. Attacking the abdomen (they produce) difficulty in urinating, . . . gonorrhœa; attacking the *penis*, they produce functional troubles of that organ, *venereal diseases*, alteration of the semen, and other diseases. . . .

The text is precise: it distinguishes gonorrhœa and urinary troubles from venereal diseases, and the title indicates that all terminate by ulcerating.

. . . anum aggressi, fistulas; hæmorrhoïdes et ceteros morbos; testiculos aggressi, intumescentias. . . .	. . . if it is at the anus, fistulas, hæmorrhoids, and *other affections;* if it is the *testicles*, it will be *tumors*. . . .

This passage is too indefinite, and nothing conclusive can be derived from it; but it occurs in connection with the following one :—

. . . telam cellulosam aggressi, tubercula tumores, insensibiles intumescentias, colli glandarum tumores, ophthalmias et ceteros. . . .	. . . if it is the cellular tissue, there are produced tubercles, *tumors*, *painless swellings*, *cervical ganglia*, *ophthalmias*, etc. . . .

Here are humors that are inclined to travel, and one would not have to be tempted much to find in this paragraph a collection of lesions which could be summarized as follows: Gonorrhœa, cystitis; fistulas, tumors at the anus, orchitis (gonorrhœal, tubercular, or syphilitic epididymitis), gummata of the skin; indolent ganglia, at the neck and elsewhere, conjunctivitis, iritis, etc. The paragraph terminates by a summary description of manifestations involving the skin, the *muscles*, the *bones*, and the *feet*, which does not tend to exclude the idea of syphilis.

We will now pass on to the most important part, entitled, *Nidanast'hana*,—that is to say, *Pathology*,—in which diseases are described separately. Let us first examine Chapter II, which treats of the *pathology of hæmorrhoids.* As may be seen, the word which Hessler translates *hæmorrhoids* means, rather, excrescences, dry or moist tumors; for the Hindoo author finds them in all portions of the body. He begins by explaining that they are caused either by bad nutrition (*perversis alimentis*) or by contact with women in the sexual act (*cum mulieribus coïtione*), etc.; and that which proves, better than all the reasoning in the world, that it was not ordinary hæmorrhoids, so well known to the constipated, is the fact that Susruta describes them as occurring upon the penis, the scrotum, and vulva, after the following manner:—

Humorum vitia penem aggressa, carnem et sanguinem vitianda, pruritum generant; illic ob pruritum ulcus oritur; in hoc ulcere carunculæ, a vitiata carne ortæ, purulento sanguine fluentes, oriuntur ad pubem, in medio aut superne. . . .

When the corrupt humors attack the *penis*, they *vitiate* the flesh and the blood, and produce itching; from this itching there springs an *ulcer;* in this ulcer come *excrescences* due to the poisoned flesh, and flowing a *sanious pus*. These products are found at the *pubis*, either above or below the middle. . . .

It is impossible to recognize either simple or phagedenic chancres from this description; the latter, as we know, destroying more or less, with or without burrowing under the skin, but never accompanied by *excrescences* with sanious suppuration; what characterizes them, however, is loss of substance. But let us continue:—

. . . testes et vulvam aggressa, mollia, male olentia purulento sanguine fluentia et fungosa excrescentia generant. Hæc sursum profecta, in auribus, oculis, naso, et ore hæmorrhoïdes producunt; . . . in ore, gutture, labiis aut palatio. . . .

. . . if the *testicles* and *vulva* be attacked, there are produced fungous *excrescences*, soft, *smelling badly*, and running purulent blood. If these be in the *upper portions*, they produce hæmorrhoids in the *ears*, *eyes*, *nose*, and mouth; . . . in the mouth, the *throat*, on the *lips* and palate. . . .

Does this not read like a condensation of the symptoms of the secondary period? What are these *corrupt humors*, if not a virus which takes its point of departure from the penis, where it first manifests itself as a *local itching*? There is scratching, then an ulcer (infecting chancre); then, at the same place, more or less elevated mucous patches. From that time, papulo-hypertrophic syphilides appear upon the pubic region or upon the integument of the scrotum. If it be in a woman, these same syphilides occur preferably at the vulva, where they are juxtaposed and symmetrical; a fetid ichor escapes, the same occurring in the scrotal syphilides of men, where there is also juxtaposition. Let us call attention to the fact that the author, who had observed that the syphilides at the pubis were almost dry, does not state that they have a bad odor. So much for the genital region. We shall now see the disease, which has become constitutional, occurring in the cephalic region. We find external otitis, mucous patches of the nostrils, of the lips, of the mouth, and of the palate; syphilitic angina; and, later, tertiary lesions, probably included in the lesions of the nose and palate by the author, for he refers at two different times to the affections of the mouth. M. Proust, who has written an interesting article on syphilis in the

"Traité de pathologie externe"[1] of Follin, would, perhaps, have done better to analyze this chapter of the *Nidanast'hana*, rather than confine himself to a passage from the *Chikitsitast'hana* (therapeutics) in regard to the suppurating bubo, which furnished him with no argument in support of the view he was endeavoring to defend.

We believe it useless to demonstrate to the reader, who has read what precedes, that the word *hæmorrhoïdes* is to be translated by the phrase: *enlargements of the form of hæmorrhoids.* At all events, we will state that this was the opinion of the translator of the Ayurveda, for we find the following note respecting the extracts from the second chapter, which we have just given. "There is no doubt that the symptoms described in these two passages are much rather to be looked upon as connected with *venereal* diseases and *syphilitic* ulcers than with hæmorrhoids."[2]

We will observe similarly in regard to Chapter V, which treats of *leprosy*, according to the title. As we have already remarked in regard to the Hebrews, this word was an indefinite term, very convenient to designate a group of morbid manifestations observed by the ancients, but which they did not know to what they could attach them. The key-stone of this pathological arch was missing; and this key-stone was the virus which they but dimly perceived. However, the reader may judge, from the text, if the symptoms described are to be solely ascribed to a disease of the skin and to external diseases:—

[1] Paris, 1874. Treatise on Surgical Pathology.

[2] "Duobus, in his locis haud est dubium, quin morbosa symptomata describantur, quæ magis ad morbos venereos et ulcera syphilitica, quam ad hæmorrhoides pertinere videantur."

Nasi devastatio, oculorum pigmentum, in ulcere vermium ortus fieri potest et vocis suppressio in lepris ossa et medullam aggressis.

The *destruction* of the *nose*, the spots of the eyes, the worms which arise here in *ulcers*, the *loss of voice*, are found in leprosy which has attacked the *bones* and the marrow.

Quæ feminarum et marium, lepræ vitio in sanguine et semine virili vitiatorum, progenies ab ipsis orta est, ea etiam cognoscenda est leprosa.

When men and women are contaminated, and the virus of leprosy has affected the *blood* and changed the *virile seed*, their *progeny* is also *affected* by this disease.

According to many authors, true leprosy is not hereditary; according to others, it is hereditary, but not contagious. Without entering into an interminable discussion, we will limit ourselves to showing, in the following passage, that the heredity of the disease is distinctly shown:—

A Brahmæ uxoris vigiliarum cæde, securi capturis, et cet., facinoribus dicunt lepræ, peccato et morbo præditæ, originem.

It is said that leprosy, a *disease* and *sign* of sin, owes its origin to the horrible nocturnal mysteries of the wife of Brahma, to the shameless commerce and other acts deserving the axe.

The point to remember in this legend is that the disease originates in the bosom of debauchery; but what Latin! The sentence is almost a puzzle.

Copulatione, corporis contactu, . . . communi cubitu, . . . dæmoniaci morbi ab homine ad hominem transgrediuntur.

Copulation, contact of the body, . . . *the same bed,* . . . such are the causes which have caused these diabolical evils to pass from one man to another.

This abundantly proves that the disease was contagious. The Sanskrit word which Hessler has translated "lepræ" is *Kakanacæ*.

In Chapter XII the author states that he will consider, among other things, swellings of the testicle and then venereal diseases. Then begins a sentence which is very obscure, and of which we will only give a few selections, with their literal translation[1]:—

Deinceps, post nimium coitum aut nimiam castimoniam (*brahmacharya*), porro post viri, feminem castam (*bramahcharini*), diu desertam, menstruantem, . . . vulva impuris aquis elotâ aut illotâ præditam, vulvæ morbis affectam, sponte corruptâ vulvâ præditam aut orbatam ultra modum venerantis, . . . in coitûs fine . . . penem aggressa irritata humorum vitia, in vulnerato aut non vulnerato homine, tumorem procreant, quem morbum venereum appellant.

Then, after excessive intercourse, or a too great continence, long after, one may have to do with a chaste woman, who has not had sexual relations for a long time, and who has her courses, . . . whose vulva may or may not be bathed in *unhealthy secretions*, or become the seat of disease; if this man use excess with the woman, whether her vulva has or has not suddenly become a *focus of corruption*, . . . the unhealthy humors engendered at the end of coitus . . . may attack the penis, and, whether the man be excoriated or not, they bring forth a *pimple* which is called the *venereal disease.*

And we have omitted the useless details of this diffuse sentence! The ancient Hindoos had then noticed that the venereal swellings, which they called *upadansa*, in a general way, were found in persons addicted to sexual excesses, and that they could be contracted from women having no apparent disease. This is what we see nowadays: the lesions are not always plain; a woman may serve as a transmitting agent,—that is to say, contain the virus of a syphilitic; have time to transmit it to one or several others before her ablutions, and not be contaminated herself. The author then explains that venereal symptoms owe their variety to the different kinds of humors; and, accord-

[1] See, for comparison, in Chapter V, the beginning of the work of Hoang-ty.

ing to his theory, when all the humors act at the same time, there are seen sores of the penis (*dilaceratis penis*), in which worms breed, and which may bring on death. This description seems to be particularly applicable to the phagedenic chancre.

In the succeeding chapter (XIII) the author states that he will consider the diseases which he calls *roga:* literally, *small.* Hessler warns us that he has translated this wôrd by *shameful*, having been given the seat and nature of the lesions described. The translator was right; for, as will be seen, it is venereal diseases which are concerned,—syphilitic, for the most part,—and which the author regarded as of small importance, with the exception of phagedenic chancres, often mortal, which he described in the preceding chapter:—

Breviter quatuor et quadraginta turpes morbi sunt: . . . ulcus rotundum (*vivrita*), testitudinata pustula (*kachch'hapika*), . . . lapidi simile tuber (*paschanagardab'ha*), . . . deformis unguis, pustula in capite, bubo (*vidarika*), . . . pedum dilaceratio, alopecia, juvenum papula, . . . ani præclusio. . . .

The shameful diseases number forty-four: . . . the round ulcer, the prominent *pustule*, . . . the stone-like excrescence, . . . the alterations of the *nails*, the *pustules* of the head, the bubo, . . . the ulcerations of the feet, the *alopecia*, the *papules of youths*, . . . the stricture of the anus. . . .

We now see the palmar and plantar syphilides, exostoses, and ulcerated gummata:—

In planta et palma, in articulatione, in cervice supra claviculas, nodus formicete similis tarde colligitur, ulceribus prodolore, madore et æstu prurientibus obtectus.

On the *soles of the feet* and *palms of the hands*, at the joints, on the neck above the *clavicles*, there appear late *lumps*, like elephantiasis, covered with *ulcers*, which itch painfully, by reason of the inflammation and suppuration.

Circa aures undique et in dorso congestus et terribilis morbus existit, Nymphææ bulbæ instar.

About the ears and in the back a red and *terrible* disease is present, like to the bulbs of nenuphar.

This disease excited horror, like in the fifteenth century of our era.

Læsione corruptus qui unguis asper, niger et calidus fit, hunc deformem unguem sciat medicus nobilem esse cognominatum.

The diseased nail, which becomes rough, black, and hot,—this deformed nail,—let the physician know that it is called the *noble nail.*[1]

Is there here a concealed irony, and is it syphilitic onychia? This is to be presumed, being given the nature of the disease described in this chapter. After having noticed the axillary and inguinal buboes symptomatic of "corrupt humors," the author speaks of a lesion in which one is tempted to see interdigital syphilitic plaques :—

Madidis digitorum intervallis affectos pedes pruritu, æstu et dolore vexatos ex corruptæ carnis contractu, tanquam intumescentiam elephantiacam medicus demonstret.

When the *interdigital spaces of the feet* are the seat of itching, with exudation of inflammation with burning, and the tissues present induration, the physician will say that these lesions are like the tumefactions of elephantiasis.

Hæc alopecia, calvitium, morbo etiam efficitur.

. . . A phlegmate, ære et sanguine oriuntur papulæ juvenum in vultu quæ os contaminant.

The disease brings on even *alopecia*, baldness.

. . . The pituitary, the air, the blood, cause the *papules of youth* to appear, which show themselves upon the face, and by attacking the *mouth.*

Let us remark that Susruta describes all these phenomena as appertaining to one general disease. He ends this chapter with a description of phimosis.

[1] For further details, see the end of this chapter.

Alopecia occurring at the same time as interdigital plaques of the feet, papules of the face, and patches in the mouth force the modern diagnosis, *secondary symptoms;* and, as the author calls attention, upon several occasions, to the analogy which exists between these symptoms and elephantiasis, we will not be told that it was the latter disease. On this account, the translator cannot forbear from exclaiming[1]: "How ancient venereal disease is, and how this antiquity reduces to nothing every opinion of an origin of more recent date; this is plain even to a blind man!"[2]

There is another Hindoo work which treats of medical matters, but incidentally only. Dr. Michéa,[3] in an interesting article on "The State of Medicine Among the Ancient Hindoos," gives us a few extracts from this book, the "Sacteya Grantham," attributed to Dhanvantari himself, in which the Indian Æsculapius describes nine varieties of variola, of which three are pronounced incurable. Although the passages we are going to give have nothing to do with syphilis, we desire to quote them; for a number of persons, even among physicians, are ignorant of the fact that vaccine, among other things, was known in India a few thousand years before Christ. The Sanskrit text plainly states:—

Take the liquid of the pustules of the cow's teat, or from the arm of a human being, between the shoulder and elbow; place it upon the point of a lancet, and introduce it in the arm at the same place, mixing the fluid with the blood; the fever of variola (*Bhadvidæ*) will be produced.

This disease will be mild, like the animal from which it is derived; it need not cause fear, and requires no remedies; the patient may be given the food he desires.

[1] Notes on Chapter XII (Nidanast'hana).

[2] "Quam vetus igitur sit venereus morbus, et quam valde hæc vetustas recentiorum hujus morbi historiam destruat; id apparet etiam cæco!"

[3] Union Médicale, 1847.

You may limit yourself to one cut, or you may make as many as six. The pustule is perfect when it is of a good color, filled with a clear liquid, and surrounded by a red circle. There is a slight fever for one, two, or three days; sometimes a slight chill, a swelling in the armpit, and other symptoms, but all of a benign character, and without danger.

This discovery takes nothing from the merit of Jenner, for Europe was ignorant, for a long time, of the discoveries of Asia. Just as the monk Schwartz, who invented gun powder in the Middle Ages, has not fallen in our esteem, because he was anticipated by the Chinese. As a matter of fact, where would the artillery of the Europeans be if they had had to wait until they had diplomatic relations with Pekin to understand the use of explosives?

The sacred book of Dhanvantari also teaches us that the Hindoos were acquainted with mercurials (cinnabar, in fumigations; protochloride and bichloride of mercury, with sugar and pepper, etc., in pills); the smoke of *datura stramonium*, in asthma; nux vomica, in paralysis; the bark of the root of pomegranate, for tape-worm, etc.

In fine, if we are to believe Klein, who has devoted a work to "The Therapeutic Methods in the Oriental Indies Against the Venereal Disease,"[1] the Malabar traditions speak of the physicians Sangarasiar and Alessianambi mentioning syphilis. These physicians, who lived about 1000 A.D., treated with mercury.

The cause is understood.

[In an article[2] published subsequently to the appearance of this book, the author discusses the peculiar appearance of the nail, known as the *noble nail* in the

[1] F. G. Klein: De morbi venerei curatione in India orientali visitata, 1795.

[2] Jour. des Maladies Cut. et Syph., Sept. 31, 1890.

Vedas. It presented a *rough*, *deformed*, *black* appearance, but this scarcely justified the conclusion that it was necessarily of syphilitic origin. Dr. Buret, however, had the good fortune of observing a symptom in an old syphilitic which possesses some value; at least, in connection with the matter under consideration. The patient, a syphilitic, who was pronounced cured in the eighth year of the disease, observed somewhat later that the nail of one of his great toes had a black spot in the centre. Regarding this as probably due to some injury, he paid no further attention to it. Other toes successively exhibited this symptom, which was due to a subungual ecchymosis, caused by the syphilitic process, Dr. Buret thinks. The nails were rough and the picture presented was very similar to that of the *noble nail* of the Hindoo Vedas. While this is rather weak in the way of proof, it is an interesting condition, nevertheless, and a very rare one.]

CHAPTER X.

ΣΥΚΟΝ.

Syphilis Among the Greeks Before and After Christ.

"Many arguments might be adduced to show that it was well known in the old continent, and that it prevailed among the Jews, Greeks, and Romans, and their descendants, long before the discovery of America."—Benjamin Bell.[1]

Like India, ancient Greece had its legend in regard to the origin of venereal diseases. But here it is no longer Siva, but Priapus, who is the hero.

According to the fable, Priapus was the son of Venus and Bacchus. Aphrodite, as the Greeks called her, had not been able to resist the glory of Bacchus, returning in triumph from India. This weakness of Venus for glory resulted in Priapus, whom Juno, in a fit of anger, caused to be born with an enormous penis. Some say that Priapus was born at Lampsacus; others, that he was merely reared there. But, no matter. At all events, this god remained there long enough to be the cock of the place, and even an indefatigable cock, much to the displeasure of the husbands, who drove him out. Priapus visited upon them a vengeance similar to that of Siva upon the Hindoos; and, says Natalis Comes, "a *terrible disease* engrafted itself upon the genital organs of the people of Lampsacus":—

. . . Lampsacenos gravissimus pudendorum membrorum morbus invasuisset.[2] . . .

[1] A Treatise on Gonorrhœa Virulenta and Lues Venerea. Edinburgh, 1793.

[2] Natalis Comitis Mythologiæ, sive explicationis fabularum, libri x. Frocofurti, 1588. Mythology in Ten Books; or, Explanation of Fables. Frankfort, 1588.

These unfortunates recalled Priapus to cure them, and instituted festivals in his honor. These consisted in debauchery of all kinds. We shall see, later on, that the worship of Priapus afterward went to Rome.

The same Natalis Comes gives another history relating to the Athenians. These, it appears, not having received the images of Bacchus with great pomp, as was the custom, and whose worship Pegasus desired to introduce into Attica, "the angry god hurled a *terrible disease* upon the genital parts of men":—

. . . deus indignatus pudenda hominum morbo infestavit, qui erat illis gravissimus. . . .

They could only become cured by receiving the god with the honors due him.[1]

The important fact to remember, in all these legends, is that among the Greeks, like among the Hindoos, the Jews, the Chinese, etc., the origin of venereal diseases goes back to a time which (two or three thousand years before Christ) they could not exactly determine. Nevertheless, it is seen that, among all peoples of antiquity, these strange and often terrible diseases, for them, always owed their primal cause to the orgies and debaucheries, disguised under the name of feasts, in the honor of Venus Aphrodite, Bacchus, Baal Peor, Siva, Phallus, Priapus, etc. The ancients, then, had contagious diseases which were difficult to cure; and, in their simplicity, they addressed themselves to the gods of their country and of their time. This is why certain temples were places of debauchery at night and true *dispensaries* in the morning.

Such is the vague information furnished us by the

[1] Aristophanes, a comic poet who lived about 400 B.C., says, in one of his comedies, that "Bacchus cures the Athenians of a very serious disease of the sacred parts."

Greek fable. We will now study the scientific and literary documents, which are more precise and supplement the others. Among these writings, the works of Hippocrates and Galen stand forth prominently; and they constituted the text-books of Europe for six hundred years. The proofs derived from the ancient books which we have given up to the present will only be half-contested, we know. As a matter of fact, among the opponents of the idea we are defending, even the most violent, the majority admit, without much opposition, the antiquity of syphilis in Africa and in Asia. This is a concession made to evidence, for which we should be thankful. Astruc himself, when pushed to his last trenches, admitted that this might not be impossible. But as soon as a European nation was concerned, then the discussion recommenced, and we run up against the inflexibles. Is it admissible that, being given the wars which the Greeks waged against the Persians, the expeditions of Alexander as far as into India, the Punic wars, etc.,—is it possible, I will even say, that syphilis was arrested until the fifteenth century by the Bosphorus of Thrace and the Straits of Gibraltar? Of course not. Well, up to the present, the opposition has not yet surrendered. The reader will understand why we choose the Greek and Latin authors, and, perhaps, will pardon us for lifting a corner of the veil which conceals Roman depravity, to seek in this reeking dung-heap the pearl which can triumph over opposition; that is to say, scientific truth!

The works of Hippocrates, written either by himself or by his pupils, were composed about the middle of the fifth century B.C., for the Father of Medicine practiced at Cos in the year 460 B.C. There cannot be found in this scientific monument any description of syphilis in the strict acceptation of the term, but there exists, for him who will see them, a host of allusions, which Littré considers as all-sufficient. Follin gives us,[1] through M. Proust's pen, the cause of this apparent silence of Hippocrates respecting syphilis: "Those physicians," says he, "who practiced this art in Greece, in Rome, or in Alexandria, were more than us so situated as to misunderstand the relations of local lesions with the general manifestations of syphilis. In fact, they lived in a climate and had domestic habits which were very favorable to the spontaneous cure of syphilis. We know, as a matter of fact, that pox cures much better in elevated temperatures than in low temperatures. . . . The frequent use of baths among the Orientals and the Romans added to this happy influence of temperature.

"To sum up, if the ancient physicians have not perceived, like we have, the symptoms of constitutional syphilis, it is because these symptoms, considerably attenuated by the influence of climate, did not forcibly call their attention to the origin of the disease. Besides, it is, perhaps, too much forgotten that syphilis, in our climate, is often cured by hygiene and diet."

Some authors admit that the descriptions given by the physicians of antiquity describe, in a strict sense, the primary local lesions of syphilis; but, in their opinion, the secondary lesions, even local, never existed. The cutaneous manifestations are to be attributed to all one may wish, leprosy, for example, and not to constitutional syphilis. Such is the basis of their reasoning. And they are proud to be able to say: "You see, Hippocrates does not mention it! If syphilis had been known to the ancients, it would not have escaped an

[1] Traité élément de path. Ext., t. i, art. iii. Paris, 1874. Elementary Treatise on Surgical Pathology.

observer like he." Without troubling ourselves with these self-constituted contradictions, let us examine ourselves the passages of Hippocrates, in which affections of the genital organs are noticed; it matters but little to us that the author does not mention their cause and origin, if the descriptions agree with what we know are the modern manifestations of syphilis.

These descriptions are somewhat scattered everywhere, but they acquire value by their entirety, without any necessity, as we have already said, of *torturing* the Greek text.[1]

In the chapter of *Aphorisms* (Lecture III, section 21), we find the following passage:—

> In summer occur . . . *ophthalmias*, pains in the ears, *ulcerations of the mouth* (στοματών ἑλκώσιες), and *rotting of the genitals* (σηπεδόνες αἰδοίων).

It is plain that the ulcerations of the mouth, taken alone, are not sufficient to suggest the idea of syphilis; but their coincidence with ophthalmias and sores on the genitals leads us to seriously think. We will observe the same thing in reference to section 14 of the chapter on *Humors*:—

> Under the influence of Southern winds, there come *moist ulcers* (ἕλκεα μαδαρὰ), especially in the *mouth* and upon the *genitals* (κάλιστα στόμα, αἰδοῖον).

[1] Prosper Yvaren, in the notes of his translation into French verse of the poem of Fracastor, says that "it is only by forcing the sense of words, by straining the parts of a phrase on the Procrustean bed of interpretation, by torturing texts, by isolating them from the medium in which they are placed, that one is enabled to create a sort of imaginary and fantastic disease, presenting some analogy to syphilis." All this is very nice as a metaphor, but, in plain language, this is called floundering. If the texts which we have so far quoted appear obscure, the bone-lesions which we have shown in prehistoric man are not, and we will soon see if the descriptions of Celsus and the humor of the Latin satirists deal with a fictitious disease.

In the treatise "On the Nature of Woman," we find a few sentences too vague to be considered as confirmatory. Section 60 commences thus :—

If the genital parts are aphthous . . .

Under the name *aphthæ* the ancients designated ulcers of small extent and superficial, or pustules ; it is plain that this expression was not to be exclusively referred to ulcerating syphilides. Hippocrates recurs to this several times. Further on we read :—

Section 65. If a bad smell (δυσοδμίη) attaches itself to the genitals, if a growth (κίων) forms, and there be pain . . .

Does this mean the fetid odor of vulvar mucous patches, which might be designated by the word κίων, signifying *elevation*, *ridge?* It is possible, but not certain. In the same manner we ignore the nature of those ulcers of the vulva which impel women to scratch themselves :—

Section 66. If ulcers (ἕλκεα) form in the genital parts, and there be itching . . .

Nevertheless, those diseases which do not heal rapidly had to be taken into consideration, for the author speaks of them upon several occasions, and counsels a certain number of topical remedies and liniments for local treatment. Let us say, *passim*, that the Greeks, by the word ἄνθραξ, which we shall soon meet, did not understand modern *anthrax*, that is to say, the aggregation of furuncles which we know : by that expression the writers of the first centuries designated chancre in general, and destructive chancre in particular. In another sense this word also signified *charbon:* let us state that the authors of the Middle Ages currently employed the word *carbunculus* (small *charbon* [coal]) to denominate the chancrous ulcerations of the genitals.

Astruc held that an entire passage from Hippocrates had never been given. "A few rags of sparse phrases," says he, "are pulled out and placed end to end."

We will reproduce *in extenso* the oft-quoted paragraph of the third book of "Epidemics," the fourth constitution: the reader can then judge for himself whether the assertion of Astruc is well-founded. In this whole third book Hippocrates speaks of things having no relation with the passage under consideration: the author seems to make a digression to note a disease which has impressed him, among other things, and whose symptoms he describes in the same and only paragraph:—

> Many had aphthæ and *ulcerations of the mouth* (στόματα ἑλκώδεα). Frequent *fluxions* to the *genital parts*, ulcerations (ἑλκώματα), tumors (φύματα) within and without; swelling in the groins. Moist *ophthalmias*, which were long and painful; *fleshy growths* on the eyelids, within and without, which destroyed the sight of many persons, and which are called *figs* (σῦκα). The other *sores of the genital parts* were also the seat of *fungosities*. In summer were seen a large number of *anthrax* and of other diseases which are called poisonous, extensive *pustular eruptions* (ἐκθύματα); in many, large vesicular eruptions (ἕρπητες).

Evidently this disease became epidemic, as it did in 1494. For Astruc it is the *plague*, an appellation as convenient as that of *leprosy* or *scabies*, which were so much abused in the Middle Ages. We will soon see that the Athenian plague described by Thucidides and Lucretius was, like the Egyptian plague, an epidemic of of venereal character, in which syphilis was far from playing no part.

But why did not Hippocrates give it a name? Always the same objection advanced for the past four centuries! How often will it have to be repeated that the physician of Cos described symptoms, which was doing well for his time? Will the numerous diseases which existed in antiquity, and of which he was not the sponsor, be denied? Because he described intermittent fever without speaking of malaria, will it be contended that the appearance of malaria dates from the nineteenth century? And lead poisoning, in which he only saw colic? Do you believe that they did not *work in lead* among the ancient Greeks? In giving the symptoms of typhoid fever,[1] did he suspect an inflammatory process of Peyer's patches, with ulceration? And certainly it could not be contended that dothienteritis had only existed since the Cliniques of Trousseau!

Let us now examine Galen, who was born at Pergamos A.D. 131, and wrote his works toward the end of the second century. Like Hippocrates, he was surrounded by a large number of pupils, several of whom became his collaborators. So that the Galenical work is, like a large treatise on pathology of our times, a sort of medical encyclopædia, in which each one contributes a share, under the more or less active direction of the master spirit.

[1] We know that Littré has stated that many cases considered before him as relating to typhoid fever were nothing but pseudo-continued fevers of a remittent type. Agreed: but there is more than one which must be referred to abdominal typhus. And, although it is somewhat extraneous to our subject, we cannot resist the temptation of giving the following case from Hippocrates, which is a part of his book on Epidemics. It may be easily seen that we have to deal with a *continued fever*, although the author did not give it a name, which lasted three weeks, with a return of the fever apparently after the first food (*febris carnis*). The title is: SEVENTH PATIENT.—"At Abdera, the young girl who lived in the Via Sacra was taken with a hot fever. She had thirst and sleeplessness. Her courses appeared upon this occasion for the first time. Sixth day: Much nausea, redness, chills, restlessness. Eighth day: Deafness, high fever, sleeplessness, nausea, chills; consciousness present, urination infrequent. Ninth and following days: Same state, the deafness persists. Fourteenth day: Abundant epistaxis, deafness diminished a little. The following days: Nausea, deafness, delirium. Twentieth day: Pains in the feet; deafness and delirium cease; slight epistaxis, sweat, apyrexia. Twenty-fourth day: Return of the fever, of the deafness; the pain in the feet persists; consciousness disturbed. Twenty-seventh day: Abundant sweat, no fever; deafness has disappeared; the pain in the feet persists, but the disease is perfectly understood."

In a chapter entitled "Medical Definitions,"[1] the author explains the different Greek terms which he is to employ frequently in the course of his work. We will give a few extracts from one of the numerous Latin translations which have been made. As in Hippocrates, they are rather indefinite terms, but some of which undoubtedly referred to local phenomena of syphilis:—

Carbunculus est magis melancholico putrefacto sanguine tumor ulcerosus.	*Carbunculus* is an ulcer with swelling derived from blood putrefied by excessive melancholy.

This definition is perfectly applicable to the chancre, which is often accompanied by œdema. Literally, *small carbuncles;* that is to say, an ulcer similar to that of the carbunculous, but smaller. It cannot be ulcerated cancer, for this latter is very large, more so than the ulcer of carbuncle, and smells horribly bad, which Galen would not have failed to notice. Further on, the author gives the name θύμος to growths which, on account of their location, may be regarded as papulo-hypertrophic syphilides:—

Thymus asperæ carnis extuberatio est, quæ similis circa genitale ac sedem oritur.	The *thymus* is a rough-looking elevation, which all alike show themselves upon the *genitals* and about the *anus*.

Let us at once put aside the notion of hæmorrhoids, as the growths are found in other places besides the anus; there remain vegetations. The following sentence reduces this supposition to nothing, for vegetations are designated by a special word, ἀκροχορδών.

Acrochordon exortus est orbicularis angustamque obtinens basim.	*Acrochordon* projects, is rounded and presents a *narrow base.*

All translators are agreed in recognizing, in this

[1] Finit. med., 18.

expression, a variety of wart. The author next speaks of hæmorrhoids, of which some are simple and others of a *malignant nature* (*malignæ*). Outside of anal syphilides, we cannot see to what known affection these *malignant* hæmorrhoidal tumors could be referred. We must not forget that Hessler translated by *hæmorrhoid* a Hindoo word having the same meaning.

Further on, in a sort of *introduction*,[1] he states that "*thymus*, *callosities*, *boils*, *vegetations*, etc., may be found on the skin, and, in a general way, on all portions of the body."

Cutem totiusque corporis partes exagitant acrochordones, thymi, clavi, calli, etc.

He advises removing them with the red-hot iron or powdering them with a metallic compound (ψωρικόν) employed at that time for the itch. The physicians of Rome cut them and smiled, according to Juvenal, which proves, in the first place, that they were not of a serious nature, and also their lively origin. In another chapter, which deals of the *composition of remedies according to their locality*,[2] he gives advice "for *tubercles* which occur upon the genital organs (*ad tubercula in pudendis nascentia*)." Let us immediately call attention to the fact that the mucous patch was for a long time designated, among other names, by those of *mucous tubercle*, *flat tubercle*, etc. The author next states that resin is very good for the fissures and rhagades of the same organs (*fissuras ac rimas pudendorum juvat resina*), advocates sovereign remedies for condylomata, and describes a *psoriasis scroti*, meaning, by that, an induration of the integument of the scrotum, occasionally accompanied by

[1] Medicus seu Introduct., cap. xxviii.

[2] De Composit. medicament. secund. loc.; i, 3; ix, 8.

true ulcers. We call attention to these passages, without further comment, in order to avoid repetition.

Finally,—what is not unimportant, as it deals with an expression which has passed into several modern languages,—Archigenes, who edited that portion of the work of Galen entitled "Of Local Diseases,"[1] speaks of the peculiar pains of the periosteum, which, says he, are so deep and so constant that the patient "believes that the *bones themselves* are the seat of the pain":—

. . . ossium ipsorum veluti dolentium inducunt imaginem.

The author adds that these pains are known as *osteocopic* (ὀστεοκόποι). We will not lose our time in showing that these osteocopic pains, peculiar to syphilis to-day, were not simply rheumatic at the time when Galen lived.

Such is the information furnished us by the two most celebrated Greek physicians. There are others whose works, either complete or fragmentary, have come to us, and have a certain weight, although those authors do not enjoy the fame of Hippocrates and Galen. Among these physicians it is proper to mention Dioscorides and Aretæus, anterior to Galen; and Oribasius, Aetius, Alexander of Tralles, Paulus Ægineta, etc. These last, with the exception of Oribasius, having lived in the sixth and seventh centuries, will be analyzed in our study on the Middle Ages. Another Greek physician, Celsus, in whose work there is much valuable information, will be the first author examined in the next chapter, with the Roman writers. As a matter of fact, Celsus, who lived in the age of Augustus, was established at Rome, and his works are written in Latin.

In almost all the works of the physicians we have

[1] De locis. affect., ii, cap. viii.

just cited, entire chapters of Hippocrates and of Galen are found reproduced; and, in a general way, the sentences, or parts of them, relating to venereal diseases, are about the same in all. The expressions, chancres (ἄνθρακες, *carbunculi*), rhagades, erosions (*rimæ*), excrescences, recur at every moment; but, in order not to weary the reader, we will only give those quotations which prove the most.

Pedanius Dioscorides lived about A.D. 60. There may be noticed, in his treatise, passages imitated from Hippocrates; but, on the other hand, there are found more allusions to venereal diseases than in the work of the physician of Cos. One may see that these diseases were already better observed; and they are described with greater detail. In the first book of the "Materia Medica," in Chapter XXXIV of the Greek-Latin translation,[1] we find Dioscorides advising baths for *condylomata* and *erosions of the anus*:—

Balnei . . . rimis sedis et condylomatis perunctione prosunt.

In Chapter XLIII, he states that oil of myrtle is good against *papules* (ἐξάνθηματα), *fissures*, and *condylomata*:—

Myrteum oleum . . . facit ad . . . papulas, rhagadas, condylomata. . . .

Here papules are grouped with fissures and excrescences, and are given the same treatment. The author had probably seen these different manifestations occurring at the same time, without suspecting their cause. But let us continue:—

[1] De Materia Medica, lib. i.

Chap. lxxxi. Thus cum lactetritum et linamento exceptum sedis ac reliquarum partium maligna mitigat. . . .

Chap. lcliv. Pix liquida . . . ceræ admixta vulvæ tubercula anique duritias discutit, . . . carbunculos et putrida ulcera marginibus circumdat.

Chap. cxxxiv. Utiliter partes eâ (amurcâ) eluuntur in sedis, genitalium matricisque ulceribus.

Incense triturated with milk and made into a liniment softens *malignant ulcers of the anus* and of other parts. . . .

Liquid pitch mixed with wax resolves *tubercles of the vulva* and the *hard tumors* of the anus, cicatrizes *chancres* and unites the edges of putrid ulcers.

It (the marc[1] of oil) has a useful action on the diseased parts in the case of *ulcers of the anus*, of the *genital organs*, and of the womb.

All the preceding could very well be referred to chancres and papulo-hypertrophic and ulcerative syphilides; we cannot easily see what other explanation could be given without resorting to the imagination. We will now see the entire series of secondary and tertiary lesions unfold itself:—

Chap. cli. Quod e nucleis (mali punici) exprimitur, coctum mellique admixtum, ad ulcera facit et oris et genitalium et sedis, necnon ad digitorum pterygia, ulcera depascentia et quæ in carnibus luxuriantur, itemque ad aurium dolores et narium vitia, maxime vero ex acido punico sumptum.

The juice obtained by pressing the seeds (of pomegranate), cooked with honey, is good for *ulcers* of the *mouth*, of the *genitals*, and of the *anus*, as well as for *pterygia of the fingers*, *eating ulcers* which luxuriate in the *flesh*, in the same manner, pains of the ears, and diseases of the *nostrils* cure especially by the acid taken from the pomegranate.

There, again, a uniform treatment is devoted to multiple symptoms which were most probably observed in the same patient, either altogether or consecutively; and, if Dioscorides had added that all these phenomena were the successive manifestations of a single disease of genital origin, no one would to-day deny the syphilitic

[1] The *marc* or grounds remaining after olives have been crushed and deprived of their oil.

nature of the affection. As a matter of fact, how is it that in this succession of accidents cannot be seen buccal, vulvar, preputial, and anal syphilides, syphilitic onychia, ulcerating gummata of the muscles, perhaps even syphilitic coryza and otorrhœa? And all these morbid products were repressed by the aid of the same acid; is this not what is done in our day with nitrate of silver, or even the acid nitrate of mercury? Our way of seeing appears, to us, at least, as rational as that method which consists in cudgelling their brains and subsequently victoriously asserting, like Astruc and his imitators, that these extracts refer to I don't know what disease, which has disappeared in our days, *which resembled syphilis*, but which was not syphilis. And these things are written without so much as a smile, because it is about syphilis! And yet, what would be thought of the innovator who would come, with the aid of a similar argument, and pretend that gastric embarrassment or diarrhœa dated from the reign of King Dagobert?

The physician who appears next, Aretæus, of Cappadocia, lived about A.D. 90. Nothing touching upon venereal diseases occurs in his book. However, in a chapter devoted to the treatment of malignant affections (*pestilentium affectium*) of the throat,[1] he describes a case of loss of substance which one is tempted to refer to the tertiary period of syphilis.

He next speaks of *Egyptian and Syrian ulcers*, in which he recognizes a special throat disease:—

Quibusdam etiam columella exesa est usque ad os (μέχρις ὀστέον) palati et tonsillæ usque ad basim et epiglottidem. . . .	In some even the uvula is destroyed, even to the palate-bone and the tonsils to the roots of the tongue and epiglottis. . . .

As to Oribasius, who lived about A.D. 360, although

[1] Therapeutics, vol. i, chap. ix.

three centuries later than Dioscorides, he only gives us information as vague as that of Hippocrates and Galen, authors from whom he borrowed extensively. In the extracts translated by Darenberg,[1] we find a few expressions which seem to refer to phagedenic chancres and to the secondary lesions of syphilis. In Book IX of the *Medical Collection* we find the author recommending poultices of bread and lentils for "certain ulcers, especially of the genitals."

Chap. xxxvii. . . . *ὅπη νομαί τινες, μάλιστα ἐπὶ τῶν αἰδοίων.*

In Book X, he speaks of certain astringent pastilles used as an ointment for the "chancre and ulcers of a bad nature."

Chap. xxiv. *ἄνθραξι, τοῖς κακοήθεισι τῶν ἑλκῶν.*

We have already said that the Greek word *anthrax*, rendered *carbunculus* in Latin versions of the Middle Ages, signified *chancre* when it was located upon the generative organs. In Hindoo, the words *Nar-Farsi*, *Ateshi-Farsi*, signify *Persian fire*, a phrase signifying chancre or anthrax, indifferently. It is, if we are to believe Rosenbaum, the expression employed by the *Cabirajas;* that is to say, the physicians of India. As to the word *κακοήθης*, it has passed into the French language with the sense of *malignant* and remained until the sixteenth century; at least, since Thierry de Héry describes "ulcères cacoëths" in 1533.[2] About the same time, Rabelais[3] speaks of a "maladie cacoèthe."

In Chapter XXVII Oribasius advises different ointments for ordinary vegetations, and alum, combined with

[1] The chapters of this book are classified in a ridiculous manner, and their numbers do not agree with those of Latin editions.

[2] Malign Ulcers, Thierry de Héry, *loc. cit.* (See chap. i, description of the bubo.)

[3] A Malign Disease, Pantagruel., lib. iii, chap. xiv.

blue vitriol and myrrh obtained by pressure, " for fungosities of the anus and genitals."

. . . πρὸς δὲ τὰς ἐν δακτυλίῳ καὶ αἰδοίοις ὑπεροχὰς.

Evidently he speaks of other things than simple vegetations which had their special ointment (the text is clear), or of hæmorrhoids, as the anus was not their only seat. Outside of syphilides, it cannot be easily seen what these elevated pimples (ὑπεροχὰς) could have been. Further on the author speaks of excrescences *resembling figs* (συκώδεις), and he employs the same word,—ὑπεροχὰς.

Let us now examine the complete works of the same author, according to the Greek-Latin edition of Kühn. In the *Synopses*[1] we find, in Book VII, descriptions which may be referred to the secondary period :—

Chap. xxxix. Thymus est ulcus aspera et squalida carne excrescens. Fit autem et in ano et in pudendo.	*Thymus* is composed of uneven, rough, and *ulcerated excrescences*. It grows about the *anus* and *pudenda*.

This is truly that uneven group of mucous patches which are elevated, and which extend from the anterior commissure of the vulva to the anus. Besides, it is well known that vegetations, properly so called, are not ulcerative. Let us now go to Book IX :—

Chap. xvii. Ad rimas quæ in sede et pudendis sunt. . . .	For the erosions of the anus and genitals. . . .
Chap. xxxvii. Pudendorum anique ulcera quæ absque inflammatione oriuntur, valde exsiccantia medicamenta postulanta.	Ulcers of the genitals and anus which do not present inflammatory reaction require more especially remedies which dry.

There existed, then, in the time of Oribasius, ulcerations of the sexual organs without inflammation; that

[1] Synopseos, lib. vii, chap. xxxix ; ix, chap. xvii, xxxvii, xxxviii.

is to say, other than herpes progenitalis, furuncle, abscess, etc. As to treatment, it has not varied. Do we not, even to-day, simply place an inert powder upon syphilitic chancres to make them dry? Soft chancres would not have been satisfied with this anodyne treatment. Like Galen, the author praises resin for erosions of the genital organs (*ad rimas pudendorum*). In another part of his work, which treats of "Therapeutics of Local Diseases,"[1] he again speaks of ulcers of the anus and of the genital organs, and he gives advice for those cases in which the ulcers are *moist* (*si ulcera humida sint*). So there were some which were not, or, in other words, which did not suppurate. We will see, later on, that Celsus also distinguishes soft chancres—those which suppurate, the *moist*—from indurated chancres, which suppurate very little, or not at all,—the *pura siccaque* (clean and dry). Further on, Oribasius speaks of œdema of the genitalia (*pudendum intumescens*) and of ulcers of the vulva. And we know that the primary lesion is the most frequent cause of genital œdema,—swelling *en masse* of the prepuce or of the labia majora and minora.[2]

Such are the documents which the best-known Greek physicians of antiquity furnish us. Before taking up the philosophers, rhetoricians, historians, and poets, we will say a few words of the manners of this people, which occupied the foremost place in Europe in the arts, sciences, and literature before the Christian era. However, we will be less prolix than Rosenbaum, who, under

[1] De locor. affector. curatione, lib. iv, chap. cii and ciii.

[2] Non-medical readers will pardon us for going into such long technical discussions and for quoting so profusely. But, among scientific men who do not admit the antiquity of syphilis in Europe are a few men at the head of schools; on this account we are forced to be as complete as possible.

the pretense of writing the history of syphilis in antiquity, has really described prostitution among the different peoples, complacently dilating upon the most depraved vices of the Orientals. He spreads before us, over a space of more than a hundred pages, in a heavy and prosy style, a mountain of filth, which he could have easily compressed in fifty lines. In addition, the German author cites such a profusion of quotations that it gives one vertigo; and, as he gives them without any translation, and almost always without comment, and, as the majority prove nothing, or are opposed to that which he wants to demonstrate, the question which arises is, whether they have been carefully considered, or even well understood.

The free citizen, in Greece, had to do with three classes of women. First, the lawful wife, the mistress of the house, she upon whom devolved the care of the house and the perpetuation of the race; but she was the most neglected one. All obeyed her; many honors and duties, but little pleasure. Then came the servants, for the whim or material necessity of the time being,—beasts of burden without individuality. So much for the home. In the third place, the mistress, for pleasure.[1] The last were generally taken from among dancing girls, actresses, or hetairæ (ἑταίρας, *prostitutes*). These horizontals of primitive ages were more or less high-strung, like their prototypes of to-day. History has handed down to us the names of the most celebrated hetairæ,—Aspasia, Phryne, and Lais. Hospitality, with the last one, whose headquarters were at Corinth, was

[1] This was an admitted fact in Athens, for Demosthenes says, in one of his addresses: "We have courtesans for pleasure, concubines (servants) to take care of our bodies, and wives to give us children and supervise our homes with fidelity."

taxed at fabulous prices, whence the proverb, *Non licet omnibus adire Corinthum*, which may be freely translated, "Every one cannot afford an escapade to Corinth." These fashionable beauties generally dyed their hair yellow with saffron, a custom in which they were imitated by the honest women, just like in our century; and what proves it is that the comic poet Menander[1] ridicules them in his pieces. In our days, as a result of chemical progress, oxygenated water has taken the place of saffron. For men about town, strangers, people in general, there were, in addition to actresses and hetairæ, the *dicteriadæ*, boarders at the special bawdy houses instituted by Solon, and known as *dicterions*.

So much for physiological needs. But the ancient Greeks did not stop there; they were too close to Asia not to have been tainted by the Oriental vices which, as a matter of fact, reigned in Athens—and especially in Rome—in Pagan times. Certain low beings, the shame of their sex, did not fear to forget their manhood to place themselves at the service of the most revolting passions. They were called *cinædi* (*κίναιδοι*; in Latin, *cinædi*, *pathici*); that is to say, accommodating instruments for *Socratic love*, upon which we cannot dilate. Dioscorides, on account of one of their monstrous acts, also called them στόμαργους (from στόμα, bucca, and ἔργον, labor),[2] an expression which corresponds to the word *fellatores* of the Romans. In a purely pathological point of view, it is well to remark that Erasistratus

[1] Menander lived about 300 B.C.

[2] For those who prefer seeing in the word *στόμαργος* an Attic form of *στόμαλγος* or *στομαλγής* (who has a sore mouth), we will say that this epithet then applied to the result of the vice, instead of the act itself; the two versions are admissible, but of little importance.

gives them the name of ῥινοκολοῦροι, *who have the nose eaten;* we may suppose a tertiary lesion, with necrosis of the bones of the nose, syphilis not being incompatible with such a profession. Besides, it would appear that the cinædi recognized each other by a characteristic hoarse voice; but it did not exist in all these miserable beings. At least, this is what is clearly indicated in an indignant discourse of Dion Chrysostom, the Greek sophist of Tarsus, who lived at the end of the first century of our era.[1] He complains of the vice (ἔργον) which "dishonors and marks the city," for everywhere is heard the voice of the Sodomites (ἀκολάστοις); then he cries :—

> What virtuous man could endure this rough (χαλεπόν) and discordant (ἄγριον) voice?

And he adds, what shows very well that it concerned a pathological fact :—

> Although this quality (of voice) is not always met with and among us, it is, nevertheless, inherent in them; it is their characteristic mark (σύμβολον).

We will see later on that Martial brands, in the same way, the vices of the *pædicones* (pederasts), and makes sport of their hoarse and discordant voice (*rancidulo* or *rancidulo ore*);[2] it might very well be syphilitic laryngitis. Dion Chrysostom then reproaches his co-citizens for enduring, in their city, the presence of those foul citizens whose *nose* is attacked by a sort of *professional disease* (πάθος), which gives them their nasal voice.

> You prefer, then, this voice to all others, as if it were possible to produce good music with the nose! Such a rhythm must necessarily be followed by *something else in addition.*

[1] Orationes, xxxiii. [2] Martial, lib. vii, epigr. 34.

The rhetor of Tarsus was probably aware that the disease did not limit itself to the nose and throat. He terminates by addressing the Sodomites themselves, and he tells them positively that the disease from which they suffer was contracted in their monstrous practices.

You are ignorant of the fact that an *endemic disease* has seized upon your *noses*, in the same manner as, in others, the wrath of heaven has wreaked itself upon some particular parts, such as the hands, the feet, or the face. It is said that Aphrodite (Venus), to punish the women of Lemnos,[1] sent them a disease of the armpits; well! it is thus that divine wrath *has destroyed the nose* of the majority of you, and it is from that that this peculiar sound emanates; for from what cause could it come? It is the *sign of depravity* of the most shameless kind pushed to delirium, and to the scorn of all morality.

As for us, who have not the same reasons as the Greek orator to explain embarrassing cases, we will give, as etiological cause of this, caries of the bones of the nose, syphilitic ostitis, at least as active as the anger of Jupiter. After all, Dion Chrysostom was not the only one to see in this morbid symptom the result of the anger of the Olympian divinities, for Herodotus, who lived about 450 B.C., says, in his book entitled "Clio,"[2] that Venus revenged herself in a similar manner by visiting a venereal disease upon the Scythians who had sacked one of her temples in Syria.

The goddess sent a *female disease* (θήλειαν νοῦσον) to those among the Scythians who had sacked her temple at Ascalon, and this punishment was transmitted forever to their *posterity*. The Scythians say that this disease is a punishment for the sacrilege, and that the strangers who travel in their country take notice of the condition of those of the Scythians called Enares (Ἐναρέας).

[1] And not *Lesbos*, as is said by all authors who record this fact upon the good faith of their predecessors without having referred to the Greek text. We desire to remark the same thing of Herodotus, whose story is entitled *Clio*, and not *Chio;* of Plutarch, who speaks of the goddess *Syria*, and not *Syra*, etc.

[2] Chap. cv.

Certain commentators have seen gonorrhœa in this disease of sexual origin. We will restrict ourselves to calling attention to the fact that the gonorrhœal flow is not hereditary, and is not accompanied by external manifestations visible to those passing by; whereas syphilis corresponds much better to the symptoms described by the Greek historian.[1]

At all events, intelligent men of those times had little faith in these good legends for the populace and which they propagated by their writings. In fact, Plutarch,[2] another historian who lived in the second century of our era, says, maliciously, that there are "superstitious persons who believe that the goddess Syria *eats the legs*, covers the body with *ulcers*, and makes the *liver melt* in those who eat herrings and gudgeons."

At Syriam deam superstitiosi potant si quis mœnam aut apuas edat, ejus crura (τὰ αντικνήμα) corrodere (διεσθίειν), corpus ulceribus (ἕλκεσι) opplere, jecur (το ἧπαρ) colliquare.

It may be seen that Plutarch has another opinion, which he keeps to himself; having no reason to irritate his reserve, or purpose to explain these symptoms by tertiary, visceral, and subcutaneous lesions.

A third historian, Thucydides,[3] who lived in the time of Pericles (fifth century B.C.), and was, conse-

[1] This passage of Herodotus, which bothered the good Astruc, has furnished him with matter for a harrowing discussion. Rejecting (this goes without saying) the idea of venereal disease, he states (entirely satisfied with his discovery) that the θήλειαν νοῦσον was the loss of virility; and, without seeing the enormity of his mistake, he concludes that the Enares were . . . *eunuchs!* If the great "novelist" of syphilis was not dead for more than a century, we would simply ask him—for the text of Herodotus is formal—where and when he has seen people who were eunuchs from *father to son.*

[2] De Superstitione, section 10.

[3] Histor. belli Peloponnesiaci. History of the Pelopponesian War.

quently, a contemporary of Herodotus, relates the history of the plague at Athens; in this description we find the following sentence:—

The disease also attacked the *genital parts* (τὰ αἰδοῖα), the hands, (χεῖρας), the feet (πόδας), and several, having lost their parts, escaped death.

Lucretius, in his poem on "Nature," describes the same symptoms in relation to this epidemic, as we will see in the next chapter.

Let us now examine the light poets, whose works, unfortunately, are partly lost. Among the fragments which have been found and collected under the name of *Anthology*, there may be met here and there allusions to syphilis which are more or less vague. So, not to weary the reader, we will merely quote one poet, Eubulus, who wrote for the theatre about 375 B.C. One of his comedies is worthy of our attention; there remain nine verses which we will analyze. But, as our interpretation is sure to be called into question, we will discuss each word after the other, giving the Greek text and the Latin version which accompanies it. In the piece entitled *Nannion*, the author pities the one who hides himself in order to give himself up to his amorous diversions.

"Is it not more simple," says the character, "to go in open daylight to see the pretty girls which the countries on the banks of the Eridon furnish us! One's choice can be made in complete safety; they are arranged side by side, entirely naked, or clothed in a transparent tunic." . . .

Eubulus simply advises his fellow-citizens to go to the *dicterions.* It is probable that these establishments were kept supplied by the girls born in the countries irrigated by the Po, for the text states: "The girls whom the Eridon nourishes in its sacred waves."

. . . ὅσας
Ἠριδανὸς ἀγροῖς ὕδασι κηπεύει κόρας.

This figure of speech is frequently employed in ancient poetry. The author is cynical when he advises going to the brothel in open day, but he reasons logically, as will be seen from the last three verses:—

μικροῦ πρίασθαι κέρματος τὴν ἡδονὴν,
καὶ μὴ λαθραίαν κύπριν, αἰσκίττην νόσων
κασῷν διώκειν, ὕβρεος, οὐ πόθου, χάριν.

. . . nummulo emere voluptatem, neque clandestinam venerem, turpissimum morborum omnium, persequi, superbiæ, non amoris, causa.

. . . there for the smallest coin (one may) buy pleasure; no risk, like in secret adventures, of finding, at the same time, the *most shameful of diseases.* Do not tell me that it is love you seek in your pleasures; it is the satisfaction of your self-love.

We have given as broad a translation as possible, in order to make it explicit; now we will take the Latin, which is literally rendered from the Greek, word for word. The most disputed phrase is plainly that in which it is literally said: . . . "while he may go and see; . . . buy pleasure, etc., and not run after (*persequi*) clandestine pleasure, and the most shameful (*turpissimum*) of all diseases (*morborum*), on account of self-love, and not for love." It may be objected that there is but a single verb, διώχειν (to pursue), for the two things which may be reaped,—the pleasure and the disease; next, that no conjunction connects the two parts of the sentence, which permits the second one to be regarded as qualitative, and to translate thus: . . . "pursue secret pleasure, the most shameful of vices." . . . We will answer, first, that the word νοσος (*morbus*, in Latin) may sometimes signify *vice*, figuratively and by extension, but that it is much more simple to give it its usual meaning, *disease*, than to look for the exceptional meaning it may have in certain cases. We will say next that this last interpretation would not be well understood, for, in a general way, and being given the person in the play, it cannot be understood why he should be more ashamed of a secret adventure (*obscuras nuptias*) with any irregular woman than to go in broad daylight, with a disregard of all shame, into an establishment for that purpose, and choose merchandise in consideration of money (*nummulo*). On the contrary, with the meaning we propose, it is easily seen that the character of Eubulus warns young Greeks against clandestine prostitution, more dangerous, as in our days, than legalized prostitution,—that which is regulated. The author is not giving a course in morals; he gives hygienic advice, and his warnings may be summed up as follows: " In wishing to gain the illusion of a conquest one is more exposed, for then all possibility of restriction is suppressed." As to the conjunction *et* (*και*), which should join the two parts of the sentence, it may very well have been omitted designedly, on account of the metre, especially as it is not indispensable for an understanding of the text. Conclusion: there were more chances in Athens before Christ, like in Paris in the nineteenth century, of acquiring syphilis with the unknown women who are met [" street-walkers "], who call themselves virtuous, than with the inmates of public houses,—human cattle which could be examined in broad daylight (*ad solem*).

We do not have to seek whether it is poetic to risk, prosaic to avoid, or moral to abstain, our subject not including this variety of studies.

We now arrive to the time of Christ. Christian martyrology itself (who would have believed it?) will furnish us proofs; but we must be believed on the word of the Fathers of the Church. Here a little history is necessary; let us review, in a few lines, the principal benefits of Christianity,—a social result which we make it a duty to proclaim loudly.

The work of Christ was to teach humanity that it should respect itself. The religion which he founded placed a curb upon the torrents of ancient corruption, the infamous practices of Pagan religion, and that lubricity which the populace exhibited in a manner that might be called official,—as at Rome, for example. But, as Dufour observes,[1] it required not less than three centuries of contention, sermons, and especially of example, to overthrow the haunts of prostitution; that is to say, the temples of Isis, of Priapus, of Ceres, of Venus, of Flora, and of other divinities whose worship was merely a pretext for the most monstrous debauches. But Christianity soon fell into the opposite excess; it required absolute continence. Exaggerations are the inevitable consequence of all religions, political or moral revolutions. Each one has its fanatics who go beyond the object. Let us interrogate history. In the Middle Ages, some fanatic monks tortured in the name of Christian charity; in 1793, the populace assassinated in the name of liberty; in the first days of Catholicism, the apostles proscribed sexual relations in the name of dignified manhood; and, by dint of imagining that it was agreeable to the Creator to condemn to rest the organs which he had given for a purpose diametrically opposed (*crescite et multiplicamini*),[2] the fact was lost sight of that the end of the world would have been the

[1] Hist. de la Prostitution. Paris, 1851. History of Prostitution.

[2] "Cross and multiply," said the Lord to the children of Noah, when they left the Ark. (Genesis, chap. viii, v. 17.)

inevitable result of a practical application of this theory. But, happily for the history of nations, there were dissenters. We may readily assume that Saint Paul was not a very warm partisan of conjugal union, for he says to the Corinthians: "It is well for your daughters to marry, but better for them not to."[1] His doctrine was adopted by the first Fathers of the Church and by the Councils. "From this horror of incontinence," says Dufour, "Christian celibacy was to inevitably result."

It did result, in fact. Celibacy was adopted in principle, and existed *de facto*, but much later for the members of clergy. The theory was absurd, from a natural point of view, since it is opposed to physiology, but excellent for the object which a militant sect of the sixteenth century proposed. This object consisted in putting different members of the association in groups, and it was a complete success without having made nature lose any of her rights. In fact, the *is pater est quem nuptiæ demonstrant*[2] of the *Code Civil* levels all difficulties which could arise. Loyola, born shrewd, immediately saw the advantages he could derive from a principle which produced power. By the sole fact of the existence of "regulation" celibacy, society, from an intellectual point of view, is not in danger; but there are pathological consequences for this disregard of nature imposed by the canons. For certain cold or sufficiently strong natures the battle is possible, if not easy; but how many tottering minds in a contrary case![3]

[1] Epistle I, chap. vii, v. 38.

[2] The law recognizes no father but the husband.

[3] We disclaim being looked upon as a "devourer of priests," for we have no hatred for members of the secular clergy, the greater part of whom are men of integrity, and our friends are among them. The rôle of the physiologist is to observe and draw his conclusions without seeking to please or offend; that is, by keeping aloof from religious or political quarrels, for which he does not care.

Then may be explained unnatural vices, rapes, the monstrous acts, which but too frequently occupy our courts of law. Or, in the case of women, it is nerve-troubles in all their forms, mystic or libidinous, or that erotic furor which fed the funeral piles of the Middle Ages, under the name of demonomania. In the nineteenth century the exstatics are called *saints;* in convents, those *preparatory schools for hysteria*, the brains of unfortunate girls, who may or may not be so predisposed, are too frequently unsettled by such spectacles, re-inforced by appropriate teaching, and who, not having been successfully enrolled, later on will bear, instead of strong and well-balanced citizens, enervated and stunted beings.

After what we have said, it will be understood why it was that Christian women held to their virginity above all, at the time of the martyrology ordered by the Roman emperors. And one of the first cares of the consuls or governors of tributary provinces was to send them to a brothel to be given over to public prostitution. The inhabitants were notified of the fact by a placard affixed to the house of prostitution. Then they proceeded to a series of tortures which varied according to the inventive faculties of these cowardly persecutors. Are we to see retaliation in the horrors of the Inquisition, the massacres of St. Bartholomew and the Dragonades? If so, what other conclusion can be drawn but that the human being is born bloodthirsty, and that circumstances alone make him victim or executioner? It is true that many centuries separate us from these historical dishonors, and that it is said we are civilized; let us not forget, however, that it was but yesterday that one dared cry, in the face of Europe: "Might is right!"

Some of the martyrs, say the Fathers of the Church, were saved from defloration by divine intervention. Those who wished to touch St. Agnes, for example, fell dead, according to St. Ambrose. Another, at Corinth, conceived, to save herself, a means which very few—at least, we hope so—virgins of our time would imagine. From the stand-point which interests us the event proves that venereal diseases were known by everybody, for the virgin in question knew a great deal for a young patrician. If we are to believe Palladius, Bishop of Helenopolis, in Bithynia (Asia Minor), who lived about A.D. 400, she was sent, like the others, to a brothel.[1] Immediately the libertines arrived, upon seeing the placard.

. . . Illa autem virgo honestissima et imprimis veneranda, et verba ad deceptionem deflectens, suppliciter eis dicebat, rogans: Habeo ulcus (ἕλκος) in loco occulto (*κεκρυμμένον*), quæ mirandum in modum male olet (*ἐσκάτως .ὄζει*), et timeo ne ros meî odium capiat propter ulcus aversandum. . . .

. . . But the virgin, who was very honest, and, above all, venerable, being disposed to deceive them, implored them to listen: "I have," said she, "an ulcer in a *hidden place*, and which *smells very badly*. I fear that you would hold me in aversion if you came to *catch my ulcer*." . . .

Palladius says that he read this account in a *very old book* written by one Hippolytus, who was intimate with the Apostles. Without entering into an interminable discussion upon the nature of the disease, we note the fact that there was at Corinth, in the first century of our era, and it was notoriously known, an affection characterized by one or more *ulcerations of the genital parts, contagious*, spreading a *fetid odor*, and not apparently interfering with the general health. For a mind which

[1] Palladius, *loc. cit.*, chap. cxlviii: *De femina nobilissima quæ fuit semper virgo.* (Of a young patrician girl who always remained a virgin).

is unprepared, this is a good description of vulvar syphilides.

The same Palladius also relates the story,[1] so often quoted, of a pious hermit, called Ero, who did not know how to resist temptation, prickings, longings, etc., as well as St. Anthony, the incorruptible, who was immortalized by Gustave Flaubert. It would appear that, in spite of the sermons of St. Paul, the devil is not always unsuccessful. But let us leave our Bithynian bishop speak :—

> . . . Finally, feeling the influence of some malice of the demon, and being no longer able to remain in his cell, he left for Alexandria. . . . There he frequented the theatres and equestrian games, and became a frequenter of taverns. He gave himself up to the pleasures of the table and indulged to excess in spirits, which led him to the shameful desire for woman. Being resolved to sin, he had repeated relations with a dancing girl, and finally found himself attacked by an ulcer (ἕλκος). In consequence of his debauchery and as a divine punishment, there appeared a chancre (ἄνθραξ) upon the glans. He was ill six months, then his sexual organs mortified and dropped off. When he became somewhat better, he returned to his solitude. . . . The operation not having been made in time, he succumbed a few days afterward.

We have quoted this passage because it has been given by a large number of authors ; but, for us, the disease of Ero is a typical form of phagedenic chancre, to which syphilis was absolutely foreign.

In conclusion, to terminate this study on Greece, we will say that we are much inclined to see, like Follin and Rosenbaum, exostoses of the skull in those *horns*, so frequent in the inhabitants of the Island of Cyprus, who were designated in that country under the name of Κεραστία. This information emanates from Xenagoras, cited by Natalis Comes.[2]

[1] Chap. xxxii. De Erone.

[2] Mythologia, lib. iii.

. . . Deinde dicta (Cyprus) Cerastia, ut inquit Xenagoras in libro secundo de insulis, quod illam homines habitarent qui multos tumores tanquam cornua quædam in capite habere viderentur, cum cornua κέρατα dicta sint a Græcis et κεράσται cornuti.

. . . Then Cyprus was called *Cerastia*, as Xenagoras says in his second book on islands, and this because the inhabitants, having numerous *tumors* on the head, appeared to have *horns*, as the Greek for *horns* is *kerata*, and, for those who are horned, *kerastai*.

It must also be remembered, from an etymological point of view, that one of the most venomous serpents is called *Cerastus*, on account of the two small horns which it carries on the head, but which, of course, have nothing to do with syphilis. The horns, properly so called, which are found in certain persons [*cornu cutaneum*], are rare in occurrence; and, for it to have been frequent enough in the Island of Cyprus to have given the country a significant name, it must be that this lesion had a current disease for its cause, and this disease, we fear, will continue for a long time yet.

CHAPTER XI.

FICUS.

SYPHILIS IN ROME UNDER THE CÆSARS (BEGINNING OF THE CHRISTIAN ERA).

"Il est impossible de méconnaître que la depravation des mœurs avait multiplié chez les Romains le germe et les ravages des maladies de Vénus."—P. DUFOUR.

[It is impossible to ignore that the depraved customs of the Romans had multiplied the germ and the ravages of the diseases of Venus.]

WE now approach the most interesting as well as most delicate part of our work. The most interesting, because the authors from whom we will quote seem in some sort of a way nearer to us, and are more familiar to us. As a matter of fact, every one does not read Sanskrit, Chinese, Japanese, Hebrew, hieroglyphics, Copt, Persian, even Greek; whilst Latin is familiar to all who have finished their studies, even incompletely; and, providing that the translation be given with the text, one can to a certain degree compare the proposed interpretation, instead of taking the author's word for it. For all the idioms brought forward, upon which we have had to depend, the reader has almost inevitably preserved a doubt. With Latin we have nothing of the sort. We have said that this work is a delicate one. Alas! yes; for the cause of our object, the more value our proofs have, the more licentious are the works from which they are derived. We find ourselves face to face with a difficult problem; we must analyze in acceptable prose the most immoral poetry of antiquity. And to say that this poetry was a faithful picture of Roman customs! It is quite consoling for our much-abused epoch, but it does not solve the problem. On the one hand, we would feel grieved to have our intentions so misunderstood as to lead to the belief that we have tried to give a course of lectures on pornography; on the other hand, we cannot resign ourselves to leave in obscurity the best materials for our argument. And, while asking the reader's pardon for leading him into these literary cloacæ, we will do all that is humanly possible to mitigate the fetidity of the text. At all events, we are persuaded that the intelligent reader will have the good sense to forget the nauseating after-taste of these free poems, and only see in them the irrefutable elements of a thesis which it is difficult to sustain. So, laying aside conventional prudery, which should disappear in a scientific territory, he will bow, like we, before those ineffaceable documents which antiquity has transmitted to us, and which confirm the first sentence of the Bible, according to Ricord: *In the beginning God created the heavens, the earth, man, and venereal diseases!*

Let us first study the authors who touch upon the medical art, more or less; that is to say, physicians and naturalists. The most celebrated physician of Rome whose name has been handed down to us is Celsus. He was of Greek origin, but lived in Latium during the Augustan period.[1] It was at about this time that physicians worthy of the name were *tolerated* at Rome. Several Greek practitioners, who had imbibed the works of Hippocrates, and who were faithful followers of his teachings, had already attempted to establish themselves in Italy; but, if they were borne, so to speak, in times

[1] First century B.C. Celsus lived at the beginning of this century.

of epidemics, they were, on the other hand, dismissed with contempt later on. Afterward—that is to say, in the course of the second century before Christ—a second attempt was made, but by a new generation of Greek physicians. They had come to treat the venereal diseases which the consul Cneius Manlius had imported to Rome (183 B.C.) after his victory over Antiochus the Great, king of Syria. Syria being a constant hot-bed of syphilis, the young Syrian girls who accompanied the army of Manlius on his return to Italy became excellent agents for its propagation. Syphilis at that time took on the epidemic form, as it did in the fifteenth century. The poet Lucilius cries: "Let us send back to the enemy this *pestilence* and scourge which the lame Manlius [has brought] to us."

. . . Hostilibu' contra
Pestem perniciemque, catax quam et Manliu' nobis.

But he does not say: "Let us be treated." Superstitious practices took the place of rational therapeutics. The physicians were compelled to give way to dislikes, bad dispositions, and vexations of all kinds; they returned to Greece.

At that time all venereal diseases were confounded under the same term,—*shameful disease* (morbus indecens, turpis morbus, etc.). Ignoring the nature of the *Proteus of a thousand shapes*, the Romans did not suspect the diathesis, and employed different terms to designate the syphilides, according to their appearance, size, number, or location. Thus, the *mariscæ*[1] which occupied the anus were voluminous, obstructed the opening, and spread about its neighborhood; this description applies well to papulo-hypertrophic syphilides. The

[1] A species of large fig.

papular, vulvar, or preputial syphilides,—not so large, —and all syphilides in general were designated by the word *ficus* (fig). The word *fi*, or *fix*, in the Middle Ages, then *fic* (French for fig), which remained in the French language until the eighteenth century, but deviated somewhat from its primitive meaning, are directly derived from this word *ficus*. And what proves that this was the term used by the Romans is that it has furnished an adjective, *ficosus*, and even a superlative, *ficosissimus*, currently employed to designate the victims more or less affected by this notoriously venereal and evidently contagious disease. The origin of this term (*ficus*, *fici*, 2d decl.) is the reddish and granular appearance of the fig (*ficus*, *ficûs*, 4th decl.) when cut in two, and whose resemblance to the eroding papular syphilide of the genitals, the classical *mucous patch*, can be perceived by any one. At other times an epigrammatic poet will say, ironically, to a courtesan that she has pimples on her sexual parts (*aliquid prominet*,—something projects). Roseola and other exanthemata or pustules of the secondary period are designated by the expressions *maculæ* (spots), *pustulæ lucentes* (shining pustules), *sordidi lichenes* (foul eruptions), etc. As general terms, we find *scabies*, a word which has been translated *itch*, but which is most often employed in the sense of *ulcerated pustules*, and its adjective *scabiosus* (rotten), which indicates a more marked degree, and especially manifestations which are more generalized than *ficosus*, probably ulcerated gummata. It is also noticeable, in the same order of ideas, that the epithet *putridus* (putrid) was hurled as an insult. The *triste mentum*[1] designated the disease localized on the chin and

[1] Grünbeck or Gründpeck, who issued in 1496 the first printed book on syphilis, appended as title, *De Mentulagra*. . . . Wendelin Hock

lower lip; the *ulcus putre, acre in ore* (putrid ulcer, virulent in the mouth), buccal syphilides; the *cæcum vulnus* (hidden wound), the *ulcus turpe* (shameful ulcer), had in view localized ulcerating syphilides of the genito-anal region, but especially those of the sexual organs. And ulcerated gummata of the vulva are to be suspected in the expression: *cunni vermiculos scaturientes* (crawling worms of the vulva.)

Venereal diseases, although "thrown in the shade," as Dufour says, "by the Greek and Roman physicians and naturalists," were none the less very numerous, always very stubborn, and often terrible. The author mentioned supposes, and with apparent reason, that religious motives prevented ancient authors from apparently classifying with the others these diseases of the genital organs which recognized debauchery as their cause. Æsculapius, the God of Medicine, was not to appear to engage in an open warfare with Venus by trying to neutralize the effects of the vengeance of the goddess; so that the patients, as if they had been loaded with infamy, concealed themselves for treatment, and addressed themselves either to Priapus or to Isis (Venus), or to magicians or venders of philters. Therapeutics was at that time reduced to prayers or to the use of a few plants. Certain patients preferred death to an acknowledgment of their disease. For ordinary physicians, the ancient Romans had slaves who were beaten if they did not cure and freedmen who paid a fine if unsuccessful; consequently, all refused to treat diseases

(1514) called his small work *Mentagra*, etc., which proves that the physicians who were contemporaneous with the epidemic knew the meaning of this Latin word. They were far from suspecting that the dermatologists of our time would appropriate the term *mentagra* to apply it to a skin disease localized in the same place (sycosis), but entirely removed from syphilis, for which the Romans had created it.

which did not appear to be able to get well in a short time, and notably venereal diseases. As to the physician, properly so called, it was quite an affair to call him in. As there were no hospitals, the clinic took place at the home of the client. The practitioner, if we are to believe Martial, arrived with ten, twenty, thirty, and sometimes one hundred scholars, according to his renown, who *all* examined the patient after their master. It is easily understood that the venereal individuals of ancient Rome, in view of this procedure, did not much care to contribute to the advancement of medical science in this way. Besides, the treatment, as we will soon see, was not always very mild. As to women, the principal sources of infection, it was a crime for them to uncover before any other man than their husbands, had it even been for a difficult labor. Strange prudery among a people in which obscenity presented itself officially. All these causes, taken together, sufficiently explain why sexual diseases were surrounded with so much mystery in antiquity. Celsus, who has described local symptoms, of which many refer to syphilis, has carefully refrained from employing the expression, *morbus indecens;* still, he knew, much better than the satirical poets of his time, that there existed a disease of genital origin,—with many forms, it is true, but always the same, and which was contracted in the same manner. The Romans were too proud of their robust health, as Dufour explains to us, to acknowledge these secret troubles; besides, it would almost have been offending Venus to devote, in a medical work, a special chapter to those diseases contracted in her worship. Celsus may have had cause to repent: and we see him, instead of openly treating of the disease of Venus, describe, as if unconsciously, some manifestations localized upon the organs of generation, without drawing any conclusions as to the origin of these troubles. For Martial it was quite different; he was not a physician. His caustic epigrams were addressed to but one class of individuals, the debauched of both sexes; whilst Celsus, by christening the disease with a special name, scientific or ordinary, would have seemed to attack all Rome, and Rome would not have easily pardoned him. At that time, at least, the little buildings [urinals] to which Vespasion affixed his name had no cause to blush: they did not yet bear upon their inner walls, as a mark of shame, the pseudonyms of the professors of occasion, more or less diplomaed, who sell orvietan under the cover of the laws in the midst of the nineteenth century!

This is how Celsus approaches the subject:—

> Now come the diseases which affect the shameful parts (*quæ ad partes obscœnas pertinent*). The Greeks, to treat of this subject, have more appropriate expressions, which are besides consecrated by usage, as they are almost always employed by physicians, either in their writings or in their daily language. Ours are more shocking, and have not even the excuse of being occasionally found in the mouths of those who speak with decency; so that it is not an easy task to maintain the precepts of the art and respect propriety also. Nevertheless, this consideration has not been sufficient to prevent me from writing, first, because I desire to transmit entire the useful teachings which I have received; and because it is desirous to inform the people of the treatment of those diseases which are never exposed to another except against one's will (*quæ invitissimus quisque alteri ostendit.*)[1]

The diseases called *secret* were evidently known in Rome under the Emperors, but we see that Celsus promised himself to be reserved. He next gives a clear description of paraphimosis and of phimosis caused by preputial œdema; he employs none of these terms, but, as they are phenomena which almost always occur independently of syphilis, no one protests. The author also

[1] Aurelius Cornelius Celsus: Medicina, lib. vi, cap. xviii.

describes soft chancres, those which suppurate (*ulcera humida et purulenta*), and the *other kind* of chancres, which are dry and without suppuration (*pura siccaque*); finally, the phagedenic chancre, which is designated in full (φαγέδαινα). "When it is possible to bring the prepuce back," says the Latin text, "ulcers situated upon the internal surface of the skin are found, as well as upon the glans or on the organ itself; these ulcers are naturally clean and dry, or moist and purulent."

. . . ulcera vel in cutis ulteriore parte, vel in glande ultrave eam in cole reperientur; quæ necesse est, aut pura siccaque sint, aut humida et purulenta.

Those ulcers which are found when the œdema of the prepuce has disappeared are simply indurated chancres accompanied by soft chancres; and what proves that the first (*pura*) are not the second which have healed is that the author suggests a treatment for each one of these varieties. Celsus then gives the formula of the astringent treatment which he employs for ulcers of the natural parts, and he adds:—

. . . Eadem autem compositio tonsillis, uvæ madenti, oris nariumque ulceribus accomodata est.	. . . This preparation may also serve for ulcers of the tonsils, of the uvula, of the mouth, and of the nostrils.

These ulcers of the mouth were probably of the same nature as those of the genitals, as the author remembers them in giving his treatment, which he sees no reason to change. A little further on we read:—

. . . Tubercula etiam quæ φύματα Græci vocant, circa glandem oriuntur.	. . . There are also seen around the glans those tubercles which the Greeks call *phymata*.

The author takes care to observe, subsequently, that the symptoms he has described respecting ulcers "do not apply to gangrene, which is known by its black color in its inception."

. . . Hæc citra cancrum sunt. . . . Incipit a nigritia.

He then gives the conduct to follow in this last; then describes a variety of chancre in which it may become serpiginous (*serpit*). In such a case, "when the ulcer extends irregularly in all directions," it must be excised :—

Si vero ulcus latius atque altius serpit . . .

As opposite, he describes, in the following paragraph, a small, *hard* pimple, almost *indolent*, and whose excision[1] he likewise counsels :—

. . . Occalescit etiam in cole interdum aliquid; idque omni pene sensu caret; quod ipsum quoque excidi debet.	. . . There is found something on the penis, in addition, which is *callous* and which is almost entirely devoid of *sensation;* this should also be excised.

In sections 9 and 10, the author speaks of certain diseases of the anus, such as hæmorrhoids, etc., and of others situated at the vulva; then he adds, in section 11 :—

Fungo quoque simile ulcus in eadem sede (anus vel os vulvæ) nasci solet.	An ulcer resembling a fungous growth may also occur in these same parts (the anus or entrance of the vulva).

This certainly refers to papulo-hypertrophic syphilides, for the vegetations are not ulcerated. And it cannot be cancer, which Celsus describes quite well in a separate chapter of Book V, stating that it is rarely observed, except in the old (*cancer fit maxime in senibus*).[2]

There certainly exists great confusion in the descrip-

[1] Excision of the indurated chancre has been practiced at several periods, and notably about ten years ago, but not, as among the Romans, with the object of a local cure. It was proposed to prevent secondary infection; unfortunately, this attempt was not crowned with success. To-day some still contend that it is successful.

[1] Lib. v, cap. xxviii, sec. 2 and 3.

tion we have just read; but the theory of the duality of the chancre with the distinction of each virus can certainly not be exacted from the author. He states what he has seen—and it is quite creditable to have been able to see—before the Christian era: that there were phagedenic chancres; that is to say, circumscribed, with much suppuration; then, again, others do not suppurate, and, finally, those whose principal characteristic is hardness and insensibility. To these last he even refuses the name of ulcers, for he frequently observed that this symptom is often less than nothing. The patients of our times, who come to tell us, as a simple precautionary measure, that they have *something on their penis* (aliquid in cole), do not express themselves differently from Celsus. It only remained for the Roman physician, to be twenty centuries in advance, to reduce these species, which he believed distinct, to two fundamental types.

Let us now consult the elder Pliny, or the Naturalist[1] who lived about A.D. 80. He gives us scientific details on the *triste mentum* and the *sordidi lichenes*, which Martial only barely mentions.

The author states that, at the time he was writing his works, diseases of the face, absolutely unknown before, were observed in Italy. It appears that they were disgusting affections of the face, showing themselves under various forms. The severest of all received the Greek name of λιχήν (*lichen*, dartre vive); but, "as it generally began on the chin, the Latins, as a joke, at first gave it the name of *mentagra* (from *mentum*, a chin), a name which it preserved."

. . . latine, quoniam a mento fere oriebatur, joculari primum lascivia, mox et usurpato vocabulo *mentagram*.

[1] Caius Plinius Secundus: Histor. natural., lib. xxvi, sec. 1 and 2 *et seq.*

This disease did not remain localized in the face, for Pliny adds that it "also descended upon the neck, the chest, and the hands, leaving dirty, *furfuraceous* [branny] *crusts*."

. . . descendentem vero et in colla pectusque ac manus, fœdo cutis furfure.

They were probably pustulo-crustaceous syphilides. As to the contagiousness of this mento-labial affection, it is clearly indicated by the following phrase: . . . . "propagating itself especially by the *rapid contact* of a kiss."

. . . proceres veloci transitu osculi maxime.

We hardly know anything but indurated chancres or mucous patches of the lips which are capable of transmitting themselves by this procedure. Besides, this disease must have been cousin-german to the *ulcer of Egypt*, for the author says that "specialists from that country, *the parent of affections of the same kind*, were sent for, and that these physicians did not attend to anything else."

. . . adveneruntque ex Ægypto genitrice talium vitiorum medici, hanc solam operam afferentes.

Let us remark that Pliny is astonished, just as they were in the fifteenth century, at these morbid symptoms, unknown from all antiquity (*ab omni ævo priore incognitos*). It might, perhaps, not be rash to conclude that syphilis has shown itself, in different places and at different times, as epidemics, in which one of its thousand and one symptoms predominated. Endemic among all nations, it passed, unperceived in ordinary times, in the midst of the different skin diseases which the Orientals and the Romans treated by hydrotherapy and sweating. Then, under an influence which has escaped us, it manifested itself with such violence that the nation which suffered from the scourge believed it a disease unknown up to that time. This is why the Roman naturalist expresses his astonishment at two different recurrences, for he adds, a little farther on: "This *contagious disease* did not exist in the time of our fathers or forefathers."

Non fuerat hæc lues apud majores patresque nostros.

Was this not what the physicians contemporaneous with the epidemic of the fifteenth century said, in the same terms, but in a Latin much less pure? Pliny contends that the disease was brought from Asia by a Knight of Perusa, about the middle of the reign of Tiberius. Was it not also said, in the Middle Ages, that the Crusaders brought *leprosy* from the East? —Asia; this is the central focus of syphilis. In conclusion, let us cite the expression *gemursa*, a name which Pliny applied to a disease consisting of ulcers *between the toes*, which recall interdigital mucous patches.

Pliny the younger, a nephew of the other, wrote toward the end of the first century. He gives, in one of his letters, a story which tends to prove that certain Romans were not free from tertiary lesions. This letter, which is often quoted, was addressed to a certain Macer:—

Maritus ex diutino morbo circa velanda corporis ulceribus putrescebat.	A married man, *in consequence of an old disease*, had, in those parts of the body which should be kept hidden, *putrid ulcers*.

The wife of this unfortunate, born curious, insisted upon seeing this disease, and we must believe that she did not see anything re-assuring, for she despaired (*desperavit*) of any cure for her husband. She proposed suicide to him, and, to convince him, employed a means which would, probably, be very little to the taste of women of our times, especially under analogous circumstances. "For," says the author, "she bound herself to her husband and threw herself in the lake (of Como), dragging him with her."

. . . Nam se cum marito ligavit, abjecitque in lacum.

We conclude from this story that the person of whom Pliny speaks had ulcerated gummata. Everything militates in favor of this hypothesis. In the first place, the author states positively that these sores were the result of a former disease, which was chronic; then, the lesions must have been grave and curable with difficulty, when we take into consideration the extreme measures adopted by the woman; and a phagedenic chancre would have healed without any deleterious recurrence, or could not have been concealed at the beginning of marriage. Then, there must have been a period of apparent health between the two manifestations of disease; and, among diseases of the sexual organs, syphilis is the only one which acts in that manner.

According to Herodianus,[1] the Emperor Commodus ended by contracting, in the midst of his debauches, "large *tumors in the groins* and numerous *red spots* on the face and eyes." While syphilis may be suspected in the vicious and cruel monarch, it cannot be affirmed.

Valerius Maximus (consul in A.D. 254), who wrote a few of the notable events of his times,[2] mentions a case in which syphilis is said to have played the principal part, according to some authors, who quote the passage

[1] Herodianus: Histor. romana. Roman History. He lived in the third century.

[2] Valerius Maximus: Facta dictaque memorabilia, lib. iii, cap. v, sec. 3. Collection of Events and Sayings.

without discussing it. It concerns a young man of the name of Pulcher, who simply died of indigestion (*intemperentia*), but, according to some commentators, in the course of a *chronic disease* characterized by *spots on the skin*, having lasted some time, and by a *cachectic state*, already well marked at the time of his death. Here is the text :—

Pulcher, præterquam quod enervem et frigidam juventum egit, perdito etiam amore vulgatissimæ meretricis infamis fuit, mortisque erubescendo genere consumptus est.	Pulcher, although having passed a quiet and cold youth, one day led a scandalous life, for he fell insanely in love with a low prostitute. (*He contracted a disease in which the body is covered with red spots, and died in a state of consumption.*[1])

The author adds that death was caused by an *indigestion of pork paunch* (abdomine avide devorato); the glutton could not assimilate this mass of fat, and *gave up the ghost* (spiritum reddidit), together with the bacon.[2]

No doubt it may be asked why the author employed the expression *consumptus est*, which implies a slow death by gradual waste, when it was so simple to employ one of the numerous Latin expressions which signify *to die* (mortuus est, abiit, interiit, morti occubuit, cecidit, etc.). But this is not the question. This so-called proof of the antiquity of syphilis rests upon a beautiful misconstruction, and we are surprised that none of the partisans of the American origin has noticed it.

[1] We have placed this sentence in parenthesis, because we give a translation in conformity with the idea of authors who have quoted the Latin text without understanding it, as we will show farther on.

[2] Like Captain Tripet, of whom Rabelais speaks (Gargantua, chap. xxxv), who was killed by Gymnastes. " . . . wherewith he fell to the ground, and, in falling, gushed forth above four pottles of pottage, and his soul mingled with the pottage."

These latter will not be able to apply that reproach of Human. "We would be tempted to believe," says he,[1] "that it is a weakness, common with all authors, to suppress truths which are opposed to the opinions they uphold." If Valerius Maximus had said *erubescente genere* (present participle), it could be translated: *of an eruptive form, characterized by redness;* but he has *erubescendo* (future participle), which means: *of which one should blush* [redden]. So that this Pulcher, given up to all the debaucheries, among them those of the table, "died in a disgraceful manner," a victim to his gluttony; and nothing warrants seeing a medical allusion on the part of the Latin author, if a strict translation be made. There could be no more legitimate or probable opinion than that the debauchee, of whom he speaks, had syphilis; but our impartiality leads us to look upon it as a duty to state that, from all appearances, the expression of Valerius Maximus did not imply this disease.

To end with medicine and history, we will give a few verses of Lucretius,[2] regarding the plague of Athens, which go to confirm the information transmitted to us by Thucidides. The Latin poet sung nature about 55 or 60 B.C., and in his description may be seen a few details having reference to venereal diseases, and, perhaps, to the tertiary lesions of syphilis. The victims of the scourge were not always attacked by the plague properly so called; there were *other manifestations* no less terrible; for, says Lucretius, positively (verse 1204 *et seq.*), "Did they avoid this impetuous torrent of

[1] Nosographie des malad. vénér. [Paris. Nosography of Venereal Diseases. The pseudonym Human conceals the name of a certain Dr. Michu, who wrote, it seems, about the year 1838.

[2] T. Lucretius Carum: De rerum natura, lib. vi. On the Nature of Things.

poisoned blood, the disease then threw itself upon the nerves, the joints, and even the *generative organs* of the body. And, fearing the terrible threshold of death, some lived by giving to the iron the remnants of their virility."

> Profluvium porro qui tetri sanguinis acre
> Exierat, tamen in nervos hinc morbus et artus
> Ibat, et in partes genitales corporis ipsas,
> Et graviter partim metuentes limina lethi,
> Vivebant ferro privati parte virili.

Before touching the free poems (elegies, odes, satires, and epigrams), it will be necessary, in order to understand the allusions, the jokes, the sarcasms, and especially the play upon words which they contain, to draw a rapid sketch of Roman customs under the Emperors; that is to say, during the first centuries of the Christian era. As our subject alone requires many explanations, —much more than we suspected, at first,—we are obliged to glance very rapidly at these accessory bits of information, which are, nevertheless, very useful. Those who desire to be fully edified concerning the incredible manners of our ancestors of the Latin branch can read with interest the works of Dufour, Villemont, Rosenbaum, and especially the most recent, that of Dr. Dupouy.[1] They will there find, concerning the Cæsars, who gave the tone, and the citizens, who imitated them, details that make one shudder, and in comparison with which the London scandals, reported by the *Pall Mall Gazette* (about 1885), appear as insignificant peccadilloes. Compared to ancient Rome, prudish Albion is yet more chaste than she would have us believe her. And to excuse ourselves of this rather

[1] La Prostitution dans l'antiquité. Paris, 1887. Prostitution in Antiquity.

shady study, which is, nevertheless, indispensable, we will say, with our immortal Molière[1]:—

> Au moins je vois toucher une étrange matière,
> Ne vous scandalisez en aucune manière.
> Quoi que je puisse dire, il doit m'être permis;
> Et c'est pour vous convaincre, ainsi que j'ai promis.[2]

Rome, which had subjugated the world, and for centuries had given an example of civic virtues, did not fail to let itself be invaded in turn, as St. Augustine says, by "Asiatic luxury." The monstrous debaucheries of the Orientals, which, at Athens, had only gangrened society in a relative manner, found a well-prepared soil in Latium. The people, intoxicated with conquests, thought of nothing but pleasure, and, finding, in the tribute and taxes imposed upon the vanquished, resources more than sufficient for their material wants, they wallowed in voluptuousness. Leaving the Greeks far behind them, the Romans distanced even the Asiatics, their masters. Every one knows the famous cry of the populace,—*panem et circenses* (bread and the circuses)! But it must not be believed that the Roman arenas were only used for gladiatorial combats and the repasts of fierce beasts fed upon human victims. There were other performances, in which lubricity was not only spread out with all the refinements of vice, but was clothed with an official character! We are speaking of the Floral festivals, whose origin and nature it is necessary to explain.

A courtesan, of the name of Flora, who had become

[1] Le Tartufe, act iv, sc. iv.

[2] The following lame rendition is offered with apologies:—

> At least a strange matter I'm going to touch,
> And may ye all not show horror, I pray.
> It should be permitted, e'en if I say much;
> It's just to convince you, as you've heard me say.

wealthy in the exercise of her profession, had liberally met, out of her own pocket, an important deficit in the public treasury. As a mark of gratitude for such disinterestedness, the representatives of the State instituted in her honor the annual festival which bore her name and recalled the origin of the *large sum* she had given. As a matter of fact, at a signal of the ædiles, the courtesans sprang into the circus, undressed themselves until they were naked, and assumed lascivious attitudes, amid the plaudits of a delirious populace. Amid the blare of trumpets, naked men jumped into the arena, and, says Dufour, "an awful *melée* of prostitution was publicly accomplished, amid the transports of the multitude." But there were men of austere manners, who were far from approving of these debauched irruptions of their fellow-citizens. The elder Cato, it appears, had ventured into the circus once, on one of the days they were celebrating the Floral games. Upon the notice of the ædiles, who warned him that they would begin, despite his presence, if he did not retire, he left, veiling his face. It must be acknowledged that, if syphilis had not already secularized itself by that time, it would have lost a splendid opportunity of making its entrance among the Europeans.

Religion also was a pretext for orgies. There were, in Rome, a number of temples which drew the debauched of both sexes, under the names of Temple of Isis (Venus), of Venus Volupia (voluptuous), of Venus Salacia (lascivious), etc. The gardens of Priapus were also much frequented. This god was represented with a rigid penis of enormous proportions; this phallus was almost always made of wood, and that which was preferred was sometimes cypress, but generally that of the fig-tree (*ficus*, in Latin). We need not explain the concealed meaning which influenced this choice. It was customary in Rome for intended brides to repair to the gardens of Priapus, before the nuptial ceremony, and sacrifice their virginity to the god, but in form only; so there was no actual defloration; nevertheless, the young betrothed was obliged to sit upon the enormous phallus in such a manner as to place its extremity in contact with her external genital organs.[1] There was, to tell the truth, nothing but simple contact, generally very short in duration, but sufficient, nevertheless, to propagate venereal diseases. They were virgins, you will say. Agreed; but, in answer, I will say that the contraband virgins, who, in our days, assume the more orange-blossoms the less worthy of them they are, must not have failed, in Rome, to make the obligatory pilgrimage to the gardens of Priapus, and there consummate, for the benefit of all, a contact which it was impossible to deny. Imagine one of these *ficosissima* (strongly contaminated), and the true virgin, who had come later, hearing Celsus saying, some time after, to the surprised husband, furious at having a chancre: *Occalescit* (It is hard)!

Men offered to Priapus the first fruit of their gardens, and addressed themselves to him to cure them. Then there were suspended about the statue *ex-votos* recalling the form (*consimilis*) of the organ; that is to say, a phallus. The women who had recourse to Isis

[1] This fact is reported by several authors, and notably by St. Augustine, in his book, Civitas Dei, lib. vi, cap. ix. [City of God.] This custom is certainly derived from India, for Duquesne reports (Voyages dans l'Inde [Travels in India]) that he *saw*, in a pagoda in the environs of Pondichery, newly-married women coming to the god to offer the sacrifice of their virginity. They were made to sit on a Lingam (the Indian Priapus) made of wood or of iron. But it appears that there were pagodas that were *more advanced;* for in those, says the author, "the priests, more adroit, robbed this god of his function which was so valuable."

filled her temple with analogous *ex-votos*, representing the organs of their sex. So that, as we have already said, the temples served two purposes,—sexual orgies in the evening, mystic treatment in the morning. It may be well to add that the male or female empirics, sellers of drugs, and peddlers of philters, overran with their business stands the approaches of these temples.

At all events, there were honest divinities. Venus herself possessed, in the twelve quarters of Rome, more suitable altars, under the names of Venus Placida, Venus Calvities, Venus Victoria, and many other Venuses who did not encourage prostitution. "They hardly tolerated it," says Ménière, "in the priests, who gave themselves up to it secretly." Considering the state of the manners of the Roman people, these divinities could be considered modest.

Considering these public dissipations authorized by law and religion, an idea may be formed of what private debauchery must have been. Here it is no longer luxuriousness, properly so called. It is not only the absence of all moral sense; it is the aberration of the genesic sense, and monstrosity in the glutting of abnormal desires. Would it be believed that pederasty was of daily occurrence in Roman aristocracy? In our days, the head of a family who respects himself and desires to be respected has the appearance of ignoring what are the dissipations of his growing son. He will occupy himself, to restore order, only upon that day when its abuse is made manifest, or it becomes a social danger. At Rome, on the contrary, it was the custom, in patrician families, to give to the young man who had arrived to puberty a [male] slave of the same age for a bed-fellow, so that he could satisfy, according to the expression of Dupouy, his first genesic impulses! This pseudo-mistress was called a [*male*] *concubine* (*concubinatus*). This is so monstrous that it would be incredible did not Catullus say so in good Latin.[1] It makes one wonder if he is dreaming! So we will return to our quotations.

The poet, relating the marriage of Julia and of Manlius cries, addressing himself to the young man: "And thou, perfumed husband, it is very nice to say that thou regretfully givest up thy *beardless pets;* but thou must abstain."

Diceris male te a tuis
Unguentate glabris marite
Abstinere: sed abstine.

It may be concluded that these abnormal habits became inveterate; in truth, they persisted but too often after marriage.[2] Whose fault was it? Catullus himself acknowledges that the young married man is excusable; since, he adds: "You have never known, as we are aware, *any but pleasures which were permitted;* but a spouse should no longer taste of them; there are others."

Scimus hæc tibi, quæ licent,
Sola cognita: sed marito
Ista non eadem licent.

Then, what are to be the duties of the concubine in the future? Catullus will inform us. The poor concubine can no longer expect the caresses of his master; his only rôle after the nuptial ceremony consists, from that time on, in throwing nuts to the children: "Give nuts to the children, thou useless concubine."

[1] Caius Valerius Catullus, lx, *In nuptias Juliæ et Manlii.*

[2] This is clearly indicated in an epigram of Martial (lib. viii, ep. 44), in which the author advises the miser Titullus to live joyously instead of amassing money, for he will have to leave all behind on the day of his death: "Then, whether you wish it or not, your bereaved son will sleep with your *concubinatus* the first night."

"Tuoque tristis filius velis nolis,
Cum cuncubino nocte dormiet prima."

Neu nuces pueris neget.
Desertum domini audiens
Concubinus amorem.
Da nuces pueris iners
Concubine . . .

It was the custom in Rome to throw nuts to the children when the bride entered the house of her husband. A trace of this custom may, perhaps, be seen in the baptismal confections thrown to children, in French country villages, upon leaving the church.

Will we be astonished, now that a Roman citizen, Callistratus, publicly married another of the name of Afer? "O, Rome! cries Martial, is it enough? Are you waiting for the fruits of such a union?"

. . . nondum tibi, Roma videtur
Hoc satis! expectas numquid ut et pariat?[1]

They only imitated the Emperors, who, believing that everything was permitted to them, furnished the example of all the crimes. Murder, adultery, incest, and prostitution protected themselves beneath the imperial purple! Was not Curio, quoted by Suetonius[2] in his history of the "Twelve Cæsars," enabled to say that the conqueror of the Gauls was "the husband of all the women and the wife of all the men?"

. . . omnium mulierum virum et omnium virorum mulierem.

Would any one dare describe the monstrous acts of Tiberius, which did not even respect infancy? Was not the infamous Nero seen wedding, amidst great pomp, young Sporus, whose virile organs he had caused to be previously removed? Was it not the same crowned lunatic who ravished, in the midst of a religious ceremony, the

[1] Marcus Valerius Martialis, lib xii, epigr. 42.

[2] C. Suetonius Tranquillus: Duodecim Cæsares; J. Cæsar, lxx.

two officiating priests?[1] Was not Heliogabalus, who did not go beyond the passive rôle, willing to give an empire to a slave of athletic form, whom he, also, had solemnly married? Let us stop, for it might be believed that we had drawn from a treatise on mental alienation, and not from the annals of the Roman Empire!

The reader, it seems to us, is sufficiently edified upon the moral state of the Latin people in Pagan times. It remains for us now to call attention to a few expressions which recur at every moment in the verses of the epigrammatists. These authors, as Darenberg remarks, always suppose a general knowledge of the fact in those who read them; and then, without a suspicion of the medical deductions which would be drawn from them sixteen centuries later, they limit themselves "to bringing out some conspicuous, ridiculous, and satirical point." Little mattered it to Martial that the debauched Nevolus had or did not have a contagious affection in the anal region; if the poet has spoken of this disease, it was because he was forced to in order to impress the fact that this personage was what is now in medico-legal parlance known as a *passive* [pederast]. In reality, this was the only thing considered degrading in Rome. One could act, but not submit, this latter condition being reserved for low slaves and cinedæ, to whose level one was reduced in imitating them. In an opposite condition, being given that pederasty was committed in Rome, we could not grasp the biting force of that epigram of the same Martial, the fierce raillery of which

[1] According to Suetonius, these were two brothers attached to the same altars. Nero, who noticed them, did not even want to wait until the end of the sacrifice to satisfy his revolting passion, and, as the brothers mutually twitted each other on their taint, the imperial monster caused their legs to be broken.

we will only hint at as to its meaning. The author reproaches a certain Amillus with leaving all his doors open when he receives large boys at his home; the conclusion is that Amillus likes to be surprised in the midst of his villainous occupation. "He who, in such a case, wishes to prove that he is not the patient, often does at another time that which may be accomplished without a witness (or without a testicle)."

> Reclusis foribus grandes percidis, Amille,
> Et te deprendi, quum facis ista, cupis;
> * * * * * * * *
> Non pædicari se qui testatur, Amille,
> Illud sæpe facit, quod sine teste facit.[1]

There is here a play upon words, easy to understand, between *testatur* and *teste*, the word *testis* meaning either *testicle* or *witness*. As to the terms *percidis* and *pædicari*, which could not be translated except by words of a revolting obscenity, they will give to the educated reader an idea of the energy of the satirical style of that time. The Latin language, with manners such as we have depicted, was, perforce, rich in terms concerning the different acts of current debauchery. The French (or English) language—at least the acceptable—does not possess all their equivalents, and the majority could only be rendered by periphrases difficult to employ, as Celsus says, and at the same time observe propriety. But, when one cannot approach an obstacle from the front, a flank movement is made; and, in the case which concerns us, scientific terms will be of great help when we cannot avoid a word of the greatest importance in our interpretation. So, like the physician of Rome, "we will not condemn ourselves to silence," just because we

[1] Lib. vii, epigr. 62.

have a difficulty to conquer; for the legend of the American origin of syphilis must be destroyed once and forever! It is our *delenda est*, and we cannot throw away the most valuable texts.

Sodomites were designated, in ordinary language, by the expressions *cinædi*, *pathici*, *pædicones;* they were the passive instruments of the unnatural lubricity of the debauched Romans. They had still another attribute,—active, though,—expressed by the word *fellare*, and then they took on the name of *fellatores;* the feminine *fellatrix* was applied to the courtesan who was sufficiently degraded not to recoil at these revolting acts. The verbs *irrumare*, *cunnilingere*, and *lambere* designated, according to the expression of Ricord,[1] "a certain prelude to the virile act;" whence the names *cunnilingus* and *irrumator*, given to the individual who gave himself up to these practices. So far as women were concerned, this last condition was, without doubt, much rarer in Rome than in the island of Lesbos, for Martial mentions but one strumpet, Philenis:—

. . . plane medias vorat puellas, [2]

says he, in a Latin which is too picturesque to dare translate it. Now, when we will have added, in order to terminate these edifying inquiries, that the Roman fish-ponds were open to all, and that men and women bathed in them promiscuously, without the smallest shred of covering or rag, we think the nauseated reader will have learned all that he should know to remain convinced that the Romans had syphilis. And we will add that they fully deserved it.

The oldest of the satirical poets is Caius Lucilius, an author very little known to us, but of whom Horace

[1] Lettres sur la Syphilis. Letters on Syphilis.

[2] Lib. vii, epigr. 67.

makes much ado. Lucilius was born about 148 B.C.; there remain of his poems but a few fragments, which are unconnected, and of which many have been collected as quotations in the works of authors who wrote after him. At all events, a few medical allusions of importance are found in them. In speaking of a decrepit old man, worn out by debauchery, he says that he may be seen "blear-eyed, the *pimples* and the *red eruptions going up* to the eyes."

> Illuvies scabies oculos huic, deque petigo
> Conscendere. [1]

We do not pretend to force the idea of syphilis from these verses; but it is interesting, in this respect, that he peremptorily demonstrates that the word *scabies* is not always applied, whatever may be said, to the itch proper.[2] In another passage, the general sense indicates that *scabies* designates a bad disease of the skin, and not the itching caused by the acarus. The author, speaking of women of a revolting appearance, says that he has seen a woman of the people "all squalid and covered with crusts." [The English "scab" and "scabby" are from the same root, *scabies*.]

> . . . squalitate summa, scabie summa. [3]

It is probably not simple itch, either, that is to be seen in that unfortunate, "exhausted, eaten by ulcers, and covered with crusts."

> Tristem, et corruptum scabie, porrigini' plenum.[4]

Here we have a physician speaking to his patient: "fearing that a *bubo* will form in the groin; not to be

[1] Satires, lib. xx, 6. This must be construed *depetigoque*. *Deque petigo* is a poetical license.

[2] The itch has *never* been seen on the face; so it cannot "go up to the eyes."

[3] Sat., lib. xxvi, 5.

[4] Sat., lib. xxx, 70.

inconvenienced by *papules, tumors, swellings of the legs.*"

Inguen ne existat ; papulæ, tama, ne boa noxit. [1]

The end of the sentence being missing, the verse of itself is sufficiently vague ; but we may be permitted to think of syphilitic lesions,[2] for the patient, a little further on, says to the physician : " This white spot annoys me, but it does not hurt."

Hæc odiosa mihi vitiligo est, non dolet, inquit.

Is this the pigmentary syphilide, the pseudo-vitiligo of the neck? Dupouy, who has published an interesting study on the Latin poets,[3] concludes for syphilis from this passage of Lucilius.

Catullus, who lived about 50 B.C., outside of his elegies and epithalamia, has also written some trenchant epigrams, in which are found allusions to syphilis. He apostrophizes a thievish courtesan in a manner whose medical meaning can be understood by everybody : " *Rotten* faggot, return me my tablets !"

Mœcha putida, redde codicillos. [4]

Further on, he brands the manners more than loose of Julius Cæsar, after the conquest of the Gauls. " They are well made to understand each other, those two frightful Sodomites, Mamurra the passive and Cæsar. For truly—the one at Rome, the other at Formiana—both have contracted a *disease* whose *marked*

[1] Fragments, xxii and xxiii.

[2] It is probably in this sense also that the sentence of Seneca, which has become a proverb, and which is analogous to the beam which is always seen in the eye of a neighbor, should be interpreted. "The *papules* in others shock you, when you yourselves are covered with *ulcers*." (Papulas observatis, obsiti plurimis ulceribus.)

[3] Médecine et mœurs de l'ancienne Rome. Paris, 1885. Medicine and Manners of Ancient Rome.

[4] Epigr. xlii.

spots have left upon their bodies stains which *will not disappear*. Both *infected*, and together in the same bed."

> Pulchre convenit improbis cinædis
> Mamurræ pathicoque, Cæsarique.
> Nec mirum : maculæ pares utrisque
> Urbana altera, et illa foramina,
> Impressæ resident nec eluentur.
> Morbosi pariter, gemelli utrique ;
> Uno in lecto. . . .[1]

Such is the Latin text, with its inconvenient clearness for the partisans of the American origin, who cannot change it. Let it be translated in any manner, the words are there, clear and limpid ; to try to demonstrate that this roseola, contracted in the bosom of debauchery, was of syphilitic nature, would be to cause a loss of value in the verses of Catullus, which are sufficiently eloquent of themselves. Let us add, for the delectation of the public, that the poet, when asked to dine by Cæsar, accepted the invitation and discontinued his invectives.

Tibullus, an elegiac poet who wrote a few years later (42 B.C.), addresses a prayer to Isis, which attests a venereal disease, without our being able to determine which one. "Now, Goddess, help me, for thou canst *heal* me; the many paintings hung in thy temple teach this."

> Nunc, dea, nunc succurre mihi : nam posse medere
> Picta docet templis multa tabella tuis.[2]

We have already stated that the temples of Isis, like those of Priapus, were filled with votive paintings, and that these paintings represented solely the sexual organs which were cured. The faithless Delia had, doubtless, left poor Tibullus a painful *souvenir*. And this invoca-

[1] Epigr. lvii. [2] Albius Tibullus, lib. i, Carmen 3.

tion of the poet proves pretty well that there existed in Rome diseases of genital origin common to both sexes, and apparently transmissible. Otherwise Tibullus would not have addressed himself to Isis, whose temples contained only feminine *ex-votos*. He knew then that the goddess was competent in his particular case, the difference in organs having no influence upon the nature and progress of this venereal disease.

About the same time (40 B.C.) appeared the works of Horace, the most celebrated of the Latin satirical poets. In one of his odes, in which, as a Roman citizen, he rejoices at the death of Cleopatra, we find verses which lead one to think that the soldiers of this African had contagious diseases. "Whilst a queen, having assembled a horde of vile soldiers affected with a *shameful disease*, insanely prepared to reign over the Capitol, and already attended, in hope, the obsequies of the empire."

. . . dum Capitolio
Regina dementes ruinas,
Funus et imperio parabat
Contaminato cum grege turpium
Morbo virorum.[1] . . .

The word *contaminatus*, meaning *besmirched*, *withered*, can hardly be explained otherwise than by syphilis, a *disease* sufficiently visible to be noted in a group (*grege*) of individuals whom it *besmirched*. We know that the conception of withering was only applied, among the Romans, to venereal diseases, and that they were easy on the score of morality. It really requires good will, or the previously made opinion of Astruc, to regard the word *morbus* (disease) as being always in a figurative sense, and translate it always *vice* when it is suspected to be related to the genital apparatus. "The

[1] Quintus Horatius Flaccus, Carm., lib. i, 31.

warriors of Cleopatra," says he, "were sodomites, and this fact alone does not prove that they had the pox."[1] We agree, but neither does it prove the contrary.

In a satire of the same author, we see a clown twitting a certain Cicirrus about a disease upon whose nature there has been much discussion. The Roman of whom Horace speaks had upon the left side of his forehead a disgusting scar, which disfigured him:—

> . . . Illi fœda cicatrix
> Setosam lævi frontem turpaverat oris.[2]

The word *turpaverat* (had disfigured, soiled) has for its root *turpis* (shameful), which implies the idea of debauchery, so far as it relates to the origin of the trouble. The author proceeds to give us the name of this venereal disease: "Having joked him a great deal about his *disease of Campanum* about his face."

> Campanum in morbum, in faciem permulta jocatus. . . .

If we do not lose sight of the fact that Campania became later the kingdom of Naples, it will be apparent, as many authors have pertinently remarked, that those who, in the fifteenth century, called syphilis the *Neapolitan disease*, in fact, translated the expression *morbus Campanus*. Platner, a German author of the eighteenth century, wrote a monograph[3] to prove that the Campanian disease was syphilis. Dupouy specifies the nature of the disease, and sees in it the modern *corona veneris*, which is quite admissible.

Finally, in the *Ars Poetica*, in verse 453, is found the word *scabies*, employed to designate the most terrible contagious disease,—the one to be most feared:

[1] Astruc: De Morbis Venereis. Lutetiæ Parisiorum. On Venereal Diseases. Paris, 1740.

[2] Sat., lib. i, 5.

[3] J. Z. Platner: De morbo Campano ad verba Horatii. Lipsiæ. On the Campanian Disease of which Horace Speaks. Leipzig, 1732.

"Just as one flies from and takes good care not to touch a man having *bad pimples.*"

Ut mala quem scabies. . . . urget,
. . . tetigisse timent fugiuntque.

Above this, in verse 417, children were seen to use this expression, which has become a proverb: "The dirty pimple for the last!"

Occupet extremum scabies. . . .

Juvenal, who was not yet born when the preceding poets had already died, wrote abaut A.D. 42. He affords us but one document relating to venereal diseases. He becomes indignant at a hypocritical cinædus in one of his satires: "Darest thou rail at obscenity, thou, the best-known cess-pool of the Socratic band! The male exterior, it is true, and those hairy limbs lead to the belief of a virile soul; but the physician who cuts off the tumefied *mariscæ* of thy epilated anus smiles with a mocking air."

. . . Castigas turpia, cum sis
Inter Socraticos notissima fossa Cinædos:
Hispida membra quidem, et duræ per brachia setæ
Promittunt atrocem animum; sed podici lævi
Cedundur tumidæ, medico ridente, mariscæ.[1]

These anal products, especial to passive sodomites, were evidently contagious, since they excited the smiles of the physicians, who divined their origin. Hæmorrhoids have nothing laughable about them; as to vegetations, they are not contagious, and it is known that they may show themselves, even abundantly, in the most honest woman, under the sole influence of pregnancy. In man, want of cleanliness, an irritating cause, may equally suffice. *Mariscæ* answer much better for hypertrophic (*tumidæ*) syphilides than anything else. On

[1] Decimus Junius Juvenalis, sat. ii.

the whole, the treatment of the Romans was brutal. It has been more willingly abandoned in our days, as internal treatment would suffice, in case of necessity.

Twenty years later, under the reign of Nero (about A.D. 65), we see the works of the two satirical poets, Perseus and Martial, appearing almost simultaneously. Although the style of Perseus is entirely different from that of Martial, and that obscenity in the language of the former is as rare as it is frequent in the other, there may, nevertheless, be caught on the wing, so to speak, a few caustic allusions, which certainly refer to venereal, if not syphilitic, lesions. And we are certainly astonished not to see them noticed by any of the authors who are partisans of the ancient origin. Dupouy, alone, has noticed in the second satire an allusion to the *rotten race of Messala* (Messalæ lippa propago[1]). The word *lippa*, which is applied to a disease of the eyelids, recalled to the mind of the author a shameful disease which apparently affected a certain Cotta Messalinus, a descendant of Messala. This Cotta, according to Tacitus and Titus-Livius, and even of Cicero, had exhausted himself by all "the excesses of debauchery; he carried its *shameful traces* upon his face; his eyelids were eaten by humors, and they turned out." It is on account of this testimony that Dupouy thought himself justified in translating the word *lippa*, which literally means *having eyes full of humors*, by the adjective *rotten*. Besides, the illustrious general, Messala, had no luck with his line; it was also from him that the famous Messalina descended. This nymphomaniac empress, deserting the couch of Claudius, the imbecile Cæsar, passed all her evenings in the "smoky antrum of a brothel," under the

[1] Aulus Persius Flaccus, sat. ii.

alias of Lycisca, and only left with regrets," says the poet, "exhausted, but never satisfied."

Et lassata viris, sed non satiata recessit.[1]

In Satire III of Perseus, verse 113, we find the part of a sentence which, being given the general tone of the discourse, relates to a disease which was not acknowledged, and which may lead to a suspicion of a secondary lesion: "Thy tender mouth conceals a *putrid ulcer*."

. . . tenero latet ulcus in ore
Putre . . .

We are surprised that Dupouy did not see in this word *ulcus* anything but *aphthæ* of the mouth; it is true that he forgot to translate the word *putre*, or he would have immediately observed that aphthæ, which never infect, could not render the thought of the author. We would have more easily understood the diagnosis *ulcero-membranous stomatitis;* but this special disease of children, which is relatively rare in the adult, does not warrant the ironical tone of Perseus. In the same way, in verse 43 of Satire IV, the author alludes to an ulcer of venereal origin, but situated this time on the genital organs. "Thou hast a *secret wound* lower down than the hips."

. . . Ilia subter
Cæcum vulnus habes. . . .

Here, again, the mocking tone of the whole satire proves very well that this implies what is called, in our days, using an analogous metaphor, a *kick from Venus* below the belt. In verse 57 of Satire V, the poet designates general infection of the organism. "That one is *rotten* by debauchery."

. . . ille
In venerem est putris. . . .

[1] Juvenalis, sat. vi.

Finally, in Satire II, this part of a phrase is met: "He is covered with *ulcers;* an acrid bile swells him."

> . . . namque est scabiosus, et acri
> Bile tumet. . . .

We will see further on, respecting Ausonius, what the pathological value of the expression *scabiosus* was, for the Romans.

Let us now examine Martial, one of the most licentious authors of antiquity, but one whose works furnish us with the richest collection of documents. The reader now knows, after the short sketch of Roman manners which we have given, what he may expect. Nevertheless, we will make it a rule, in translating, to be correct in the medical sense of the word, while forcing ourselves, at the same time, in being persuasive, from the point of view of the thesis we are sustaining. We will first examine the texts which treat of venereal diseases without prejudging their nature. In this line of ideas, we first find the oft-quoted epigram concerning a passive sodomite, who transmited contagious lesions to a youth: "Thy young slave *ails in his penis;* thou, Nævolus, it is at the *anus;* I am not a magician, but I know thy habits."

> Mentula quum doleat puero, tibi Nævole, culus:
> Non sum divinus, sed scio quid facias.[1]

This disease, which Martial mentions solely to prove the *passiveness* of his personage, may be referred either to syphilitic lesions or to soft chancres. The puerile objection may be made to us that the allusion is to a pain of the irritated parts, but the text itself proves the contrary, for contagion is manifest.

[1] Marcus Valerius Martialis, lib. iii, epigr. 71.

Further on the reference is to a courtesan celebrated by her sculptured beauty, and whom Martial denounces as dangerous for idle youth; but he does not specify the nature of the *professional* disease which she had. "I recommend you, Rufus, to beware lest Chiona read my little book. She is *wounded* by my verse; but she also *can wound.*"

> Ne legat hunc Chione, mando tibi, Rufe, libellum.
> Carmine læsa meo est; lædere et illa potest.[1]

It is the same case with that other play upon words, which is a little more complicated, in which the author speaks of a disease of the penis, whose nature he does not specify. "The Greek Baccara confided to a physician, his rival, the care of *curing his penis;* Baccara will become a eunuch (or a Gaul)!"

> Curandum penem commisit Baccara Græcus
> Rivali medico; Baccus Gallus erit.[2]

The *finesse* of this rests upon the double meaning of the word *gallus*, which means *priest of Cybele*, *castrated*, or *Gaul*. This Greek was going to change his *nationality* in losing his *virility*, as a result of his imprudent confidence, just as a horse who has been castrated takes on the name of a Hungarian horse,[3] although he may never have left the soil of America. We hope that our apparently trivial comparisons will be pardoned, but we are forced to make them in a way, for a pun in a foreign language is always difficult to understand; and Martial, who is accustomed to this, affords us others which are more obscure, and which we will explain later on.

Now, are we to see terrible lesions of tertiary syphilis or an ulcerated epithelioma in that horrible disease which led a Roman knight to suicide? Either opinion

[1] Lib. iii, epigr. 97. [2] Lib. xi, epigr. 74.

[3] In French a gelding is called a *cheval hongre*, whence the above.

may be defended. "The throat shamefully attacked by a *cruel* and devouring *disease*, which made fatal progress in his face, Festus, without shedding a tear, consoled his weeping friends and resolved to visit the banks of the Styx."

Indignas premeret pestis quem tabida fauces
Inque ipsos vultus serperet atra lues;
Siccis ipse genis flentes hortatus amicos
Decrevit Stygios Festus adire lacus.[1]

We do not receive any more information as to the nature of the malignant virus which caused the death of Demetrius, the *confidant* slave of Martial. "When the *impious disease* consumed its victim."

Ureret implicitum quum scelerata lues.[2]

Further on, it is *tumors* of which Martial reproaches a debauchee. They were certainly venereal, and they were chiefly found in the *priests of Cybele*, eunuchs who submitted themselves to passive sodomy.

It appears that these tumors were *ulcerated;* and, as they have taken the name of the country whence they came (Syria), papulo-hypertrophic syphilides, or, rather, ulcerated gummata, may be seen in these. "I have not said, Coracinus, that thou wert a sodomite. . . . I swear it by thy *Syrian tumors;* . . . what I have said is a notorious fact, which thou thyself wilt not seek to deny; I have said that thou wert a *cunnilingus.*"

Non dixi, Coracine, te cinædum;
* * * * * * *
Juro per Syrios tibi tumores,
* * * * * * *
Quod notum est, quod et ipse non negabis;
Dixi te, Coracine, cunnilingum.[3]

One thinks immediately of that special perfume of

[1] Lib. i, epigr. 79. [2] Lib. i, epigr. 102. [3] Lib. iv, epigr. 43.

syphilitic angina for the bad odor of the mouth which Martial has noted in *fellatores*, *cunnilingi*, and *pædicones;* these individuals were, as a matter of fact, more often at the source of the disease than others. The author addresses a certain Fabullus: "Thou sayest that pederasts have a *bad breath.*"

Pædiconibus os olere dicis.[1]

The author had already attacked a certain Zoilus, to whom he certainly owed a grudge, and at whom he had flung this burning insult: "Thou sayest that lawyers and poets have a bad breath; but, Zoilus, it is still worse in the *fellator!*"

Os male caussidicis et dicis olere poetis;
Sed fellatori, Zoile, pejus olet.[2]

Precocious tertiary lesions might be surmised for the disease of the young Canaca, the beautiful child whose epitaph Martial wrote. The age of this young victim of the debauchery of the time excludes all idea of cancer.[3] "Here the manner of death is more mournful than the act itself. A *horrible disease* has destroyed her face; it has located itself upon her delicate mouth; the *cruel disease* has devoured that place of kisses and snatched from the funeral pile almost entirely her childish lips!"

Tristius est leto leti genus: horrida vultus
Abstulit et tenero sedit in ore lues;
Ipsaque crudeles ederunt oscula morbi
Nec tota sunt nigris tota labella rogis.[4]

[1] Lib. xiii, epigr. 87.
[2] Lib. xi, epigr. 30.
[3] In 1881, we had occasion to observe in the Hôpital de Lourcine (salle Astruc), acting as substitute for an interne, a girl of 20 affected with an ulcerating syphilide, which had destroyed the alæ nasi. The tertiary lesions had shown themselves a *few months after the chancre*, and the cicatricial contraction ended in atresia of the nostrils. The patient remained in the hospital several years. We will hasten to state that it is the only case of the kind, so far as the grave nature of the lesions is concerned, which we had an opportunity of studying since we have seen syphilitics: that is, since 1873.
[4] Lib. xi, epigr. 91.

The following epigram fixes us as to the nature of the term *ficus;* it can be well seen that the principal manifestation of the disease consisted of venereal ulcers, and that the infected individual (*ficosus*) was a danger to his neighbors. In this *syphilitic family*,[1] the virus spread like a train of powder: "The wife has *figs* (I should say, *syphilides*); the husband has *figs*, the daughter has *figs;* the son-in-law and the grandson also have them. The steward, the farmer, the farm-hand, and the plow-man are all attacked by this *shameful ulcer.* Thus all, old and young, have *figs;* this is quite surprising, for there is not a *fig-tree* in their field."

DE FAMILIA FICOSA.

Ficosa est uxor, ficosus est ipse maritus,
Filia ficosa est, et gener atque nepos.
Nec dispensator, nec villicus, ulcere turpi,
Nec rigidus, fossor, sed nec arator eget.
Quum sint ficosi pariter juvenesque senesque,
Res mira, ficos non habet unus ager.[2]

Martial, according to his custom, relates this pathological case merely to have an opportunity of perpetrating a pun. The humor lies in the words *ficus*, a fig-tree,

[1] Unfortunately, cases of this nature are not rare. In 1874, being attached to the service for venereal diseases at l'Hôpital St. Sauveur, at Lille, we had occasion to cauterize the anal and buccal syphilides of an individual, and, at the same time, those of his son, a lad of 10 or 12 years, in the same ward. Upon questioning the man as to the origin of the child's syphilis, he informed us that his wife and little daughter, 5 years of age, were in the same condition. The same sponge was used by the entire family! The syphilis had passed from the father to the mother, and from her to the children. On the other hand, our colleagues at l'Hôpital St. Antoine, in 1879 (service of M. Duguet), must certainly remember a woman, aged 65, who had, just beneath the nose, a beautiful indurated chancre, followed by roseola, etc. She was a snuff-taker, whose upper lip, irritated and frequently fissured, presented a favorable surface for the absorption of the virus which her son, whose sores (of syphilitic nature) she dressed, very innocently transmitted to her. She had forgotten to wash her fingers before taking her snuff.

[2] Lib. vii, epigr. 71.

which produces *figs*, and *ficosus*, he who has *figs*, the fruits of an imaginary but productive tree, which is called in our days the *syphilitic virus*. An epigram, in which Martial makes Priapus speak, justifies this manner of seeing the matter: "I am not of fragile earth, and this rigid column is not of a wood taken at haphazard; it is made of a cypress full of life. . . . Whoever thou art, O, miserable one! Beware of it; for if thy rapacious hand wound, in ever so little, one of the branches of this vine, the cypress will, in spite of thee, graft a *fig-tree* on thy body."

> Non sum de fragili dolatus ulmo;
> Nec quæ etat rigida. . . .
> De ligno mihi quolibet columna est,
> Sed viva generata de cupresso;
> * * * * * * *
> Hanc tu quisquis es, ô malus timeto:
> Nam si vel minimos manu rapaci
> Hoc de palmite læseris racemos;
> Nascetur, licet hoc velis negare,
> Inserta tibi ficus a cupresso.[1]

This *point*, as it was called in the time of Louis XIV [and in ours, among English-speaking people], may be explained as follows: The fictitious *fig-tree*, grafted on the profane man, will make him gather a crop of actual fruit which will be not figs, but *figs* [condylomata]. Ode 42 of the *Priapidæ*, whose translation we will give later on, and the new pun of Martial, which we will notice, prove that the two meanings we have given to the word *ficus* were really in the minds of the Latin poets. "Because I have used the expression *ficos* [condylomata], you laugh at me, Cecilianus, as if I had committed a barbarism, and you pretend that *ficus* (contraction for *ficues*, figs) should be used. We will call *ficus* (figs)

[1] Lib. vi, epigr. 49.

the fruit which grows upon the tree we know (the fig-tree); but for *those which grow upon thy body* we will employ the word *ficos* [condylomata].

> Cum dixi *ficos*, rides quasi barbara verba,
> Et dici *ficus*, Cæciliane, jubes:
> Dicemus *ficus*, quas scimus in arbore nasci:
> Dicemus *ficos*, Cæciliane, tuos.[1]

The vulvar pimples of the vulva, which the author attributed to the courtesan Laufeia, must have been analogous *fruit;* and, if she refused to go to the bath with him, it was doubtless out of fear that he should see them. And Martial asks himself if this is ill founded prudery, "or if her ulcerated groins show a gaping hole, or if she has not upon her genitals *something which projects.*"

> Aut infinito lacerum patet inguen hiatu,
> Aut aliquid cunni prominet ore tui.[2]

Those who wish to contradict will not fail to see falling of the womb, with procidentia of the uterine cervix, in that "something projecting at the labia majora." But prolapsus uteri is something exceptional in courtesans, who rarely are parturient, and, at all events, is quite incompatible with their mode of living. Martial, who has reviewed the physical imperfections which this member of the *demi-monde* might present (pendulous breasts, wrinkled skin, etc.), then begins the list of diseases, the buboes of the groins, and the eruptions of the genitals. In the mind of the author, it must have been a venereal disease which Laufeia did not wish to expose, for obvious reasons. The paraphrase of Martial indicates hypertrophic mucous patches. As to warts, they are too small a matter to be compared with the "gaping wounds of the groin;" so that it is

[1] Lib. i, epigr. 66.

[2] Lib. iii, epigr. 72.

more rational to think of *ficus*, the classical disease. And we are quite sure that Laufeia, in reading this biting epigram, did not ask herself a second time what these *pimples* were which the poet might attribute to her.

Here are now a series of expressions which designate divers groups of cutaneous syphilides, of which some are localized in the face and chiefly in the mouth. With what the elder Pliny has informed us, considering the depraved manners of ancient Rome, and on account of the mania for kissing which then held sway, there is room to believe that more than one indurated chancre of the lips was the prelude of this varied symptomatology. The satirical poet, like Molière, becomes incensed at these "givers of frivolous busses;" but, if these produced, in the reign of Louis XIV, nothing but the indignation of Alceste, they had, in the days of Martial, somewhat more serious consequences. "There is no way, Bassus, of escaping the givers of kisses. . . . Neither the *malignant ulcer*, nor the *shining pustules*, nor the *mournful disease of the chin*, the *disgusting eruptions*, . . . or the congealed drop from the nose, can prove a sufficient obstacle for them."

> Effugere non est, Basse, basiatores.
> * * * * * *
> Non ulcus acre, pustulæve lucentes,
> Nec triste mentum, sordidique lichenes,
> * * * * * *
> Nec congelati gutta proderit nasi.[1]

When everything which precedes has been read, can any one decently, like certain authors, see a cancer of the tongue in the *shameful disease* of Manneius. That libidinous individual, whose exploits we will pass by in

[1] Lib. xi, epigr. 98.

silence, only to retain the pathological fact, evidently contracted a venereal disease which was directly transmissible; and cancer has never been contagious, nor considered venereal. We will not produce entire the too forcible text of Martial: . . . "A *shameful disease* has condemned to rest that insatiable organ; now Manneius *can no longer be pure* or impure."

> Lingua maritus. . . .
> Partem gulosam solvit indecens morbus:
> Nec purus esse potest nec impurus.[1]

Here again we find a pun, which the author cannot resist making; it is between *purus* and *impurus:* the debauchee can no longer be *pure*, physically; that is to say, healthy, which implies a vitiated blood, a *general* infection of the organism. He cannot continue to be impure, morally; that is, shameless, since the *local* manifestation of the disease stops it short. So that those who have seen a paralysis (*solvit*) in this disease have made a contradiction, for one may have a labio-glosso-laryngeal paralysis without ceasing from being healthy (*purus*). Now, as the chancroid is not seen in the cephalic region,—or, at least, never has been, in a positive manner, outside of experimental inoculations[2] made to verify this fact,—we are compelled to conclude that the *indecens morbus* of the Romans was syphilis. Was it not an analogous adventure which happened to Zoilus, who has already been mentioned, that emulator of Manneius whom the poet pities in such an ironical manner? "An evil star has suddenly *struck* thy tongue, Zoilus."

> Sidere percussa est subito tibi, Zoile, lingua.[3]

[1] Lib. xi, epigr. 61.

[2] Conf. Follin: Traité de path. ext., t. i, p. 639. Treatise on Surgical Pathology. Nadau des Islets: De l'Inoculat. du chancre mon à la région céphalique. Thèse de Paris, 1858. On the Inoculation of Chancroid in the Cephalic Region.

[3] Lib. xi, epigr. 85.

In order to make an end of Martial, we will explain two more puns in which the word *ficus* naturally plays the principal part. "Labienus has sold his gardens to buy young slaves; now Labienus has but one *orchard of fig-trees* (or *field of figs* [condylomata])."

> Ut pueros emeret Labienus, vendidit hortos,
> Nil nisi ficetum nunc Labienus habet.[1]

To appreciate the meaning of this satirical quip, it must not be forgotten that these young boys were destined to the same end as the pets (*mignons*) of Henry III, but with this difference: that the Roman slaves were forced to submit, whereas the assassin of the Duke de Guise only had the embarrassment of a choice among the young lords who surrounded him. It was as to which one, among the *court butterflies*, as they were called, would offer his complaisance to the royal pederast. Labienus, to arrive at the same result, had to sell his land. Martial, in a joking way, tells him that he exposes himself to another harvest. As a matter of fact, the word *ficetum* changes its meaning according to its root; if it is derived from *ficus, ûs*, it will signify, like *ficaria*, plantation of fig-trees; if the root is *ficus, i*, the dictionary translates it: "body covered with figs."

We know that *ficus* is a warty, rounded, ulcerated, and contagious excrescence. This is the appearance of the ordinary mucous patch; and still one cannot, and for a good reason, wonder excessively that Martial did not use the expression "syphilide." In the mind of the poet, the concubines bought by Labienus for a low purpose might, on account of their repelling duties, become, like prostitutes in our times, the *ficetum;* that

[1] Lib. xi, epigr. 33.

is to say, centres of syphilis. The allusion is still more obscure in the following epigram, which would mean nothing to us if it were not picked, so to speak, word by word: "If thou dost not cease, Hedylus, to be carried by two joined *goats*, thou, who wast only a *fig-tree*, wilt become a *wild fig-tree.*"

> Gestari junctis nisi desinis, Hedyle, capris,
> Qui modo ficus eras, jam caprificus eris.[1]

The pun bears upon the double meaning of *ficus* (*condyloma*, or *fig-tree*) and of *capra*, which means *goat*, or *prostitute.* In our days, the language of the streets also designates these unfortunates by the names of animals. At Rome, in Latin slang, they were called *lupa* (she-wolf), whence *lupanar* [brothel], a word which has become French, and *capra* [French, biche; Anglicé, doe, cat], etc.; so that the meaning which is understood is as follows: "If thou dost continue, Hedylus, to live constantly with two low girls, thou (fig-bearer) who hast already seen venereal buds (*ficus*) grow upon thy person, wilt not delay in reaping a virus of slums (*caprificus*); that is to say, everything that is grave among diseases contracted in crapulous debauchery." Such is the interpretation we propose to make; it seems difficult to express otherwise the meaning of this sentence, which would mean nothing, translated literally, according to the classic meaning. Our terms are sometimes somewhat raw, but it will be perceived with us that, the subject being given, it is very difficult to make puns understood in an idiom no longer spoken, by limiting one's self to the language of *salons.* The majority ignore the antiquity of syphilis, many deny it, whilst we, with

[1] Lib. iv, epigr. 52.

a few others, uphold it. Proofs are wanted; we give some.

We will now examine the *Priapeia*,[1] which supplement, in a sort of a way, the epigrams of Martial, and furnish us with valuable information. The *Priapeia*, an anonymous work, constitute a collection of light poems addressed to Priapus by numerous authors, and which were composed at different epochs. On the whole, they were inscriptions found upon stones which ornamented the gardens of Priapus, or on the base itself of the statue of the god. The Padua edition, which we refer to, is one of the most complete.

One of these odes, in which the author makes Priapus speak, bears witness to the habit which poets of the time had of making verses for the god of the gardens. "Let every one of those who come here become a poet, and let him dedicate light verses to me. He who fails will walk *covered with figs* among poets who are expert (in erotic subjects)."

> Quisquis venerit hic, Poeta fiat:
> Et versus mihi dedicet jocosus.
> Qui non fecerit: inter eruditos
> Ficosissimus ambulet Poetas.[2]

Here is an alternative clearly laid down: anacreontic verses or a severe syphilis; choose! The following ode, in which is found a pun of which we have already spoken, might be Martial's, for it is in his manner and style: "The farmer Aristagoras, delighted with the success of his vines, offers the waxen fruits. But thou, Priapus, who art content with the image of the fruit which is sacred to thee (the fig), contrivest so that this peasant carries upon his body *genuine fruits* (*ficus*).

[1] Priapeia: Sive diversorum poetarum in Priapum lusus. . . . Patavii, 1664. Priapeia; or, Lusus of Different Poems on Priapus.

[2] Carmen 14.

Lætus Aristagoras natus bene villicus uvis
De cera facta dat tibi poma, Deus.
At tu, sacrati contentus imagine pomi,
Fac, veros fructus ille, Priape, ferat.[1]

These *fruits* were no doubt analogous to those of Cecilianus, of which Martial speaks. (See page 193.)

In another place we find that the treatment was often terrible, and still that the disease, upon a prayer to Priapus, that is, when left to itself, could cure spontaneously. Evidently diet and hygiene were the cause of the cure, without receiving any credit therefor; but this is a way in which syphilis often acts. It is an *ex-voto* whose inscription we give: "You ask why the organ which has procreated us is represented on a votive tablet? When my penis was *seriously damaged*, when, unfortunate, I feared the *hand of the surgeon*, I did not dare address myself to those of our gods who are connected with medicine, such as, for example, Apollo and his son Æsculapius. They are too awful, and it seemed very presumptuous in me to ask them to *cure my penis.*"

VOTI SOLUTIO.[2]

Cur pictum memori sit in tabella
Membrum quæritis, unde procreamur.
Cum penis mihi forte læsus esset,
Chirurgique manum miser timerem,
Dis me legitimis nimisque magnis,
Ut Phæbo, puta, filisque Phæbi,
Curatum dare mentulam verebar.

The unfortunate patient then addresses himself to Priapus, and asks him to remedy the organ which, in his statue, is represented as equal in size to the rest of his body, and of which he is the tutelary deity: "If thou curest me *without amputation*, I will cause to be painted the organ which thou hast relieved, and I will

[1] Carmen 42. [2] Carmen 37.

dedicate the picture to thee. The representation will be similar to the original in every respect, not only as regards size, but also form and color." The god promised, made a sign of acquiescence, and "*fulfilled my wish.*" Any other god would have moved the head, but in Priapus this was not the most important part.

Qua salva sine sectione facta,
Ponetur tibi picta, quam levaris,
Parque, consimilisque concolorque
Promisit fore : mentulam [1] movit
Pro nutu deus, et rogata fecit.

A lover's prayer demonstrates to us in a peremptory manner that, among the venereal diseases, *ficus* was the reigning one, and the one to be most feared. Besides, it is always this which Latin authors put forward when it concerns a divine threat, an injury, or a contagion to be feared, in frequenting intimately the women of the *demi-monde* of the *Via Appia*, the Boulevard des Italiens of ancient Rome. The young adorer of the female in question is in for the expenses of his gallantry ; as he is amused with fair words, and the psychological moment never arrives, he begins to think that there is something mysterious underlying it all. He then asks himself if she is not in *full syphilitic bloom*, which would explain everything. "Is it not your opinion, Priapus?" he cries. "This young beauty, who makes me jump around, must be *covered with figs*, for she grants me no favor, telling me that she will not always refuse. In the meantime, she finds some pretext each time to put me off to a later day."

[1] Whence the word *mentule* [yard], which is so often found in writings of the Middle Ages: "And drawing out his mentule into the open air, he so bitterly all-to-be-pissed them that he drowned two hundred and sixty thousand four hundred and eighteen," etc.—*Gagantua*, chap. xvii.

Quædam, si placet hoc tibi, Priape,
Ficosissima me puella ludit,
Et non dat mihi, nec negat daturam;
Causasque invenit usque differendi.[1]

As, despite all, he is much taken up by her, he promises Priapus crowns of flowers if he succeeds, without fixing the date. This would seem to imply that *ficus* was curable, and that the disease ceased to be contagious at a certain time. Those venereal ulcers in which worms occur can hardly be explained, except as ulcerated gummata of the genitalia or as phagedenic chancres. The anonymous author addresses himself to a prostitute given over to all the debaucheries: "Daughter of the streets, thou who art not more sincere than a Moor, but more depraved than all the sodomites." He ends by saying that it would require at least ten handfuls of garden-rocket[2] to clean the holes which he has in the groins and scrape out the *worms which crawl* in her genitals.

O non candidior puella Mauro,
Sed morbosior omnibus cinædis.
* * * * * *
Erucarum opus est decem maniplis,
Fossas inguinis ut teram, dolemque
Cunni vermiculos scaturientes.[3]

A satirical poet, Ansonius, who lived A.D. 340, that is to say, nearly three centuries after Martial, has left us a few light poems (free epigrams), among which we have noticed one which we are surprised not to find noticed by any author. When we examine it closely, and without any preconceived idea, a generalized syphilis may be detected in it. All translators have rendered the word *scabies* by *itch*, without noticing that frequently—and

[1] Carmen 50.
[2] An aphrodisiac plant sacred to Priapus.
[3] Carmen 46.

especially in this particular case—they found themselves in the face of a generic term concerning a disease whose principal symptoms were characterized by true ulcerated tumors, and even by loss of substance in certain localities. Never did the itch produce *putrefaction of the limbs*,—a phrase of Ansonius which applies much better to ulcerated gummata than to anything else, being given, as we will see, that the limbs were not the only parts attacked. Varicose, scrofulous, and other ulcers have their sites of predilection either on the limbs or in the lymphatic glands, etc.; cancer localizes itself; itch itself respects the cephalic region; syphilitic manifestations alone can manifest themselves everywhere at the same time under the most varied forms,—vegetating, pustular, crustaceous, or ulcerating. Besides, the adjective *scabiosus*, according to the dictionary, signifies, primarily, *rough*, *pimply*, sometimes *scabby*, and, most often, *rotten*. We see it, as a matter of fact, applied by Latin authors to individuals covered with tetter, crusts, and ulcers. We will translate as follows: "Against Polygitonus, the *rotten*. When Polygitonus has been seen, seated in his bath-tub, bathing the *ulcers* of his limbs *gangrened by the virus*. . . . He moves his arms, his chest, his legs, his sides, his belly, his thighs, his genitals, his calves, his back, his head, his shoulders, and the soiled opening of his symplegada (his anus); the *cruel disease* invaded these *different* regions, going from one to the other."

IN SCABIOSUM POLYGITONEM.[1]

Thermarum in solio si quis Polygitona vidit
Ulcera membrorum scabie putrefacta foventem,
* * * * * * * * *
Brachia deinde rotat. . . .
Pectus, crura, latus, ventrem, femora, inguina, suras,
Tergum, colla, humeros, luteæ symplegadis antrum:
Tum diversa locis vaga carnificina pererrat.

[1] D. Magnus Ansonius: Epigrammata, 108.

Among the Romans, who employed general terms to designate groups of skin diseases resembling each other in their entire appearance, certain benign cases of syphilis must have often been confounded with itch, properly so called, and *vice versâ.* Certain ecthymas, in filthy individuals having the itch, must certainly have been considered as manifestations of the *indecens morbus* upon the least indication that the sheath of the penis, as is the rule, was the seat of pustules. On the other hand, many light roseolas must have passed for insignificant forms of the itch, the expression *mala scabies* being reserved for malignant forms of syphilis. Besides, let us remember that, in the Middle Ages, syphilis was called the *bad itch;* so there must have been a degree of similarity, but rather complicated. A trace of this is found in the saying which everybody knows: "You may drink out of my glass, I haven't got the itch!"[1] If the disease produced by the acarus was alone concerned there would be no *raison d'être* for the popular saying, for, we repeat it, itch is *never* found upon any part of the head. Those who, under similar circumstances, employ the term, certainly are ignorant of its origin; but it had reference in the beginning—let us not doubt it—to a contagious disease of the mouth, and especially of the lips. This disease may have been called *scabies*[2] by the Romans, but, at all events, it had no relation with the sarcoptes.

[1] Tu peux boire dans mon verre, je nai pas la gale!

[2] One thing which cannot be denied is, that the majority of the authors of the fifteenth and sixteenth centuries employed this word to designate the *new* (to them) disease, which was the great event of the time. Ulsenius (1496) designates syphilis under the name of *scabies epidemica;* Fallopius (1564), under that of *Gallica scabies;* he was an Italian physician. Bourdigné (*de Morb. Vener.*, 1529) says that "the French called it the *great pox* and *itch of Naples*," etc. Besides, let us not forget that the translators of the Bible have employed the word *scabies* to express the sense of a Hebrew word meaning contagious, hereditary pimples difficult to cure,

To terminate our study on the venereal affections in Rome, we will examine a poet who is little known, and who came after Ansonius. This is Claudianus, who wrote about A.D. 395. In a long diatribe against a certain Rufinus, the author imagines his character going to Hades before the famous tribunal. There Eacus reproaches him with being tainted by all the crimes. "The *spots* impressed upon thy chest are a blighting mark, which constitute a *proof* of thy vices."

. . . in pectus inustæ
Deformant maculæ, vitiisque inolevit imago.[1]

A detailed clinical description cannot be required of a poet; but, outside of syphilis, we cannot see what could be the disease capable of proving the debauchery of an individual by showing itself in the form of spots upon the chest!

Claudianus, however, does not furnish us only more or less debatable allusions. But, as he has affected more particularly the epic style, and as his detached poems are epithalamiums, epistles, panegyrics, or idyls, and his epigrams relate more especially to political events, no one has noticed that, among the last, there was *one* in the style of Martial. It is one of the rare documents upon which no one has depended to demonstrate the antiquity of syphilis, and it is, perhaps, the only one which defies all objections. Last year, one of my friends who succeeded me at Lourcine in 1879, and with whom I was discussing the manner of interpreting the epigram against

and seated at the margin of the anus (Deuteronomy, xxviii, v. 17). And is it *itch* which "goes up to the eyes" of that old man of whom Lucilius speaks (v. *supra*). As to the familiar expression which Roman children employed to excite themselves in races (occupet extremum *scabies*), it recalls this exclamation, so frequent in Rabelais: "May the fire of St. Anthony burn you!" . . . We will see later on that St. Anthony's fire and the disease of the burning (feu *des ardents*) were syphilis.

[1] Claudianus: Invectives Against Rufianus, lib. ii.

Manneius, said: "It is very probable that you are right; Martial wished to designate syphilis by his expression *indecens morbus.* For me, as well as for many others, the antiquity of the disease is not doubtful. But it will be objected to you, and with force, that in this case it is cancer of the tongue; and you will not be able to refute this opinion with any possible reply, seeing that there is only a local lesion present. If the author had said that this disease of the mouth had been followed by lesions of a similar character in other remote regions, it would be another thing!" Well, my dear D., meditate upon the case of Curetius, and conclude.

The epigram of Claudianus, which is composed of two parts, alludes to a disease gotten by a single contact and developing itself in two opposite places. At all events, we will limit ourselves to a simple medical discussion of this pornographic text, for the least timid modesty would recoil in terror before a complete translation. Latin sometimes braving honesty too much, we leave it to the caution of the reader to read between the lines. Claudianus recalls to his fellow-citizens that a certain Uranius, who was an augur, had amassed riches by deceiving his contemporaries by means of the organ of speech; and, says he, "it is with the same organ that his son dissipates them." In truth, this Curetius often gave himself up to intimate gossips with expensive young women (*meretrices*), the hetairæ of Rome; and this life, if we are to believe Claudianus, had its inconveniences. . . . "The son has in his mouth a *disease* which is the *just punishment* (pænam merito filius ore luit)." It may be objected that here the word *pænam* signifies *punishment*, and nothing else, and that we may translate thus: "punishment by the mouth," which changes the meaning, and constitutes a *moral* chastisement; that is to say, the ruin which cannot fail to cap the climax. Besides, what would seem to re-inforce those who contradict us is the final verse: . . . "ruining his house by his prodigalities and shameful debaucheries."

Consumens luxu flagitiisque domum.

But let us abide our time. Between the two verses which we have just quoted there is another one which explains in energetic terms where this *contagious disease* may have been acquired; and one reason which appears peremptory to us, if the punishment should have consisted in the loss of fortune, there would have been *meritus* instead of *merito.* It is the guilty part which bears the punishment; hence, it is a local disease. Put in *meritus*—which in no wise changes the metre—and we will acknowledge that nothing but a total ruin can be thought of; but as soon as there is *merito*, even if the author did not say more, it is that Curetius had either a chancre of the lip or buccal syphilides; this cannot be avoided. However, here are the three verses alluded to in the order in which they follow each other:—

Et pœnam merito filius ore luit:
Nam spurcos avidæ lambit meretricis hiatus,
Consumens luxu flagitiisque domum.[1]

Spurcos hiatus literally means *infectious openings;* but these orifices are infectious because they have been *infected*,[2] and the proof of it is in the revenging virus (*pœnam*) which attacked the *ore merito* of Curetius. It is exactly the history of Manneius, as related by Martial, but with this difference, that Claudianus notes a second stage in the history of his character.

[1] Epigrammata, In Curetium.

[2] Guillaume de Salicet (1270) employed the word *fœda* (spoiled) in the same sense applied to a woman capable of transmitting a contagious disease.

In the second part, addressing Curetius himself, the author states that he will be more sincere than his father Uranius, and that he will indicate to him the stars under whose influence have been engendered his vices and diseases. He owes his madness to Mars, and it is Saturn which causes him to dissipate his riches; "as to the *shameful disease* which is situated in his *anus*, where may be seen the signs of premature age, it is the work of Luna and of Venus, female stars."

> Quod turpem pateris jam cano podice morbum,
> Femineis signis Luna Venusque fuit.

This disease, which first appears as a contagious affection of the mouth, as we have seen in the first epigram, and which afterward reacts upon the organism in such a manner as to show itself similarly at the *anus* (podice); this *shameful* (turpem) disease, what can it be except syphilis? There is not even a means of invoking the possible coincidence of another local contagion, such as chancroids, for example; for, if Curetius had been a sodomite, Claudianus would not have hesitated to reproach him with it. On the contrary, he says plainly by what means his character has contracted the disease: *lambit hiatus.* He even insists upon this etiological cause, for he recurs to it in his second epigram. As a matter of fact, in the last verse, he asks himself to what star Curetius can owe this habit, and he designates the *hiatus* by its name.

> Hæreo, quæ cunnum lambere causa facit.

As everything must be expected, perhaps there will be chicanery about the expression *jam cano* (already white), which accompanies *podice.* Those who contradict us will certainly see in this discoloration of the hair (premature age) an indication of passive sodomy in

Curetius. We will content ourselves by replying that it proves precisely the contrary; for we know, from the testimony of authors of that time, that the *pathici* (and there were enough in Rome!) epilated themselves to more conveniently ply their degrading traffic. "For whom epilatest thou thyself, Labienus?" cries Martial.

Cui præstas culum, quem, Labiene pilas?[1]

In another place, the same poet ridicules Chrestus the Bald, who has the "head more polished than the rim of the anus in sodomites."

Et prostitutis lævius caput culis.[2]

Was it not from an epilated anus (*podice lævi*) that the physician of whom Juvenal speaks excised large mariscæ? Quotations could be multiplied, but those given are sufficiently demonstrative. Hence, if the incriminated region could have whitened on account of its abnormal functions, it would have been impossible to observe it, and Claudianus would not have written *jam cano*. Q. E. D.

Such are the documents, mostly secular, which we have been able to obtain after three years of research, which was at times laborious. We will feel compensated for our endeavors, and will have fully attained our purpose if the reader finds himself drawn to the following conclusion, which is our deepest conviction: SYPHILIS DATES FROM THE CREATION OF MAN.

[1] Lib. ii, epigr. 62.

[2] Lib. ix, epigr. 28.

CHAPTER XII.

CONCLUSION.

Rational Treatment of Syphilis in the Nineteenth Century.

Guéris du soir au lendemain,
Et content du syphilicure,
Les dieux donnèrent à Mercure
La bourse qu'il tient à la main.

—Sacombe.[1]

Cured from eve till morn,
And with this satisfied,
The gods to Mercury have borne
The purse that to his hand is tied.[2]

Syphilis, the daughter of prostitution, was born as soon as Commerce, chasing Love, presided over the exchange of caresses. The venereal virus must have marked the first step of the human race on the highway of civilization. This is what leads us to believe that India must have been its cradle. The race of Aryans, a migratory people which furnished inhabitants to Persia, Palestine, Arabia, and Egypt, spread itself over Europe. It required many centuries for these erring hordes to become organized into nations, to cultivate the arts, sciences, and letters; but syphilis continued to remain among them in an endemic state. For, if a few thousand years sufficed to wear off their savage source, nothing availed against the venereal disease, which is, in a sort of a way, inherent to our species. Will syphilis become a quantity to be disregarded at that day when each one, armed with the hereditary principle, will oppose to it a soil

[1] La Vénusalgie. Paris, 1814.

[2] The indulgence of readers is asked for this attempt at rhyming on the part of the translator. The translation, however, is approximate.

inaccessible to the reigning virus? Is it destined to become extinct by the very fact of the succession of beings? These are theoretical problems whose verification could not be made materially possible except outside of the human species, and animals are almost always refractory; but even here the final word cannot be given, perhaps. Happy the scientific man who, advancing beyond the works of his time, might endow his century with the *true* vaccine of syphilis!

But, while waiting for the discovery of this liquid,—much more useful than that of Brown-Séquard [or of Koch, we are tempted to add],—syphilitics must be treated. And on this account we are going to examine the different methods of treatment actually employed, discussing their merits, and point the most effective and practical.

Syphilis, like all constitutional affections which are accompanied by external manifestations, requires general treatment; that is to say, an internal treatment and a local or external treatment.

GENERAL TREATMENT.

The treatment which addresses itself to the entire economy is by far the most important; since, if, necessary, as we have already said, it would be sufficient. As a matter of fact, it is the only one directed against the virus, as it is destined to be absorbed and carried to all the tissues by the torrent of the circulation. We have already stated (Chap. I) that the two great therapeutic agents, *mercury* and *iodine*, constitute the basis of treatment. We will now explain how the metal and the metalloid act, under what forms they can be administered, and we will then give formulas recognized as the best in the actual state of science.

Without entering into the discussion brought up by certain dissenters, who, in a spirit of contradiction, or from calculation, have declared themselves as antimercurialists, we will say, once for all, that *mercury* is recognized, nowadays, as the *only specific* remedy for syphilis. When we study the sexual pathology of the Middle Ages,[1] we will see that this metal was employed as a remedy from the epidemic of Naples (1494), and many years before the *thick itch* (ad scabiem crassam), which was nothing else but classic syphilis. This fact is related by Fracastor, a contemporary of the epidemic, and that physician supports himself upon an old manuscript of the first centuries of the Christian era. The preparations of iodine are next in point of importance; then come the tonics and hygiene, excellent adjuvants. Let us follow the three periods, and let us see what course should be pursued in general and in certain particular cases.

The First Period.—This is characterized, as has been seen, by the appearance and evolution of the primary lesion; that is to say, one or sometimes several indurated excoriations, which persist for one or two months. We will repeat that there is an object in beginning mercurial treatment as soon as possible; that is to say, as soon as a diagnosis can be made in a certain manner. Then hygiene is recommended to the patient, and his moral state is to be taken care of also, if it is necessary. The most *tempé* man always experiences a disagreeable mental sensation when the physician tells him that he is syphilitic. The legend, which is not very re-assuring, although exaggerated, and which attends the word *pox*, and especially the prospect of a treatment always long; the social consequences; the

[1] F. Buret: La Syphilis au Moyan Age. Syphilis in the Middle Ages 1891.

worries of a being who ceaselessly fears an irremediable catastrophe,—all this is not calculated to bring peace to the soul. So that the duty of the physician is, first of all, to re-assure his patient as to the consequences of his disease. He should, without making a course of syphilography, which would be tiresome, enumerate the principal possible symptoms of the disease. He will call the attention of his patient to the fact that the word *terrible* is seldom applied, nowadays, except to the lesions modeled in wax and carefully preserved in the museum of the Hôpital St. Louis; that one is not forced, fortunately, in his quality of a syphilitic, of posing as a model of the genus by presenting on his person the entire series of venereal manifestations; finally, that he is to make up his mind in reference to the matter, and that he is far from being the only one of his kind. When the patient has acquired the certainty that he cannot walk the boulevards without encountering hundreds of syphilitics who are not so badly off; when he has exchanged confidences with his friends situated as he is, and whose appetite, muscular strength, etc., are unimpaired, he will take courage and be treated, which is the essential thing.

If you have to do with a debilitated, lymphatic, or strumous individual, predisposed to cachexia, tonics are indicated in the form of a maceration of gentian or of quassia amara (a wineglassful before each meal). This medication is simple and cheap. For those who cannot take anything bitter, we prescribe very advantageously the following :—

℞ Vini gentianæ,
Syr. cort. aurant. amar., . . . āā p. æ.
Ft. sol.
Sig.: A small wineglassful ten minutes before each meal.

Then, *after* eating,—and not before, to avoid cramps, —it will be well to take a liqueurglassful of wine of cinchona made by a good pharmacist. Good food, in sufficient quantity, exercise without fatigue, regular habits, and sobriety in all things, are the indispensable adjuvants of a well-directed treatment.

Let us now see how specific treatment may be given. In the sixteenth century the first thing employed was rubbing in mercurial ointment. This treatment, based upon cutaneous absorption, is still employed to-day, and it is useful in certain cases in which rapid effects are desired, but rarely at the beginning of syphilis. Several drawbacks are connected with it. It is not pleasant, as it soils a great deal; it rapidly starts up a local irritation and mercurial stomatitis, with salivation; and only the approximate quantity of mercury employed can be estimated. The stomatitis, which was considered useful in the sixteenth century, caused troubles of a serious nature, which largely contributed to the discredit in which mercury is held. We will study this interesting question later on, when we occupy ourselves with the syphilographers of the three centuries preceding our own. Mercury has also been employed in fumigations, in the form of cinnabar, which was roasted, as it is still done by the Chinese; but this method has been entirely abandoned in our day.

Many years later, ingestion by way of the stomach was tried, and, if we are to believe history, it was Francis I who, in France, took the first mercurial pills.[1] These were very mercurial in composition, but are completely neglected nowadays. The best known are

[1] He obtained their formulæ from Barberossa, a celebrated Algerian pirate. This new treatment was especially begun and praised by Paracelsus, a renowned physician of that time.

Belloste's pills, the *blue* pills, and Sedillot's pills. Later on, mercurial salts were caused to be absorbed, and this method was based upon the reasonable assumption that mercury, to be absorbed, must be first combined with the gastric fluid or intestinal secretions in such a manner as to produce, if not a *salt*, chemically speaking, at least a soluble substance. A flood of preparations then arose. The principal are protiodide of mercury, in the form of pills; the biniodide of mercury, most often combined with iodide of potassium (Gibert's syrup); protochloride of mercury, or calomel; and the bichloride of mercury, or corrosive sublimate. The cyanide and the tannate of mercury have also been suggested; but these two latter preparations do not enjoy the popularity of the others, of which we will speak more in detail.

The protiodide of mercury owed and still owes its use in current practice to Ricord. Although adopted by many syphilographers, we never prescribe it, for the following reasons: In the first place, it almost always brings on enteritis; this irritation of the intestines manifests itself in the form of severe colics and diarrhœa; besides, it often causes mercurial stomatitis. It is only by giving opium and chlorate of potassium that it can be tolerated; some patients are forced to abandon it. Another reason makes us prefer corrosive sublimate. As it is proven that mercury, no matter in what form it is administered, does not pass into the circulation until after its change into bichloride, it has appeared to us—as to many others—more rational to give it in that form, which obviates the work of a laboratory on the part of the digestive via. The best method consists in giving the sublimate in solution in the proportion fixed by Van Swieten, the Dutch pysician. Bichloride rarely excites stomatitis; as far as we are concerned, we *never* saw a case; this is a point of some importance. Besides, it does not bring on colic, except in large doses. But, eventually, it irritates the stomach, a complication which may be avoided by the addition of opiates in very small doses. Van Swieten's liquor (a 1-to-1000 solution) is the simplest, the most economical, and most employed solution. It is given in tablespoonful doses daily after some meal. Unfortunately, it leaves an after-taste which is disagreeable, which patients state is *coppery;* so that we prescribe a solution of half the strength, of which we give two tablespoonfuls daily, which amounts to the same thing.

℞ Hydrargyri bichloridi, ...	0.25
Alcoholis (90°), ...	50.00
Ext. thebaici, ...	0.35
Aquæ destillat., ...	450.00

Ft. sol.

Sig.: A tablespoonful at each meal in a half-tumblerful of water.

If necessary, the following may be employed, which patients find to be almost agreeable:—

℞ Hydrargyri bichloridi, ...	0.12
Alcoholis (90°), ...	25.00
Syrupi codeini, ...	50.00
Syrupi florum aurantii, ...	175.00

Ft. sol.

Sig.: A tablespoonful in a half-tumblerful of water before each meal.

If, despite these expedients, the syphilitic experiences an insurmountable disgust, the classic pills of Dupuytren[1] are given, which we advise, in the interest of the stomach, to modify as follows:—

[1] Dupuytren's pills each contain three-twentieths of a grain of bichloride, three-tenths of a grain of extract of opium, and three-fifths of a grain of guaiac.

℞ Hydrargyri bichloridi,
Sodii chloridi, ... āā 0.60
Ext. thebaici, ... 1.00
Gluten. recent., ... q.s.

M. ft. pilulæ no. lx.
Sig.: One pill before each meal.

Solution, mixture, pill,—all are combined in such a manner that the patient takes three-tenths of a grain of bichloride daily.

About ten years ago it was proposed to cause the absorption of mercury by hypodermatic means. Martineau advocated this method and abandoned Van Swieten's liquor in his service at Lourcine. All the syphilitics were treated by means of subcutaneous injections of ammonio-peptonate of mercury. No abscess or mercurial stomatitis occurred; and, as the injections are in the back, they are not painful. This method may be regarded as not very practical, requiring the *daily* attendance of the physician. Nevertheless, it may be a valuable resource in cases where the stomach is profoundly wrecked, and in which, for some reason or other, we might not wish to prescribe mercurial frictions. This treatment, which is rarely employed—in private practice, especially—except in a temporary way, is of the greatest value in certain malignant cases of syphilis; it is for the enlightened physician to judge of its necessity. For our part, we owe several successful treatments to this method, used in unfortunate cases, in which ordinary means had not materially changed the condition of the patient.

Second Period.—This is characterized by more or less numerous manifestations, which show themselves upon the skin and mucous membranes; as we have enumerated them in Chapter I, we will not repeat them.

The internal treatment is exactly the same as in the primary period; if it has not already been begun, it should be done immediately.

In a general way, the patient can easily stand his bichloride treatment for three consecutive months. At all events, the physician will do well to watch the digestive functions and suspend medication for a few days upon the slightest indication of impaired nutrition. At the end of these three months, if the cutaneous manifestations or those of the mucous membranes are decreasing, a *therapeutic rest* of three weeks or a month may be prescribed, for it is well to know that the physiological action of mercury continues for a certain length of time after its use has been stopped, as it is eliminated little by little by way of the secretions. Then the solution or pills are taken again for two months with two other months of rest, and so on for a year or two, according to the case. In a general way, the first year of the syphilitic requires six months of treatment and six months of rest, which time he uses in fractional parts, alternately. It is plain that we are not speaking of those exceptional cases, in which the physician is the sole judge as to any modification of this method, which is the rule. The second (or third) year is generally devoted to the mixed form of treatment, also given in an intermittent manner, and which consists in the use of the combination of mercury and the iodides.[1]

One of the best preparations employed for this pur-

[1] Mixed treatment is indicated during the first year if precocious tertiary lesions are seen, this being a rare occurrence. [I have seen gummata of the iris appear two months after the roseola.] It is also useful in certain cases of very intense cephalalgia, which appears most often during the evolution of the chancre or at the beginning of the secondary period. Still, it is well not to abuse the iodides; and, most often, mercurial treatment can be continued with advantage up to the third or even fourth year of the disease.

pose is, without doubt, the syrup of Gibert, which contains in each tablespoonful (a dose for a day) one-sixth of a grain of biniodide of mercury and nearly eight grains of iodide of potassium. Frictions with blue ointment may also be used, giving, at the same time, iodide of potassium or of sodium, in doses of from eight to fifteen grains a day. Iodides are given in solution or in the form of a syrup :—

1°. ℞ Potassii iodidi,		
Melissæ alcoholat. comp., ...	āā	ʒiiss.
Aquæ fontis, ...	q. s. ad	℥x.

M. ft. sol.

Sig. : A tablespoonful contains gr. viiss of iodide (to be largely diluted in water).

2°. ℞ Potassii iodidi, ...	ʒiiss.
Syr. cort. aurant. amar., ...	℥ix.
Aquæ destillat., ...	℥j.

M. ft. sol.

Sig. : To be taken like the solution.

For the succeeding years, unless there are indications to the contrary, the treatment should be limited to two months at each change of season. The patient must not permit himself, as so often happens, to be lulled into a deceptive security, for he is always exposed to disagreeable relapses ; and, upon the slightest indication, he should consult his physician, who will judge, from the nature of his symptoms, if the disease has entered upon its tertiary phase.

Third Period.—The tertiary period especially demands the iodides, given in doses of fifteen, thirty, forty-five, or even ninety grains daily, according to the gravity of the lesions. As a general thing, it is sufficient to take fifteen grains daily for two months, in spring and autumn.[1] But, in the presence of a gumma (ulcerated or not), the physician may, when necessary, carry the dose up to three-fourths or a drachm daily. He should add mercurial frictions, if it is a gumma of the brain, which manifests itself either by paralyses (hemiplegia, aphasia) or by epileptiform attacks. Exostoses also require mixed treatment (Gibert's syrup or mercurial frictions and iodides internally). In those cases, which, happily, are rare, of necrosis of the bones of the nose and of the palate, and of rebellious ulcers, it is the iodide which is indicated, in doses varying from one to one and one-half drachms (Ricord). It is understood that the patient is to be toned up by all possible means, without forgetting local treatment, of which we are going to speak. And, to conclude with general treatment, we will simply mention cases of benign syphilis, sometimes so benign that a treatment which is too prolonged would fatigue the patient more than the disease itself.[2] These consoling cases are far from being rare.

LOCAL TREATMENT.

First Period.—We have already said that the indurated chancre cures spontaneously, and that it is sufficient to powder it with some inert substance. After pouring a little lukewarm water upon this small lesion, morning and evening, it is simply to be covered with calomel powder. In some cases, such as mixed chancres, for instance, other means will have to be resorted to. Those who are desirous of knowing all the details

[1] We give the method which is most generally followed. Although mercury is really less efficacious at this period than at the beginning of syphilis, we are of the opinion that the patient would do wrong to abandon it entirely as soon as the third period begins.

[2] The opposite extreme should not be adopted by discarding all treatment.

in regard to this are referred to special treatises on the subject.

Second Period.—The lesions which characterize the secondary period are cutaneous eruptions and lesions of multiple forms, called *mucous patches*, which are found either upon the genitals, the anus, the mouth, or in all three regions simultaneously :—

℞ Potassii chloratis, ...	ʒj.
Syrup. idææ, ...	℥j.
Aquæ fontis, ...	℥v.

M. ft. sol.
Sig. : A tablespoonful every two hours.

Mucous patches of the mouth are seen upon the lips, inside the cheeks, and especially in the throat, on the tonsils, and anterior pillars of the velum palati. They should be cauterized every two or three days with stick nitrate of silver, and, unless the lips alone be involved, gargles containing chlorate of potassium should be added. In certain cases, knowing that this salt is eliminated by the saliva, it may be additionally prescribed in solution or lozenges.

The patches or syphilides of the ano-genital region should be lightly cauterized with nitrate of silver every third day, if they are papular or not abundant; every other day, if they are papulo-hypertrophic and confluent. Patients, especially women, whose genital lesions are generally more abundant, on account of the form of these organs, will derive benefit from the *permanent* application of compresses wet with the following solution :—

℞ Hydrargyri bichloridi, ...	gr. iij.
Ammon. muriat., ...	gr. xv.
Aquæ destillat., ...	℥xiiss.
Aquæ rosæ, ...	℥iiiss.

M. ft. sol.
Sig. : For external use.

Labbaraque's solution (of hypochlorite of soda) may also be employed for the same purpose, or a solution of chloral (2 per cent. to 4 per cent.).

All these methods are more practical, and especially more clean than that of applying mercurial ointment to eroded syphilides. Nevertheless, this latter is good, since it acts locally and in a general way by absorption. However this may be, it can scarcely be employed, except in a hospital, where patients have but one object, that of being cured as rapidly as possible, and where the necessity of wearing immaculate linen is not so much felt as outside.

Baths are good adjuvants during this period. In the first place, from the point of view of cleanliness, for water carries off irritating liquids, whose corroding action alters the neighboring tissues and transforms them into a propitious soil for the propagation of syphilides; then, from a curative point of view, on account of the composition of these baths, some of which act in both a local and general way.

At the beginning, certain syphilographers prescribe sulphur-baths, which have a general tonic action, and act locally by irritating the skin. Their object is, so to say, to attract the whole anger of the virus on the part of the integument. The cutaneous manifestations are not handsome, it is true, but they are less inconvenient than those upon the mucous membranes. The former, being dry, cannot be communicated, while the latter are highly contagious. Let us haste to add that practice does not always confirm theory, and that the two most often occur simultaneously. Nevertheless, there may be some advantage, from the stand-point of the future, in forcing the virus to explode at once; but it is without doubt related to the Phœnix, for it rises but too often from its ashes! In the same manner, advantage may be derived from steam-baths, providing that the *proper way of taking them is known.*

The first thing to do is to select a hydro-therapic establishment provided with steam-stoves, dry sweating-rooms, spray douches, jets, circular showers, etc., where treatment can be pursued according to medical directions. First condition: to be entirely free in one's actions and squarely send about his business the attendant who wishes to impose *his method.* You first enter the first hot room, having a temperature of about 50° C. (122° F.); there you walk around for a few minutes, and arm-movements are made to promote perspiration. This room being generally provided with gymnastic apparatus, it is well to take advantage of this. Then you go to the next room, heated to 70° or 80° C. (158° to 176° F.); you should walk up and down for five or ten minutes at most. General rule: go out as soon as the least discomfort is felt, and direct yourself to the douche apparatus. The first to take is the *cold* shower-bath, which is merely transversed; the first impression is permitted to pass off, and then the shower is permitted to fall on the body for a few seconds. Then a true state of well-being is experienced. At the end of one or two minutes the douche in a jet is taken in front, from behind, and on the sides; then the shower-bath is sought once more. From time to time the skin of the body and the forehead should be felt; as soon as there is a return to the normal temperature, the hot rooms or the vapor-bath may be sought, following the rules given above. Generally three or four trips are made from the heat to the cold water, and inversely, which requires altogether about one hour. 'With practice, one may pursue it for several hours, but it is not of any use. If care have been taken to get weighed in coming and leaving, it will be surprising to see that over two pounds have been lost, being about *one quart* of sweat charged with excrementitious and noxious principles. Mercury is equally eliminated by this way. And, what may appear surprising *à priori*, the majority of patients subjected to this treatment become more vigorous and retain their average weight; some even increase in weight. As a general thing, one vapor-bath is taken a week; sometimes two, according to the directions of the attending physician.[1]

We will merely mention sublimate-baths, which are good, but not practicable outside of a hospital, for it is necessary to get a small package from the pharmacist and have a *wooden* (or porcelain-lined) *bath-tub*, which is rather expensive. The following is the formula of the little package, for those who may wish to use it :—

℞ Hydrargyri bichloridi,
Ammon. muriat., . . . āā ℥ss.
M. Sig.: For one bath (of at least thirty gallons).

Third Period.—The principal lesions of the tertiary period which necessitate local treatment are exostoses, gummata, necroses, and ulcers. Upon exostoses are to be applied blue ointment, or, better still, *emplastrum de Vigo.* The same may be said of old ulcers, in which it may occasionally do good to stimulate them by topical remedies, whose description would lead us too far. The emplastrum de Vigo may also prove useful in gummata as long as they are not ulcerated. But, as soon as they form a sore, it will be necessary to modify the treatment, and, above all, to be conservative in cauterizing, if this be deemed necessary. These lesions being generally

[1] Unless there be special indications, this treatment is only applicable to robust or obese persons. [The custom in America is to take Turkish baths, which answer the same purpose; at least, in my experience.]

very painful, many patients will be relieved by the daily application, morning and evening, of an ointment containing cocaine:—

℞	Cocaini muriat.,	gr. ij.
	Vaselini albi,	ʒvj.

M. ft. ungt.

At the end of ten or twelve days, when the sore has changed its character under internal treatment, this can be alternated with an iodine ointment, which will finally be applied alone:—

℞	Potassii iodid.,	ʒss.
	Aquæ destillat.,	q. s.
	Adipis,	℥j.

M. ft. ungt.

For necroses, if they are of the bones of the nose, irrigations of Van Swieten's solution are to be made twice daily, and once or twice with a 1-to-1000 solution of permanganate of potassium, on account of the terrible smell which the patients spread. If there be perforation of the palate or ulcers of the throat, Ricord's gargle should be prescribed:—

℞	Tinct. iodini,	ʒiss.
	Kali iodidi,	gr. xv.
	Aquæ destil.,	℥vj.

M. ft. sol.

Such are the broad lines of antisyphilitic treatment, which we have indicated in as succinct a manner as possible. It has seemed useful to us to conclude our first volume with a formulary, accompanied by some explanations. We do not pretend to offer it as a substitute for the masterly works on the subject, and, still less, to render useless the advice of the intelligent physician. We even believe that we can say that he who reads our work will only follow the counsels of his physician the better, for he will know why and with what he is treated. In the next place, we hope to have reconciled many of the timorous with mercury, while preventing them from falling in the clutches of charlatans; those who exploit a fear which they are the first to awaken. We have said what we thought of this social fester, against which the law seems to be impotent. We cannot share in the too complacent philosophy of Maynwaringe, who consoles himself by saying: "*Populus vult decipi*, they love the imposture; they will not be informed, so let it go on."[1] On the contrary, we are of the opinion that the victims should be instructed by showing them things in their true light. When patients will only hearken to the counsels of men of science, the dealers in "magical" powders will have to close their shops. Then the walls of Paris[2] will no longer have the shame of testifying that there still exists, at the approach of the twentieth century, individuals capable of forgetting that medicine is, above all, a sacred trust, and that, if it be permitted to earn a livelihood by it, it should never be absorbed into the ranks of trades which cannot be acknowledged!

[1] Maynwaringe: The History and Mystery of the Venereal Lues. London, 1673.

[2] And the newspapers in general.

Medical | Medicine